Praise for
To Carry Wonde

This is a must-have . . . A treasure trove of valuable information, resources, and references that focus on the physical and mental health of women during each stage of pregnancy and the first months after giving birth.
—Cheryl Tatano Beck, DNSc, CNM, FAAN
Distinguished Professor, University of Connecticut, School of Nursing

[Parker shares] the experience of pregnancy and postpartum . . . [with] a whimsical and personal tone [and] valuable educational content that is well-researched and up-to-date. She takes complex topics and illustrates them for readers in an approachable way. . . . I was particularly pleased and impressed to see both the breadth and depth of information on mental health topics that are frequent during this vulnerable perinatal time. I would highly recommend this as reading for anyone planning a pregnancy, currently pregnant, or in the early postpartum stage.
—Anna Glezer, MD, Certified Integrative Psychiatrist
Associate Professor of Psychiatry, UC San Francisco
Founder of Women's Wellness Psychiatry

Informative, with up-to-date medical information, yet lighthearted with plenty LOL moments. You will feel like you are in a book club with your best pals while gaining valuable knowledge. . . . I will definitely encourage my patients to read this book, not only for the educational value but to assure them that their symptoms are experienced by many and overcome by most. Wish I had this book when I was expecting!
—Lexie Morales, MD, Obstetrician-Gynecologist

Informative and poignant. With humor and candor, Emese walks readers through the weeks of pregnancy in an easy-to-read format. This is an invaluable book for those who are pregnant and their partners.
—Heidi Collins Fantasia, PhD, RN, WHNP-BC, FNAP, FAAN
University of Massachusetts Lowell School of Nursing

To Carry Wonder is a unique blend of earnest memoir and technical week-by-week pregnancy guide. [Parker's] ambitious compendium is packed with tips and resources and is especially useful for the person navigating pregnancy for the first time. [It] acknowledges the vast spectrum of feelings and experiences women may have as they go through the prenatal stages, and . . . makes accessible some critical topics around body image, sex, and mental health. Parker's is a supportive and encouraging voice to have along on your ever-changing pregnancy journey.

—Miriam Schultz, MD
Clinical Associate Professor, Stanford School of Medicine,
Department of Psychiatry and Behavioral Health

This is a great resource for mothers and partners . . . [and] could be useful to doulas, student midwives, and antenatal teachers. While aimed at a U.S.-based audience, much of the content could easily be transferred to other countries.

—Dianne Garland, FRCM, SRN, RM, ADM, PGCEA, MSc
Midwifery Today

A well-written guide . . . filled with colorful illustrations depicting diverse women and babies. . . . The stories are interspersed between evidence-based nursing and medical knowledge that all women making this journey need. As a women's health nurse practitioner with 25+ years of experience providing care to women, I highly recommend both the book and guide.

—Allyssa L. Harris, RN, PhD, WHNP-BC
Dean and Professor, Prairie View A&M University, College of Nursing

TO CARRY
WONDER

A Memoir and Guide to
Adventures in Pregnancy and Beyond

Emese C. Parker
RN, WHNP-BC, MPH, PMH-C

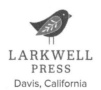

LARKWELL
PRESS
Davis, California

To Carry Wonder:
A Memoir and Guide to Adventures in Pregnancy and Beyond
Published by Larkwell Press

www.tocarrywonder.com

Copyright © 2023 by Emese C. Parker

This book is intended to nurture your well-being and empower you to have a rich, beautiful, and healthy journey through pregnancy and motherhood. The information provided is *not in any way* intended to substitute for care, delay care, or override advice by a medical or mental health professional. Rather, it is designed to equip you with the necessary information and resources to: (1) engage in meaningful conversations with your healthcare provider, (2) make informed healthcare decisions, and (3) advocate for yourself and family.

Cover illustration by Christa Pierce
Cover and book design by Carla Green, Clarity Designworks

Printed in the United States of America
First Edition
ISBN: 979-8-9864401-0-1 (paperback)
ISBN: 979-8-9864401-2-5 (hardcover)
ISBN: 979-8-9864401-1-8 (e-book)
Library of Congress Control Number: 2022911971

Publisher's Cataloging-in-Publication Data

Names:	Parker, Emese C., author.
Title:	To carry wonder : a memoir and guide to adventures in pregnancy and beyond / Emese C. Parker, RN, WHNP-BC, MPH, PMH-C.
Description:	First edition. | Davis, California : Larkwell Press, [2023] | Includes bibliographical references and index.
Identifiers:	ISBN: 979-8-9864401-0-1 (paperback) | 979-8-9864401-1-8 (e-book) | LCCN: 2022911971
Subjects:	LCSH: Pregnancy—Popular works. | Pregnancy—Handbooks, manuals, etc. | Pregnant women—Handbooks, manuals, etc. | First pregnancy—Handbooks, manuals, etc. | Subsequent pregnancy—Handbooks, manuals, etc. | Labor (Obstetrics)—Handbooks, manuals, etc. | Newborn infants—Care—Handbooks, manuals, etc. | Infants—Care—Handbooks, manuals, etc. | Motherhood—Handbooks, manuals, etc.
Classification:	LCC: RG525 .P37 2022 | DDC: 618.2/4--dc23

To my parents, Márti and Paul,
who planted within me the dream to write a book one day.
And
to my husband, Dan, and our little loves
who patiently waited for me to finish already.

CONTENTS

FIRST TRIMESTER

SECOND TRIMESTER

THIRD TRIMESTER

BABY'S EARLY MONTHS

INTRODUCTION

I couldn't believe it and maybe neither can you. Me, with a positive pregnancy test? Such a life-changing moment! Before you know it, a mix of emotions surface and a vast array of questions bombard you: What should I do? What can I do to have a healthy baby? What about my relationships, schooling, or career? Or even, how will it compare to prior pregnancies?

And just like that, you're off on a pregnancy adventure, a path well-traveled by many before you, and possibly even yourself. Whether this is your very first time or not, it doesn't take long to realize pregnancy changes everything, every time. It's not simply the physical experience of forming the life of another. It's so much more.

Pregnancy magically connects people—not just you to your baby, but also you to other mamas (and everyone else in proximity, for that matter). It's a time to face ourselves, our hopes, fears, bodies, beliefs, and choices. It is a process of becoming, of being, and of letting go—perhaps a time to be healthier, reassess our ambitions, address addictions, or even get out of destructive relationships. From anxiety to peace, isolation to connectedness, desperation to hope—the range of experiences in pregnancy and motherhood is broad and varied, from moment to moment, day to day.

Given this reality, you can imagine how incomplete (and disappointing) it would be to travel this road focused solely on the physical changes. You would miss out—on the opportunity to experience, explore, and grow in all aspects of pregnancy and motherhood. While blood pressure checks, lab tests, and medical treatments are certainly important, you're a whole being, far more complex and spectacular.

To Carry Wonder is a fun, nurturing, and engaging weekly companion—like a close friend inspiring you to journey with authenticity, boldness, and mindfulness. Maybe even a little sass. It's the culmination of my own experiences with pregnancy, my background caring for countless pregnant and postpartum women as a women's health nurse practitioner (NP*), as well as my years of contemplation and research on the subject.

My hope is that through these stories and insights, you'll find the freedom to laugh, reflect, and learn about yourself when you encounter snapshots of the raw, surprising, difficult, funny, and even awkward transformations of a woman like you—a mother-in-the-making or made anew. It's meant to be a safe space where you can let go of others' expectations and simply be. I also hope the resources in it empower you to navigate the shifting landscape of pregnancy, to advocate for your health and wellness, and to find the support you need in pregnancy and beyond.

Now, I know *To Carry Wonder* seems a little long, but don't let the book's thickness fool you! Although its stories are designed to be read in order, feel free to frolic about the book, jumping to sections that seem to connect with you the most at that moment. Go ahead and flip back to the appendices at any time. They offer you a chance to delve deeper into various compelling topics. Focus on the ones you're interested in.

As another note of disclaimer, since a good part of this book is based on journal entries, you will find references in it to things that are important to me, like friends and family, and God. My intent in including these references is not to challenge, persuade, or alienate, but to simply be true to my perspective and experiences.

So, dear friend, what are we waiting for? Join me on this expedition of growth and discovery!

Emese

---

* Nurse Practitioners (NPs) are registered nurses who have completed a master's or doctoral degree, advanced clinical training, and passed national certifying exams. In various settings, NPs focus on holistic care, promoting people's health and helping them prevent disease. When seeing patients, they diagnose, treat, and manage health problems, order lab tests, prescribe medications, and counsel people within their scope of practice. NPs also work in other areas, such as health research, leadership, health policy development, and teaching.

PROLOGUE

Eggs with an Appetite

Who would have ever guessed that a simple collection of little eggs could be such busybodies? For the past 31 years, they've been politely going about their business while I've been going about mine—but no longer.

They held off just long enough for me to earn my master's degree in nursing, and almost long enough for me to complete another in public health. Of course, as a nurse practitioner, I loved helping people with their pregnancies, but—nope—I didn't want that to be me. Determined to finish learning how to care for women of all ages effectively and creatively, I'd decided the last thing I needed was to have motherhood get in my way.

But my eggs begged to differ.

Hello up there, remember us? The time has come to drop the birth control and cooperate!

It's as if my little friends had developed a voracious appetite for sperm and were ready to par*tay*! With their persistent voices pressed into my consciousness, I soon found women with child everywhere—in the clinic, on the street, and in stores. Now, pregnant bellies follow me like spotlights, as if blindingly revealing my childlessness from every angle.

And to make matters worse, it's not only pregnant women I notice. Children, too, have caught my eyes. In the span of a glance, the breadth of a heartbeat, I find myself trying to envision what our child would be like. Would he or she have Dan's sense of adventure and my stubbornness? What would I look like pregnant? How would I parent?

This can't be right.

How can I, one completely uninterested in mothering, be experiencing these sorts of feelings? What am I to do? Would running away help?

Somehow, I've found myself smack dab in the middle of an unexpected conundrum: a love-hate relationship with motherhood. I now feel like I am running a race against my ovaries—and against myself.

Is that even possible?

Or maybe, it's against humanity: against this crazy course where time passes faster than you can blink. Where family and career seem like two ends of a pendulum swing in a world where people don't live forever and our eggs scream, waiting to be remembered. I wonder, can we women balance the notions of career, motherhood, family, and aspirations? Can the puzzle pieces even fit together?

The Itsy-Bitsy Things of Life

I seem to have become keen on little things these days. While road biking by vineyards and farms in our neighborhood streets of Santa Rosa, California, I catch myself taking second glances at fluffy ewes and suckling calves. Since we're near the famous Napa Valley wine country, it's not uncommon to see farm animals and stretches of green vineyards that transform into rich seas of red, yellow, and orange every fall. But somehow, this season is different.

Now, I'm fixated on the signs of growth and newness—on the bright green leaves peeping out from grapevines, the apple bulbs emerging from the pink blossoms on our trees, and a mother dove in the hanging basket on our porch that nests beneath a canopy of fuchsia, its blooms dancing in the breeze. It's as if some primordial instinct were trying to invade me, override my normal logical senses, and get me to start nurturing—something—*anything*. A farm animal. An apple blossom. Anything I can hold and squeeze or cradle and rock.

What?

I'll graduate this May, and my womb is now yearning for company. It's lonely, when forever, it has felt perfectly content being single. My close friend just announced she's pregnant, and somehow I found myself jealous despite the fact that Dan and I haven't even started trying. How does that make sense?

Mothers-to-be swarm the streets again, coming out of hibernation after winter, now infiltrating earth's every nook and cranny. They're impossible to escape.

For so long now, I haven't even dared look at bumps big and small, round and pointy, high- and low-set for more than a moment, for fear looking meant yearning, and yearning meant my birth control measures would immediately disintegrate.

But now I can't help it.

I want that to be me.

FIRST TRIMESTER

WEEKS 1–13

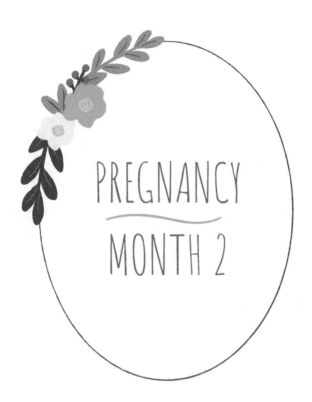

PREGNANCY
MONTH 2

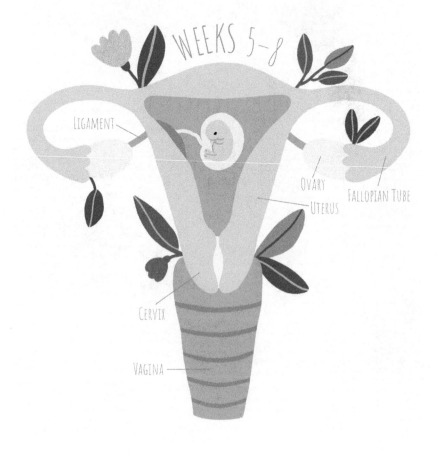

WEEKS 5-8

Ligament

Ovary

Fallopian Tube

Uterus

Cervix

Vagina

WEEK 5

Baby

- Is the size of a poppy seed.
- Starts developing the brain, spinal cord, and heart.

Mama

- Secretes progesterone hormone from your ovaries to support your growing embryo.
- Begins revving up the heart and circulatory system. Your heart rate will soon increase to provide adequate blood flow to you and your baby.

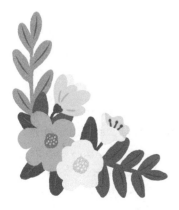

Can I Count?

I did what any reasonable woman would do when she was a few days late for her period. I plopped down on my porcelain throne, peed on that plastic wand, and waited for time to magically unroll my unknown path. Little did I know that the day before, Dan had an epiphany at his best friend's bachelor party. Apparently, our life was too ordinary, predictable, and quiet. He was ready for something new.

Funny how life goes.

I glanced down, and there was my answer. One blue line plus another one saluting beside it. Is that *two* I see? Last night I went to bed confidently knowing how to count all the way to two, and now I'm wondering if I should re-enroll in kindergarten.

I rubbed all things nighttime out of my eyes. Away soared the moon and stars. Faint now are the lingering images of last night's dream. *Okay. Let's try this again, shall we? One and two. One plus one is two. Right. So, two minus one is still one.*

Then, the dawn stretched across my horizon and my soul rose as if tied to a bouquet of balloons. I don't need to re-enroll after all. I can't believe it! In our eight years of marriage, that blessed little stick turned positive. No, we hadn't officially started trying yet, but I sensed Dan's views, like mine, were changing.

Unfortunately, it didn't take long for anxious thoughts to flow in the wake of my morning's revelation. Had I done anything to harm the baby in the past week? Anything at all? Though I'd been using prenatal vitamins for a while now, lately I've only halfheartedly followed the regimen. *Heaven forbid*, I even ate a soft cheese! Surely, I'm growing an alien cyclops.

My mind baits me with questions. Should I call Dan, or wait until he comes home from work? How should I tell him? Will this pregnancy last its full term? What will it be like?

Oh my gosh, I'm pregnant! I can't believe it.

All I want to do is bask in this moment and forget about my work that starts in an hour. There's a full day of patient visits ahead of me, with endless labs to review, emails to answer, and phone calls to make. Women will be waiting for reassurance, refills, referrals, and reality-checks, not to mention the usual prenatal checkups, endometrial or vulvar biopsies, testing for sexually transmitted infections, pap smears, breast checks, menopause conversations, and birth control prescriptions.

There's always more work than time.

But world, don't you know today is not like any other? I'm pregnant! Me. Pregnant. God plucked a little being from his imagination and sprinkled it within me. A tiny soul and body are blooming in my core.

And yet, wonder continues to mingle with worry. How will this fit into our lives? I mean, what's this going to look like? I just completed my schooling and am switching jobs. Dan's graduating from medical school residency training and starting a sports medicine fellowship in another city, so we'll soon be moving to San Jose for a year.

How will we make this work?

It's been the longest day ever, but I managed to keep my cool. *Okay, kind of.* Dan and I are home from work, and a huge, uncontrollable smile stretches across my face every time our eyes meet. I try to hide this curious reflex, telling him it's just so good to see him—which *is* true.

I'll be nonchalant and wait for the right time, *really*. Dinner will provide the perfect moment to tell him, I'd decided. I'll set the table, replace the knife with the positive pregnancy test, and then watch him like a lab rat.

But I couldn't help myself. Dan was in the shower before dinner, asked for a bar of soap, and got handed a positive pregnancy test instead. Just like that, all his movement and small talk came to a dead halt. Thick steam continued to billow out from behind the curtain, but I could hear nothing more than the shower running.

Oh no, I evaporated my husband!

I peeked behind the shower curtain and was relieved to see he hadn't disappeared in a puff of mist. He had the same confused expression I must have had that morning. After a brief eternity, his eyes grew big, his eyebrows soared to the sky, and a wide smile stretched across his face. Apparently, he really was ready for something new.

What to Call It?

They say, "Sticks and stones may break my bones, but words will never hurt me." But I don't believe it, not even for a minute. Words have the incredible power to not only reflect but also *create* levels of attachment. I remember how significant it was when I labeled someone my "best friend" in middle school, and when that undefined relationship became official.

Words embody expectations, encapsulate our hopes and fears, and when uttered or thought, they carry us along like a marionette's strings. We dangle—vulnerable—dancing to their whim. Words shape our perspective and our reality. For this reason, I can't help but wonder: What am I to call this little thing inside of me?

Should I refer to it by a medical name? "Blastocyst." It has nice rhythmic syllables. Blast-o-cyst. Official. Scientific. And better yet, conveniently void of emotion.

Or should I say "baby"? But heart activity just barely started, and what if this pregnancy only lasts a few weeks longer? I can only imagine how much harder it would be to have first imagined this collection of cells as my future son or daughter.

On the other hand, if at the end of all this I get to hold a delightfully precious child, shouldn't I, out of respect, start calling him or her by some name now?

This train of thought races through my mind, each railcar a word—compiled, combined, and rearranged—each car a carrier of meaning, heavy-laden with its cargo. Which one should I choose?

How could I possibly decide?

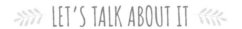

LET'S TALK ABOUT IT

Is This Normal?

Finding out you're pregnant can be a crazy and emotional experience. This can be partly explained by pregnancy hormones kicking in and your body starting to make changes to support your baby. And then again, who wouldn't have a tornado of thoughts and feelings with all the life changes and unknowns ahead? Give yourself some space to let the news sink in and take it one day at a time, remembering there is a purpose to your journey.

Pregnancy symptoms galore

Pregnant women (yes, like you, my friend) can experience all sorts of surprising and unsurprising symptoms. You may have anticipated nausea and vomiting, but did you know exhaustion, bloating, breast tenderness, and even peeing all the time are also on this list? Although these may start now or in the next few weeks, there's usually a light at the end of the tunnel around the end of the first trimester, at about 13 to 15 weeks.

While these symptoms may make you feel discouraged or like a hot mess, try to remind yourself that at least they're reassuring signs. Look at your body rising to the occasion like a champ! Enjoy your better days rather than focusing on the harder ones, and work to cultivate an attitude of hope rather than worry. Who knows, you may even be one of those lucky ladies who doesn't have any pregnancy symptoms!

So, while you're busy lying on the couch or living off of fruit, you may be happy to know this is not all for nothing. Your baby is very busy developing throughout pregnancy, but especially early on, with the organs—like the heart, brain, bones, and spinal cord—forming in the first 10 to 16 weeks of pregnancy.

Living mindfully

This exciting news also means your baby is particularly vulnerable to the outside world. What a great time to switch into protective pregnant mode by being mindful of what you put on or in your body! Watch out for undercooked eggs, meats, and seafood; unpasteurized milk and drinks; paint fumes; and cleaning products (what a great way to not clean for nine months!). Consider the risks involved in circumstances like the coronavirus pandemic and take the necessary precautions to keep you and your little one safe. It's also wise to have someone else change your cat's litter box, avoid traveling to areas with the Zika virus, and skip saunas and hot tubs since your baby's development is sensitive to your body overheating.

Yes, that also means now is the best time to stop using alcohol, tobacco products (including vaping), and illicit drugs—yes, even marijuana. Remember, it shows strength to ask for help. Support can make such a difference!

Digging Deeper

For more on how to set yourself up for a great pregnancy, mosey on back to appendix A-3a and B-4h. Here you'll find answers to common questions like:

» How do I set myself up for an awesome pregnancy? (A-3a)

» When do I notify my healthcare provider that I'm pregnant? (A-3a)

» Should I stop my psychiatric medications? (A-3a)

» Are supplements a good idea in pregnancy? (A-3a)

» Using marijuana or smoking cigarettes isn't that bad, right? (B-4h)

WEEK 6

Baby

- Is 3 mm long, head to rump.[1]
- Heart activity is detected.
- Forms the head, chest, and abdominal cavity.
- Begins growing arms and legs.

Mama

- Starts forming the placenta, the hormone factory organ, which supports your baby's growth and development.
- Pregnancy symptoms may include breast tenderness, nausea, vomiting, constipation, bloating, fatigue, urinary frequency, and cravings. Some women experience all of these, while others don't have any.

Breaking the News

It's now been one whole week since my life-changing porcelain throne revelation. Since then, I've outwardly managed to go about the normal motions of life, but inwardly, it has been a different story. I'm still in utter disbelief, rechecking the results of that sacred fortune-telling stick still displayed on our bathroom counter. Is my little whatcha-ma-call-it *really* in there, growing within me—like petals swelling and unfolding? I lean forward, hovering over my precious, plastic artifact, convinced for another few minutes—yes!

I suppose the only appropriate thing then would be to plan my grand pregnancy announcement for some very important people—airport security. Okay, my focus on this announcement is a bit embarrassing, I'll admit. Still, we're flying up to Seattle to stay at Dan's family's home and attend a friend's wedding, and what's a pregnant woman to do?

Plan it down to the minute, that's what.

I'll start by vaguely informing them I can't go through the scary deathtrap of a scanning machine and will need a pat-down instead, thank you very much. Naturally, they'll ask, "Why?" and I'll boldly announce something along the lines of "Don't mess with me, I'm pregnant." *Roar.* Sure, my body shows absolutely no outward signs, but really, I *am.*

Then it will be out. My pregnancy will be official. *Really official.*

Little did I know, though, how things would transpire. Nothing went according to plan. *Wait, where was that machine?* I asked someone on security staff, and he had the nerve to shrug it off and say they didn't have one.

What? How's that possible?

"Well good," I managed. "Cause I'm pregnant."

So there. I released the words into the greater cosmos. It was unnecessary, but they were twirling about—*real*—just like the being inside of me.

Later in the trip, however, things started to really sink in. It was over dinner with Dan's family where we had a much less official, and notably *un*planned, pregnancy announcement.

We had settled in around the long, farm-style table on their back deck. As the light faded into dusk, the shadows danced along the fine meal spread out along the board before us—the savory dishes of early summertime. A crisp breeze drifted among the pines.

I was passing a bowl of fruit salad when a question interrupted my thoughts.

"When are you two going to have kids already?"

Sure, it was a typical query, usually warranting a wisecrack comment from us in response, so I suppose we could have prepared for it. Instead, Dan and I were quiet and simply smiled.

Eyes bugged amid the silence.

"Wait, are you pregnant?"

"Yes," we admitted, voices soft.

What a mistake that answer turned out to be! Before we knew it, we were flooded with exclamations and advice. I wasn't ready for the hype at all. Sure, the excitement was legitimate—we were years "overdue," a term that always made me think of a library book. But this was too much. A cascade of well-intentioned comments doused us. Rising on the unhelpful tide were notes on how our life was going to change. *Forever.*

"Dan, no more five-hour bike rides on Saturdays," one said, or "Think you're tired now, wait until you have kids." Then, seeing our frightened faces, they tacked on, "It's definitely worth it," "It's so gratifying," and "There's nothing like having a little one look to you for love."

Wait, I don't care about that last part. What do you mean I'll be more tired than ever before? I'm already tired enough!

Oh, if only we'd been able to keep it secret just a little while longer, I thought as I wiped my tears later that evening in one of their upstairs bedrooms.

I guess I must truly be pregnant now.

Old World, New Me

Okay, so maybe I overreacted just a tad last night. But aren't pregnant women supposed to be emotional? Even logical little me? *Sigh.* I can't say I'm thrilled with this newfound sensitivity, but I suppose it's allowing me the opportunity to soak in my world with the viewpoint of a philosopher or explorer.

Take, for example, when we had landed in the Washington airport earlier. Blearily shuffling out to baggage claim at 1:00 a.m., I had witnessed an interaction—a moment between a child and her dad—that struck me.

There at a corral of black chairs between the towering glass windows, a toddler sat on her father's lap, legs curled around his waist. As we approached, she cupped his scruffy face, smashed her button nose against his, and peered through his glasses as children do through toyshop windows. They couldn't stop giggling. Then she proceeded to lift his glasses, up then down.

Up and down.

Down and up.

Up and down.

And then, once more.

She kneaded his cheeks with her roly-poly fingers and tugged on the silly putty skin draping his neck. Despite being in a foreign environment, surrounded by strangers, she was perfectly at ease. To her, "Daddy" meant *home*.

I was captivated.

She had a closeness with him that I can only hope to have with God. I wish I could yank on his cheeks whenever I needed to feel his love. As the moment passed, I wished our baby would someday be working Dan's face—or mine—like that.

But that wasn't the only intense introspection I've had lately. This morning, still wary after yesterday's dinner conversation, I had tiptoed my way over to the playroom, which was stuffed to the brim with toys for the grandkids' amusement. Surrounded by the myriad of stuffed animals, dollhouse accessories, and puzzle pieces, I sat.

In the quiet, my mind's eye greeted a montage of imagined memories—tea parties with ponies, stories shared on the laps of loved ones, and pies baked in pink, vanilla-scented ovens. As the jumbled children's toys and the overlapping chorus of kids' voices eventually faded from the projector screen of my imagination, they were replaced with a certainty that this is a haven.

The room hummed innocence, imagination, and limitless possibilities—a place where children can feel at home and conjure up great unimaginables. It was the type of place in which our child would surely thrive, I thought, as I traced my fingers along Winnie the Pooh marching down a cross-stitched log.

And then it hit me. Kids can't stay in a playroom like this forever! What was I thinking? There's a much bigger, scarier world out there—with so many sharp edges and exposed wall outlets. How can I prepare our child for that greater, un-babyproofed world out there while still providing a magical childhood? Won't that be my job as "mother"? Talk about an overwhelming thought for an amateur pregnant woman like me! How could I possibly do both?

If only I could just poke God's cheeks and remember He's with me.

⇶ LET'S TALK ABOUT IT ⫷

How to Survive Nausea, Vomiting, and Other Great Wonders

You probably never suspected how quickly your world could turn upside down from innocent little hormones—like human chorionic gonadotropin (hCG), estradiol, and progesterone—not to mention the physiological changes of pregnancy.[1] These can easily make you feel quite unladylike and wish you had never gotten pregnant. Let's be honest, things may come out when we'd rather they not (like vomit or burps) or not come out when we'd do anything for them to evacuate (such as constipation or bloating). So, for the scoop on some common gastrointestinal novelties, read on.

Nausea and vomiting

The term *morning sickness* is (unfortunately) a misnomer, since nausea, retching, and vomiting can happen *any* time of day. For many women, it's worse at night or when they're tired.[2,3] These symptoms usually start between four to nine weeks, peak around seven to twelve weeks, and then resolve by the sixteenth week.[1,3]

Now, every pregnancy is different. You may have a different experience in this pregnancy compared to a previous one, and you may even have a pregnant friend without any morning sickness. If you're in the mood, there are many potential things you can blame, such as hormones, genetics, slowed gastric emptying, evolutionary adaptation, or even infections and vitamin deficiencies.[1-3] Yet the exact cause is still unknown.

Talk to your medical provider if, because of morning sickness, you're feeling miserable and can't keep food or fluids down. It's much better to get a handle on symptoms before they become debilitating and cause dehydration or other problems. This is especially important if you experience a severe form of morning sickness called *hyperemesis gravidarum* or *HG* (think nausea gone *hyper*) since this can cause problems like dehydration, weight loss and abnormal lab values.[1] Interestingly, HG is more common among those who are carrying a baby girl, have a digestive system infection called *Helicobacter pylori*, or have a history of motion sickness, migraines, or HG.[1,2,4]

Heartburn

Now here's a bit of trivia for you Jeopardy fans—*gastroesophageal reflux* (or *GERD*) is one of the most common digestive problems in pregnancy. GERD or heartburn occurs when the stomach acid enters your food pipe (*esophagus*) and causes a burning feeling in your upper chest or throat. This tends to happen more often as you get further along in pregnancy, but yes, it can happen earlier.[1] Pregnancy hormones make it easier for the doorway (valve) between your esophagus and stomach to open and welcome stomach acid into the esophagus.[1,5] Some researchers speculate that later on, your little dumpling pushing upward could contribute to this phenomenon.[5]

Ptyalism

Ptyalism is a rarer symptom and has got to be one of the best spelling bee words out there. If you are struggling with it, you salivate more than ever before and don't know what to do with all that spit. This can make you tired, depressed, and even have a decreased appetite.[6] Sometimes ptyalism occurs alongside nausea and vomiting (HG).[1,6] The good news is it tends to resolve by the second trimester, and certainly after birth. You got it—hormones are likely at work here.

Constipation

I can't think of a more fitting way than to end this conversation with the topic of constipation and its partner in crime, hemorrhoids. Contrary to popular belief, you are not required to poop every day. However, you're probably constipated if you go infrequently, can't poop easily, only get a few measly pebbles out, or are gassy or bloated. Causes can include pregnancy hormones that slow down the digestion process and decrease water in your intestines, the iron in prenatal vitamins, and later in pregnancy, your growing uterus.[1]

Hemorrhoids

As for hemorrhoids, these are (internal or external) tender and swollen blood vessels around your anus. Typical symptoms include itching, discomfort, bleeding with bowel movements, and, if external, visible lumps and swelling. Though not inevitable, hemorrhoids are especially common later in pregnancy and after childbirth. As always, let your maternity care provider know if you are battling hemorrhoids, especially if you're in a lot of pain or notice a hard lump (which may indicate a blood clot in the area). Don't worry—hemorrhoids can improve and may resolve with time. Getting constipation (or diarrhea) under control can be game changers!

Digging Deeper

Be sure to check out the appendix, which is packed with survival-guide tips for the symptoms we just discussed. Since your body is unique, you'll find some of these tips work better for you than others, so don't give up! In A-3b, you'll find answers to questions like:

» Do I have to suffer from nausea and vomiting, or are there things that I can try to feel better?

» Can I prevent heartburn? What can I do to treat it?

» Help! What do I do with all this spit?

» What can I do about constipation and hemorrhoids?

WEEK 7

Baby

- Is 10 mm long.
- Now presents distinct sides of the brain (the right and left hemispheres), which are important for communication, math, and creativity.
- Makes 100 brain cells every minute.
- Is developing ears and fingers.

Mama

- Kidneys filter more blood to clear potential toxins, making you pee more.
- Prolactin hormone levels increase to enlarge and prepare breasts for breastfeeding. Your breasts may already feel different.

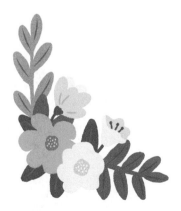

What's in a Tattoo?

Sometimes, at the end of a long day of work, there is nothing more relaxing than flipping through whatever random catalog the postwoman managed to stuff into our much-too-small mailbox. Today, it was a sports-clothing catalog, which I'm grateful to receive since it's so much more interesting than the usual tire shop leaflet or coupon to the local barbershop. What better than to check out glorious fabrics and fashions designed to aid the sports I now only theoretically love? Because let's face it, the activities I once enjoyed now seem too much to ask of the snippets of energy reserve I have left after limping through my workday.

What, on any other splendid, nonpregnant day, would have been a pleasant skim-through at my kitchen table became anything but. The catalog's pages were filled with strong, fit, and active women—a fact that would normally not have phased me one bit. But today, with every page-turn, with each successive image of toned models in fitted activewear, an unwelcome thought pressed into the pit of my stomach.

I'm not like them.

Slamming the pages shut, I tossed the offending catalog on the table, only to watch five young, muscular women in bathing suits slowly slide away from me, mocking me from their place on the front cover. Further and further away, greater and greater the distance spreads between me and these figures who exemplify the American ideal.

Our bodies are moving in opposite trajectories. While they are getting stronger, I'm expanding, crossing over, slowly joining another group of women—the *mothers*. The people who pick their babies' noses, have crumbs stuck in their own hair, and rub their kids' faces "clean" with spit. You know, those *minivan drivers*.

As an NP, I've seen firsthand how pregnancy can affect women's bodies. But everyone is different, and I can't help but wonder—*How will my body react? What will my belly look like after delivery? Will I have tons of stretch marks? Will pregnancy or labor cause hemorrhoids? Me, with hemorrhoids!?* These thoughts are all petty, I know. But it all feels so out of my control, like I'm being carried along for a ride in my own skin.

It was not too long after Dan came home from work that I blurted out my concerns. I was sitting at the kitchen table, too exhausted to budge, while Dan bustled around the room, tidying up and prepping for dinner. He was loading the dishwasher when the thought that had been festering in my mind for the last few hours would no longer be contained. Tears were gathered in the sidelines, ready to rush in and comfort me.

"I'm turning into a *mother*," I exclaimed. "A mother!"

"What do you mean?" Dan asked, moving dishes from the sink into the dishwasher.

"My body is never going to look the same again, and I'm going to get big and then bigger—I'll have nothing in common with these cover models." I choked up and welcomed in my tears.

Dan looked up, dish in hand.

"Oh, Sweetie," he soothed. "Pregnancy is a beautiful and sacred time. Your body is now a cabin, a place where our special little someone lives. It isn't just about you and your body anymore."

I sniffed and swiped a tear from my cheek.

"And isn't that part of why we wanted kids anyway?" he continued. "Look, did you notice that one of the women on the magazine cover even has *Mom* tattooed on her ankle?"

Nope, I had not. *Now that's cool.*

Maybe not all moms have to look like crap. Hmm, an athletic mother—such a person might exist? Wow! It's as if, before *this* moment, I've never *ever* run across a mother before. Nope, never met one at the clinic nor had one of my own. As I considered this concept of thriving mothers, a whole parade of images marched into my mind—images of beautiful, joyful, kind women; strong, healthy, brilliant, and wise women; gutsy, interesting, talented, and creative women. Women who all happen to be mothers.

It's crazy to me how shocking that picture is. Almost as crazy as my meltdown over image and appearance. I mean, I know it's something we all deal with to some degree—either consciously or subconsciously. We can't help it. Anyone who's a part of a society is going to be shaped in some way by its views on beauty. It's just that most of my life, I haven't consciously thought too hard about it. Until today. Suddenly, my whole world flipped upside down over the thought that this may be the closest I'll ever get to the American ideal, even though that thought is a bit preposterous. After all, I've known women to reach their prepregnancy weight around six months after their delivery. It's doable.

And while it turns out that model didn't actually have a "Mom" tattoo (Dan was just trying to console me), I realize she could have. Or, if not her, some other beautiful model whose life is not limited by motherhood. Just the fact that such a tattoo *could* exist sparked revelation: Motherhood doesn't mean you have to lose yourself. In fact, it might just be a way of delving deeper into your identity.

A Matter of Business

In the past day, I've been referred to as an incubator, a sacred sanctuary, and even a manufacturing company. Even though I'm officially very productive on the inside, outside I feel anything but. I feel more like a trash compactor. Food sounds awful. Not a single taste is enticing, and not eating simply perpetuates this cycle. What I would pay to have one—*just one!*—food craving.

So, I do my best to nibble on a small snack every couple of hours, sip freshly steeped ginger tea, and make sure I take my vitamin B6 twice a day like a good little girl. In my desperation, I even borrowed my neighbor's acupressure wristbands, taking care to cover the gray elastic with my long sleeves so patients and coworkers don't ask why I'm wearing sea sickness bands on dry land.

With the nausea and sluggishness, I haven't been in much of a mood to write. It's all I can do to go to work, come home, and drag myself on a 60-minute walk that once lasted a mere 45. I then sit down and watch some old rerun while Dan is away from the house, finishing his last week of medical residency training.

There, mission accomplished.

It seems ages ago that I felt well. Since the nausea started, I've had to find creative ways to deal with my symptoms at work. I now take a few extra seconds washing my hands with my back turned to patients, which kindly allows me to gag to my heart's content without raising suspicion of pregnancy. Handwashing is the best way to protect people against nasty bacteria and viruses, right? It's simply a matter of business. Patient safety first, of course.

And when it's time to perform a physical exam, I just hold my breath (literally) and hope for the best. Before now, bad breath, body odor, or the scent of vaginal infection wasn't a big deal, but now, smells are a killer. I'm so worried someone will send me into uncontrollable dry heaves. Women are already self-conscious, making sure their legs and bikini areas are pristine, I shudder to imagine how they'd feel if this happened!

Finally, after my last patient of the morning says goodbye, I lock my office door with a sigh of relief and thank God for lunch breaks. Not that I'm excited for the food, though I usually manage to consume a quick snack. No, I'm more grateful for rest. With the office light off and an alarm set, I crumple up my jacket into the semblance of a pillow, pull out my blanket (a sheet I'd smuggled in for the purpose), and lie down on the floor. For the next 20 minutes, I let myself doze until my alarm jolts me into reality, beckoning me to prepare for the second half of the day. As if I have energy for that.

Groaning, I roll out of my makeshift bed, my stomach momentarily appeased. *What a relief.* Sometimes, rest really can help with nausea. Flicking on my office light, I squint in the fluorescent flicker. I shove my sheet back into a pillowcase, toss my jacket over my chair, and sit at the computer to skim my patient schedule, hoping my energy will magically appear if I'm desperate enough.

Don't get me wrong, I love my job, but it would be much appreciated if, at the end of the day, it didn't feel like I just endured a long, muddy, treacherous marathon. If I had the choice, I'd rather it felt like I had completed a fun color run where I got sprinkled with an array of bright paints while pushing for 5K.

⟫⟫ LET'S TALK ABOUT IT ⟪⟪

Eating for Two

Has pregnancy changed the way you look at and experience food? If yes, you're not alone! Truly though, you have lots of freedom in how and what you eat in pregnancy. You may even find pregnancy gives you an opportunity to enjoy new flavors, textures, recipes, and restaurants (or bathrooms).

Now, for my disclaimer before we move on: If you're in pregnancy survival mode, trying to keep foods or fluids down, don't fixate on healthy eating for now. Just try to eat foods that are safe in pregnancy and sound tolerable. Be sure to check out the previous week's "How to Survive Nausea, Vomiting, and Other Great Wonders" and come back to this section when you feel better.

You likely have heard the expression *eating for two*. Nope, this doesn't mean you eat twice as much as you did before you were pregnant. Since your baby is still smaller than a strawberry, she doesn't need as much sustenance as a grown adult. Instead, let's think of eating for two as this: what you eat impacts both you *and* your baby, who depends on you to get the right amount and type of nutritional building blocks to grow.

Benefits of nutritious variety

For baby

When you eat a good, nutritious variety of food, you'll help your baby receive vital ingredients for a strong and healthy mind and body, while also setting her up for a healthier future.[1-4] If your baby is born at a healthy weight, she is more likely to have a healthy weight as a child and as an adult and also has a lower chance of developing chronic health problems (like heart disease or diabetes).[1-3,5,6] Plus, you not only keep your palate entertained but you also train your baby to get used to different food tastes in utero (yes, food changes the taste of your amniotic fluid!).[7]

For you

Nutritious eating also means you'll have more energy to enjoy pregnancy, cope with changes, and prepare for motherhood. Yes, we need all the help we can get! You'll be more likely to gain the right amount of weight in pregnancy, making you feel way better while minimizing risks for complications (like gestational diabetes, high blood pressure problems, and Cesarean birth).[8-11] Trust me, since it'll be easier to get back to your prepregnancy weight after delivery, you'll thank yourself! Yep, this mindfulness is also a down payment for future pregnancies and your long-term health.[8,9]

MEDICATIONS AND SUPPLEMENTS

Check with your maternity care provider first before starting something new, even if it's over the counter or touted by your mom, best friend, or the internet at large. This will give you a chance to talk about its safety in pregnancy and see if it's a good option for you based on your symptoms and medical history.

Next steps

Perhaps you have a hard time feeling comfortable with eating and weight gain during pregnancy, even if you hear and know it's normal. Women who may especially notice this are those who have past experiences with dieting, eating disorders, trouble relating to their bodies, or gaining a lot of weight during prior pregnancies.[*] If you can relate, ask your maternity care provider to connect you with helpful resources like an experienced registered dietician or therapist (like MFT or LCSW). With support, you'll have a much more enjoyable pregnancy!

Either way, allow yourself to think of this like an adventure. Seize the day and see what it's like to nourish yourself and your baby in pregnancy. Throughout, you may find yourself adapting to accommodate a shifting relationship with food. Embrace it. You're growing and changing every moment.

---

[*] Veronica Benjamin, RD, personal communication, August 1, 2015

Digging Deeper

Since what you eat can make such a big difference for both you and the development of your little one(s), check out B-1 for helpful tips, tricks, and other tidbits on the topic. There you'll find answers to common questions like:

» What's the scoop on eating in pregnancy? (B-1a)

» What should my eating plate look like? (B-1g)

» What are food and drink "no-nos" in pregnancy? (B-1a)

» Can you share some practical tips for mindful eating? (B-1a & b)

» I'm a busy woman. Do you have any quick grab-and-go snack ideas? (B-1e)

WEEK 8

Baby

- Is 16 mm long.
- Forms the bones of the rib cage and spinal column.
- Has distinct toes.
- Develops sweat glands.

Mama

- To have adequate oxygen flow for pregnancy, your lung capacity grows, allowing you to inhale and exhale more air during normal breathing.
- The cervix, the mouth of the uterus, begins to soften, and its blood supply increases.

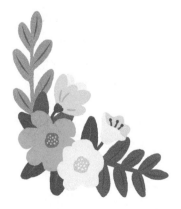

Surprise!

After years and years of taking apart, reassembling, and constructing oily motors and shiny gadgets, my brother, Palko, is graduating with his PhD, in—you guessed it—robotics. It just so happens I will be eight weeks pregnant when my family reunites, and we've been dying to figure out when and how to tell them the big news.

Of the options we considered, one stood out: a truly unique graduation present for my brother. We'd hand it over and say, "You did it! Happy graduation. Hope you like it." And then he'd rip off the wrapping paper and probably look a little confused. Maybe his eyebrows would scrunch or raise in a question. Then, as per family tradition, he'd pass around the item so everyone gathered could see the gift. From hand to hand the mysterious object would go until someone had the guts to state the obvious.

The emperor has no clothes. Or, in our case, two lines on the pregnancy test equals Meshi plus Dan having sex. Yes, I suppose we really would let people hold a stick I peed on.

I can only hope the excitement of a new child in the family—the first and long-awaited grandchild for my parents—outweighs that awkward thought we all have when we think of family members sharing bodily fluids in the name of love. Sure, it was always presumed, but now has been confirmed. *Yuck.*

Well, we chose the plan and stuck to it. After the graduation ceremony had concluded, we must have walked miles around campus to get to the outdoor seating area and the long, linen-covered banquet table where the catering crew had set up a celebratory meal for the graduates' families. Other overachieving students and their well-wishers were grouped around at tables nearby, and in the hum of conversation, we handed over the paper-wrapped stick. And waited.

Palko was at the end of the table, with my father to his right. He unwrapped the package, and they both squinted at the gift, eyebrows rumpled. They paused long enough for others to ask, "What is it?" and "What did they give?" Then silently, they handed it along down the line.

My family passed around that blessed pee stick amongst themselves until it reached my mother—who shrieked. *So. Loud.* Everyone within earshot, which was pretty much the entire graduating class and their families, looked over and stared.

She teared up and asked the only logical question left to ask.

"Meshi, how did this happen?"

Dr. Dan Parker, ready to put his inflated medical school tuition to good use, kindly started to explain.

"Well," he said, "when a man and a woman really love each other . . . "

The Pregnant Gardener

Despite how awful the pregnancy symptoms have been, I've noticed joy shine through in the most unexpected places. Somehow, I still look forward to visits with my prenatal and postpartum patients. I've always been grateful for the chance to hear women's stories and, with their permission, enter into their storyline. What an honor!

Pregnancy is much like stepping into a bubble of newness and staying there—you breathe it, taste it, feel it, and interpret the world through it—and it's a gift to be able to support pregnant women, helping them navigate their journey, while tending to their needs like an attentive gardener. I get to carefully watch pregnant women change, grow, and root (and sometimes uproot or even transplant) in response to their little growing bud within.

Just like tulips prefer full sun and bulbs need a good freeze to blossom, so every pregnant woman has her own unique environment in which she can flourish. This has got to be one of my favorite parts of my job. I love exploring how she and I can partner together to ensure she has the most nourishing climate around her.

Want more shade? Try this umbrella. Need more water? Here's a sprinkler. No room to grow? Let's weed. For a pregnant patient, this nurturing care could mean giving more information, validating her, making a telephone call, investigating a new symptom, recommending a lifestyle change, offering a medication, giving a referral or even a hug, or writing a work accommodation letter.

In this role, I often see how incredibly resilient we can be. When women flourish and grow even in tough circumstances, I'm reminded of the spread of yellow-blossomed succulents sprouting between the crags of a California shoreline. I can't help the urge to say, "There, see that flower clinging to the face of that rocky cliff? It made it! It pushed its roots down deep into the surrounding hardness and grew anyway." No matter how alone, lost, or scared we pregnant women may feel at times, there is hope to be had—another chapter to be read or an unexpected rainbow after the storm.

Now if only I could remember this for my own self.

I've spent so much time learning to tend to the needs (and the weeds) of those who walk through the clinic's doors that I forget now that I, too, am pregnant; I am both the flower and the gardener. It's as if I should walk around with a watering can and douse myself. But just as flowers can't pick their own weeds or bring over a watering can in the absence of rain, I find myself in need of a gardener—a maternity care provider who can come alongside me in this pregnancy just as I have come alongside others.

In finding a safe place, I'll get to be a patient and not a provider. I won't need to have all the answers. I could be anxious, anal, excited, demanding, and whatever my little self feels like doing during this journey of unexpectedness.

Though in Santa Rosa, I've been enjoying the care of a wonderful family physician, Ann, who also happens to be a friend. Soon Dan will finish his training, and we'll be heading south to Cupertino, near San Jose. I've found someone there who works with several midwives and fits my must-haves for a care provider—a holistic, patient-centered approach to care and a desire to minimize unnecessary medical interventions. I will certainly appreciate her wisdom, perspective, and attention.

In the meantime, I'll continue to enjoy prenatal care from Ann, who is so sweet and compassionate that she just warms the world around her. That's exactly what full-sun plants like me need. Help to bloom. Maybe even a rich dump of manure now and again.

⋙ LET'S TALK ABOUT IT ⋘

Finding Good Prenatal Care

By now, you might be wondering when it's time to officially get initiated into prenatal care. And no, there's no hazing process. Typically, prenatal care starts between seven and ten weeks *gestational age* (*GA*), or the number of weeks from the first day of your last period. You and your maternity care provider may wish to rendezvous sooner if you've had multiple miscarriages or have other pressing concerns. Either way, if you don't already have a preferred provider, it's time to look for a qualified person to care for you during pregnancy and after delivery. Let's call this person a maternity care provider.

Finding a maternity care provider who you like and who takes good care of you is not always easy. But trust me, it's worth the energy! It can dramatically change your experience of pregnancy, labor, and birth, and it will also affect the safety of you and your baby. Here are a couple of tips to get you started.

Set your expectations

Commit to finding someone who's not only well trained in maternity care but who is also excited to partner with you and engage you in decision-making. You'll save yourself a lot of angst when you find someone who has a similar approach to pregnancy and birth as you do. This approach may be called a *philosophy of care* on a website or brochure. Don't worry, though, if you don't have any strong sentiments about the subject—that's okay, too.

You'll notice there are many types of maternity care providers, all of whom have different training, areas of expertise, places they attend deliveries (like hospitals, birth centers, or home births), and ideas regarding which methods provide the best care for their patients. Based on where you

If you don't have any health insurance, check with your state's public health department to learn if you qualify for free health insurance now that you're pregnant.

live in the U.S. and your health insurance, you may have the following maternity care provider types to choose from: midwives (either nurse or non-nurse), physicians (Ob-Gyn or family), nurse practitioners (women's health or family), and physician assistants.

Do your research

Become a pregnant Sherlock Holmes. Just think how adorable you'll look when you hold up that magnifying glass to your eye. And after you've posed at the photo booth, do your detective work—don't just go off hearsay. Once you've compiled a list of potential maternity care providers, check out their websites and call their offices to see if they (1) are accepting new patients and (2) take your insurance. Be sure to find out more about the maternity care provider and his or her practice setting.

When you get tired of doing all this work (because yes, it's exhausting and it's asking a lot), remember, finding the right maternity care provider is one of the most important decisions you'll make during your pregnancy. No exaggeration. It's worth your time.

Switching providers

Now, Sherlock, let me take the pressure off a bit by reminding you that picking a maternity care provider doesn't mean you're committed for life. Sure, it's ideal and convenient to have the same person or team taking care of you throughout pregnancy, but if you must, you can change providers, even late in pregnancy. It's your right. You may switch providers because you are moving away or you feel you are not receiving good (thoughtful, informed, respectful, or culturally sensitive) care. If need be, streamline the transition to another maternity care provider by making sure your records are transferred promptly.

Now, go and see what wonderful maternity care provider options you have around you. I wonder who you're going to find.

Digging Deeper

To help you in your detective work, A-3d includes a rundown on the types of maternity care providers and what distinguishes them from one another. Some of the questions it will help you answer include:

» What types of maternity care providers are there?

» What are good questions to ask when learning about providers?

» Are there other things for me to consider?

» I had a difficult birth experience and am dreading this next one already. How can I set myself up for a beautiful pregnancy and birth?

Notes

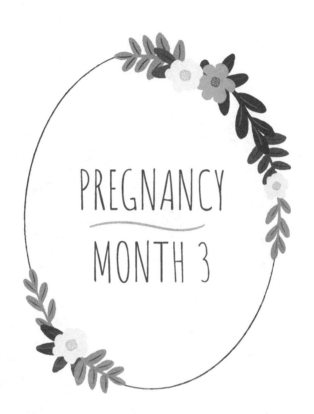

PREGNANCY

MONTH 3

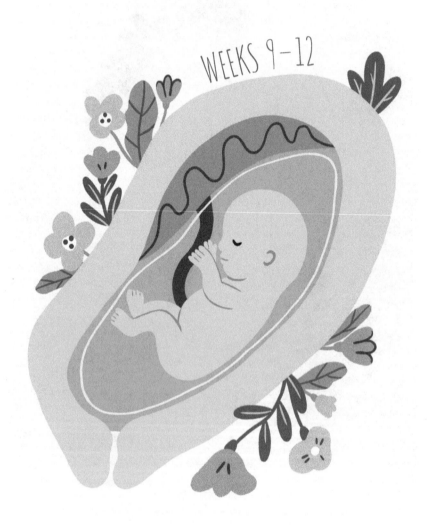

WEEK 9

Baby

- Is 23 mm long.
- Has detectable brain waves.
- Can move the hands and neck.
- Has developed ovaries or testes.
- Begins to develop the urinary system.

Mama

- Hormone-making transfers from the ovaries to the placenta.
- You may be especially tired, so make time for rest!
- Since the progesterone hormone slows food passage through the intestines, you may experience constipation.
  - It's a great time to increase your fiber and water intake.

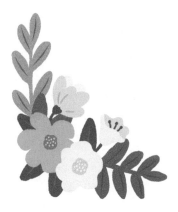

A Mother's Love

Most of all the other beautiful things in life come by twos and
threes, by dozens and hundreds. Plenty of roses, stars, sunsets,
rainbows, brothers, and sisters, aunts and cousins, but only one
mother in the whole world.
—KATE DOUGLAS WIGGIN

I don't know if there is anything more comforting than the love of a mother or a mother figure. I liken it to the crisp autumn air, a sunny day, or my great-grandmother's homemade apricot jam. It is love flowing and sweetly surrounding, reminding me that everything will be okay.

Unfortunately, my mother lives hundreds of miles from me, and so I can't drop by on a whim when I need that homemade jam. However, I can get whiffs of it in our daily phone chats and her visits every few months. She is like a dedicated mother hen who is not about to let mere miles separate her and her children. And boy am I grateful.

This trip she's come equipped for battle with several pregnancy books, some new but many saved from her own pregnancy days—which, unfathomably to me, are still her favorite times of life. From her striped tote bag, she even pulled out her floppy and weathered pregnancy folder, packed with lines of blue, right-leaning notes, handwritten in cursive. How is it possible that even then, this woman never *ever* scribbled anything, not notes, not a grocery list, nor a check? I suppose her writing echoes other aspects of her life—intentionality and beauty.

We soon settle around the kitchen table and leaf through the books in an attempt to plunge into all things week nine of pregnancy. We pored over every little detail, each comment and illustration. Get this: my little grape now has all its essential body parts, has lost its embryonic tail, and has started forming miniature teeth.

That's incredible! It's one thing to tell my patients about their pregnancy in general terms, and it's another to be realizing that these statements are now narrating my own life.

We turned page after page in wonder and delight, until my pesky companion, Nausea, started to feel excluded and had to speak up. In the span of a breath, I was carried along down that familiar, churning river, adrift in an unmanned raft. *Not again.*

Trying to calm the tide, we slice up a ripe watermelon and head to the living room to watch a movie, hoping the liquid, food, and taking a break from talking will help ease the queasiness. As my mom sits on our green couch, I perch myself on a cushion by her feet and lean back against her legs. While one scene on the screen slides into another, and the pink watermelon juice dribbles down my face, my mom brushes and braids my hair—one small section after another—and then repeats.

I'm not sure which of us enjoys this activity more. Me, feeling pampered by my mommy, or my mom sharing closeness with her baby who's growing a baby.

Regardless, by the end of the night, I contrived to look like a giant dandelion that somehow managed to grow arms and legs—thin braids poking out on my head, just waiting for someone to make a wish.

It reminds me of what children look like when zooming down that yellow plastic slide in our nearby playground, hair electrostatically projecting at every angle. *So funny!* Except, right now *I* don't feel funny—or like laughing. I don't have that elated look those kids have, because my slide seems much steeper and curvy. I can't even see the bottom. Is there even mulch down there in case I fly too fast and shoot out the end like a gumball hurled from its dispenser?

And yet, as I stare in the bathroom mirror, standing beside my mom, the image of this human dandelion fades in the light of her excited smile and attentive eyes. I forget the monumental changes and responsibilities lying ahead of me and simply bask in the reality of being my mother's daughter. She'll be there if I fall. Like those kids playing around that yellow slide who run to their mothers when they stumble and scrape a knee, I'll let my mother do what she does best—love.

Orange Chicken

That's it—Chinese food! Jackpot! I can't even remember when I last thought about that type of cuisine, let alone ate it. However, from the moment I saw someone else enjoying it—on a TV show, of all things—I could think of literally nothing else. I need it. Now. I can't bear living without orange chicken—that sweet crunchiness entwined with the pleasure of protein. I must have chicken. *Stat.*

China House, oh China House, how I thank you for your free-range orange chicken, veggie chow mein, and spring rolls. I made a special detour on my way home from work just for you—to study the diverse delights of your menu. One of each, please! Okay not really, but definitely an assortment, nonetheless. Before too long, I piled thirty dollars worth of little to-go boxes in the passenger seat beside me, envisioning the perfect dinner with Dan, as the tantalizing scents emanated from the packages and serenaded my taste buds.

Eventually, I made it home and spread out my treasured goodies on the kitchen table around me. I leaned back and proudly basked in the awesomeness of my loot. What a purchase! I then scarfed most of it down until I was stuffed to the brim and felt like a bloated dumpling.

Eating that much was not the only thing I came to regret, however. By the next morning, I was appalled to see that food in my fridge, with a revulsion that almost rivaled my disgust at seeing our teacher, Mr. Pratt, pick his nose with a paperclip in second grade. Who possibly allowed these despicable intruders into my home? *Get them out of my sight, immediately!*

Yep, thirty dollars down the drain just like that, to pamper my undecided taste buds for a moment. What a waste!

⇶ LET'S TALK ABOUT IT ⇷

Running to and from Food

Drooling for a milkshake and french fries? Sauerkraut and potatoes? Cheesecake? Want Mexican food for breakfast, lunch, and dinner (and midnight snack)? Or maybe you can't stand the thought of eggs or the smell of bacon? *Food cravings* are intense, all-consuming desires for certain foods, while *aversions* are smells or foods you can't stand.

That's right, welcome to pregnancy!

Interestingly, commonly craved foods vary by culture.[1] For example, chocolate and rice are commonly craved foods in the United States and Japan, respectively.[1] Moreover, cravings themselves can even mean different things to different people.[1] In the rural part of northern Tanzania, for instance, pregnant women indulge in food cravings—often meat, fish, veggies, fruits, and grains—believing these indicate babies' long-term food preferences and going without could lead to their babies feeling dissatisfied.[2]

> Cravings can be fickle, and the desired food may not sound remotely edible in a few hours or days. Instead of stockpiling your craved foods, try buying smaller quantities a few times a week.

So, where do studies show food cravings and aversions come from in the first place? Well, the jury is still out. Let's take a look at a few suggested reasons, shall we?

Possible reasons for cravings

Nutritional need.[1,*] Cravings may be your body's way of crying out, signaling its need for certain nutrients. For example, if you're craving ice cream, it may mean your body's craving more calcium. Hamburger cravings may indicate your budding body wants more fat. This is great news because, instead of being enslaved to your cravings, you can use them as a tip-off for what types of nutrients you may be lacking. Since your baby doesn't need that particular food so much as a key nutrient in it, you can satisfy that need with a more nutritious alternative.

Emotional need.[3,†] Foods can comfort us when we get anxious, stressed, depressed, or lonely. As with any item offering these benefits, food can be misused to give us a sense of control over our lives, provide us with an outlet for when we are angry or frustrated, or even give us something to do when we get bored.

---

* Veronica Benjamin, RD, personal communication, August 1, 2015
† Benjamin

Hormonal response.[1] Yes, hormones are always a solid scapegoat, remember? Your body is going through many changes to support your little one, and cravings are common side effects.

Regardless of the reason for cravings, this is a fabulous time to explore new tastes and sensational food combinations. Here's your chance to try what you've always dreamed of—like dipping pickles in ketchup. What a perfect treat! You'll notice that your food cravings will likely peak around the second trimester and then slowly decrease thereafter.[1]

Possible cause of aversions

Embryo protection.[4,5] As the main theory goes, aversions to smells and foods may be Mother Nature's way of keeping you away from potentially embryo-toxic foods—thereby protecting your little one from harmful substances.

As always, if you're struggling with how to best deal with cravings or aversions, or are getting stressed by them, reach out for help. Ask your maternity care provider to connect you with a registered dietician.

Digging Deeper

If cravings and food aversions sound all too familiar, welcome to the club! And if you don't have any right now, that's fantastic! Either way, feel free to peruse the B-1c and A-3f to find answers to common questions and concerns like:

» Are food cravings a problem? (B-1c)

» Help! I need tips to navigate my food cravings and aversions. (B-1c)

» What should I do if I feel like eating non-foods like ice, clay, and chalk? (B-1c)

» I'm an emotional eater. What strategies can help me cope without food? (B-1c)

» Does it matter how much weight I gain in pregnancy? (A-3f)

WEEK 10

Baby

- Is about 1 ¼ inches long.[1]
- Weighs about 1 ¼ ounces.[1]
- Begins occasional breathing motions.
- Has fully formed fingers.
- Makes urine, which becomes part of the amniotic fluid.
- Has developed about 90% of an adult body (about 4,000 separate body parts).

Mama

- Moodiness is especially common in the first trimester due to hormonal and life changes.
- Corneal thickening occurs, which may call for a new prescription for contact lenses.

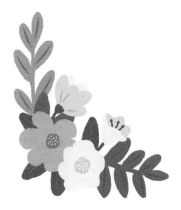

Birdsong

I can't help but think life would be lovely if there were a little bird perched at every street corner. No, not because I think ducking for cover to avoid bird droppings would be exciting. But rather, it's their cheerful songs I love so much.

Birds convey this amazing, carefree, Bob Marley–like, "Don't worry about a thing" attitude. They seem unfazed by life and trill even when things aren't so beautiful. I love how on some early mornings, while the dark sky is still studded with stars, they sing into the stillness. Have you noticed they will sing into the rain, too—even when caught in a downpour? Not much seems to get them down—a good reminder for someone like me who doesn't much feel like chirping these days.

I imagine this merry birdsong is why my great-grandmother, a Hungarian emigrant, had at least one parakeet loose in her kitchen for as long as I can remember. I can still see her, hovered over the stove in her long, button-down, pastel peach smock dress, stirring paprika-laden potato soup while her birds watched from either the curtain rod or from her shoulder where they would tug a few strands of her golden hair. Her entire 1970s-style wood-and-tile kitchen was their birdcage, which was not much of a cage at all now that I think of it.

Sometimes they managed to fly out the screen door, past the potted red geraniums planted in remembrance of her home country, past the pool where my cousins and I swam for hours, and up to a branch high in the towering palm tree. While most people couldn't conceive of allowing this level of freedom, I wouldn't really expect anything less from this graceful woman. It's as if their freedom was a symbol of the reason she chose to leave everything she knew—to spread roots in a new land and, accompanied by these joyful calls, raise a family she called *lelkem*, "my soul." Perhaps she took a cue from her birds, sharing their easygoing joy with everyone around her.

Now, as I trek along our Santa Rosa creek trail, it's as if God heard my plea. I know he's not a genie at the whim of my wishes, but now birdsong, like the tune from her parakeets, escorts me along my walk, lifting my soul with each step.

How incredible is this!

Today, this trail is even more of a haven for renewal than usual. The constant flow of bikers, joggers, and walkers bustling about both paths on either side of the stream makes me think others must agree. Though this route has long since ceased to surprise me, today everything seems to have changed. In fact, not only has the landscape seemed to change but also strange scents surround me on all sides.

Is this really the same place I know so well?

As I meander past the stream, it's as if I've been transported back to clinical rotations for my RN training, specifically to the labor and delivery room. It smells like amniotic fluid—spilling out of the earth's vagina.

That's odd.

Also, come to think of it, that would mean I'm walking on the earth's inner thigh.

Nope, *odd* doesn't fully cover it. This is, in fact, very weird.

I continue along, amid the sweet aromas of wildflowers and ladybug-speckled fennel, mesmerized by the newness bursting forth everywhere—ferns are unfurling, mustard flowers are blooming, and, if I look closely enough, I bet I could spot a butterfly emerging from its chrysalis. To think, I have joined this league of blossoming beginnings. I've now shifted from producing graduate reports and term papers to something—someone—far more meaningful and lasting. Eternally significant.

As my footsteps continue their steady beat on the pavement and cheery chirps flutter in the air, I absorb the scene as if every facet were new.

Clustered in bunches near the brook, beneath the trees' lacy branches, sheaves of wild wheat sway in perfect unison. They bend with such ease under the pressure of the wind. Their flexibility looks so effortless. How do they do it? They're not fighting the present moment at all. They're not breaking or having mini wheat-tantrums. Adaptation is woven into their core fibers, just as it's woven into the feathers of my winged friends.

Is it possible for me to be this way during pregnancy, flexible and adaptive? Can I afford not to? I sure hope the joyful trill of these little feathered friends will permeate my being, giving my core the fiber needed to flex and sway when the winds blow.

Mission Minuscule

All day at work, my mind has been silently mulling over an upcoming quest. I smile to myself, assured that the clinic staff is completely unaware of this covert op. It sure helps that my plan isn't hinging on sneaky little me going incognito. I didn't need to show up wearing all black, a cloak, or even night-vision goggles. How utterly convenient. Still, I can't help but think there should be a theme song emanating from somewhere in the background—even though this is a different type of mission, one at the most minuscule level.

Finally, I make it to the magical hour—five o'clock, on the dot. Most of my coworkers grab their purses and rush out the back door while I continue to battle my usual archnemesis, patient visit documentation. Though it doesn't feel like such a burden today because I know there's something exciting waiting for me: I'm on a mission to hear my little one's heartbeat.

Once I'm one of the only ones left, I tiptoe down the quiet hall to an exam room, determined to check, even if it's possibly too early. I climb onto the table, tuck a paper towel under my lowered waistband, tug up my shirt, and squeeze some cold gel—or "slime" as one child called it— on my belly.

I glide the hand-held Doppler machine up and down my abdomen in a slow, methodical circuit—as I do with my pregnant ladies, while explaining how the Doppler rays dive through the abdominal wall, glide into the amniotic water, and then bounce out noise from what it encounters deep down inside. I feel like I'm fishing with sound waves for extra- (or *intra*-) terrestrial life. The game of hide-and-seek continues and makes the time spent feel like eons, as if time is a blob of strudel dough, a couple minutes stretched and expanded into an impossibly thin sheet of eternity.

Amid this eternity, I hold my breath, hoping for a sign. I know the heartbeat can be audible by Doppler as early as 10 weeks, but that's not guaranteed since even at 12 weeks, the uterus is usually barely peeking out from behind the pelvic bone. As expected, I hear static. Gurgles. I'm desperate to locate any evidence of life, but I'm afraid I only hear myself. My bowels. My own comparatively slow heartbeat through my pelvic blood vessel.

Shhh, shhh, shhh.

I'm tired of hearing just me. So status quo.

If only I could will the machine to do a better job.

Sigh.

A failed mission, how disappointing. Nothing accomplished. I guess I can try listening again at the end of the we—

A faint noise.

Sh, sh, sh, sh, sh. A rhythm, way faster than my own. *Sh, sh, sh, sh, sh.*

My baby's heartbeat! *Finally*, audible, objective proof that my body is really, truly inhabited by a being, not just a blob or a whatcha-ma-call-it. I can hear our lives superimposed already, my baby's heartbeat next to mine.

⇾⇾⇾ LET'S TALK ABOUT IT ⇽⇽⇽

Prenatal Screening and Testing

As a developing human being, your little one is incredibly complex. So too are our interactions with these little ones—the ways we experience their behavior or learn about their development and attributes. For instance, in the first trimester, you can see your baby's little heartbeat on an early ultrasound and can hear it thumping away by Doppler near 12 weeks—a sound that signifies your miscarriage risk plummeting. And around 18 to 21 weeks, you'll get to feel your baby's movement as flutters for the first time.

It's such a journey of discovery!

Beyond these surprising experiences, there are various ways to find out about your baby's health—a topic that will be included in one of your first prenatal appointments. Babies routinely get a fetal anatomy ultrasound around 18 to 21 weeks, sometimes sooner.[2,3] This is a fabulous opportunity to dote on your little one while the radiology technician or perinatologist checks out the details of your baby's growth and body parts, the location of your placenta, and so on. Usually, at this time, you can also find out your baby's sex if you so choose and haven't already (though no guarantees he or she will cooperate!). While this ultrasound is one of the fundamental components in prenatal care, there are other optional tests that can be run.

Additional screening and testing

At some point early on in your prenatal care, your maternity care provider will ask whether you'd like additional tests to assess potential birth defects. I know this is a hard topic to even consider, so for starters—breathe!

A *birth defect* is a physical problem a baby develops while in utero. These problems can pertain to his or her body's structure or how it works and can be minor (like an extra finger) or more serious (like a heart problem).[4,5] Some can be identified before birth, while others only reveal themselves after birth (by a **newborn screening** blood test or physical exam).[5]

Screening versus diagnostic tests

Now, the good news is the average pregnant woman only starts off with a small (3%–5%) baseline chance of having a baby born with a major birth defect.[4,6,7] Although some of us may prefer if we had the power and technology to detect every single abnormality in utero, the complexity of human genetics—as well as the fact that birth defects are not solely caused by genetic factors—makes this unrealistic. However, it is still possible to detect certain conditions with two basic categories of tests. *Screening tests* tell you if your baby has a *higher chance* of having a specific birth defect than the general population. *Diagnostic tests*, on the other hand, tell you if your baby *has* the tested-for condition.

To get a little more specific, screening tests involve an extra one or two blood tests from your arm, and possibly another early ultrasound (called **nuchal translucency**).[3,6,8,9] This route is not too involved, nor does it carry a high amount of risk. Examples of these blood tests or *screens* include the **integrated**, **quad**, and **cell-free DNA** (which is also called *noninvasive prenatal testing/screening*, or **NIPT/NIPS**).[3,6,8,9]

On the other hand, most diagnostic testing is invasive and more involved. For example, with *chorionic villi sampling* (or *CVS*), cells may be collected from the placenta, while an *amniocentesis* (or *amnio*) test collects your baby's skin cells from the amniotic fluid surrounding your baby.[10] As with all invasive procedures, there's a slightly heightened chance of miscarriage, but for some women, the knowledge gained outweighs the risk.[8,10] Both invasive and noninvasive tests have their pros, cons, and limitations.[3]

Genetic carrier screening

Though all of this is enough to think about, there's yet a third category of testing called genetic carrier screening. This involves a simple blood test from the arm to see if you (or the baby's dad) carry changes to genes that are linked to specific disorders, such as cystic fibrosis.[11] Being a genetic carrier doesn't automatically mean your baby will miss out on living a normal and healthy life. He or she may simply be a carrier like you. How your child may be affected really depends on each specific condition.

Final thoughts

While learning about the options and deciding which (if any) to go with, the main thing to remember is this: prenatal testing is a personal choice, and while it can provide helpful information, it is not mandatory.[3,11] Not everyone will want to know everything that can be learned about their little one. Ultimately, it's your baby inside, and it's you and your partner (if applicable) who must decide which tests (if any) to run and what to do with the results. Some decide on testing because of the implications (like better preparing for a special needs baby or terminating the pregnancy). Others decline testing because they know any abnormal result would only lead to worry, but not to any further changes, testing, or termination.

If you have questions, feel free to take the time to get your questions answered. Please, do not allow anyone to pressure you into something you don't feel comfortable with. It is just as appropriate to decline testing as it is to accept it.

Digging Deeper

Though it can be a heavy topic, it is still an important one. I know it may be easy to become carried away by fears and anxieties or to avoid making a decision because it is hard to think about. My hope is that you will make an informed decision you are comfortable with, and any anxieties you may have will be replaced by peace and hope. If you're looking for answers to some of the questions below, check out A-3e.

» Where do birth defects come from?

» If I want to learn about my baby's health, but don't want to undergo an invasive procedure, what options do I have?

» What are the pros and cons of prenatal screening and diagnostic tests? What does the "low" or "high" risk test result mean?

» If I'm over 35 years old, does it mean I have to have an amniocentesis?

» I spoke to my maternity care provider but still can't decide which way to go. Now what?

WEEK 11

Baby
- Is about 1 ½ inches long.
- Weighs about 1 ½ ounces.
- Is now referred to as a fetus.
- Begins thumb-sucking, yawning, kicking, and stretching.
- Intestines and bowel descend into the abdominal cavity.

Mama
- Your expanding rib cage may require you to loosen your bra.
- Blood volume continues to increase, making you work harder to circulate blood while exercising.
- The immune system is changing to protect your baby. You may notice longer colds or asthma getting worse—or magically improving.

Starry Night

I can't believe it. I just really can't. A fact so obvious, it's been in front of me all these years, plain as day, yet somehow unnoticed. Every single person—each one—was born of another.

Brilliant, right?

But really, hear me out. If we think about it, this fact does warrant meditation and a respectful, dare I say—pregnant—pause. Sure, it might bring to mind one obvious factor. Yep, sex—lots of it—in beds, cars, pools, under bleachers, on washing machines, and in closets; possibly fertility tracking; and likely a lot of broken condoms, forgotten birth control pills, and people wishing they'd have tried the more effective intrauterine device (IUD) or implant. Beyond this, it may even bring to mind fertility treatments and the planning and intentionality they involve.

But, if we look just a bit closer, more stunningly this means that whether the conception was planned or unexpected, every single person alive today was born through sacrifice. You, me, and everyone else is here because someone else experienced a profound journey, life-changing experiences, and often pain, to bring about a life. In this, newness gets tucked inside a woman, and she is forever changed by it.

Thinking of it now, it's as if, after all these years, I finally had the fortune of encountering the original Vincent van Gogh's *Starry Night* at the Museum of Modern Art. Sure, I've often seen reproductions of the image—flattened copies of the light- and dark-blue dashes swirling above the village tucked into the hills. But now that I'm up close, seeing dimensionality in each contour and brushstroke, it makes more sense. I have a richer understanding of the true depth of the dark hues, set against the vibrancy of the brights. It doesn't matter that I've seen it a hundred times. Today, it's new.

This "born-of-another" reality is so mesmerizing that it has speckled and spanned my own world. It's my companion as I sit on my back porch staring at a horizon of rooftops, when I'm driving to work, roaming the grocery store aisles, and walking by the homeless encampments a few blocks over. It's a canopy, coloring my perspective and shaping my world, like those rolling clouds hovering over the townspeople I imagine in van Gogh's painting—the ones who look up at their *Starry Night* sky.

Each of the nearly eight billion people on earth was carried and birthed in sacrifice. How is this possible? It's perplexing and frankly outrageous. Yet, because women are tougher and more spectacular than diamonds, you end up with an earth saturated with lots and lots of new and grown babies.

How beautiful! It's as brilliant and captivating as the luminous moon and stars above.

Weathered Moving Boxes

Out come the worn, wrinkled boxes from the garage—again. They've heroically served us over the past seven years, traveling with us every-where. They journeyed to quaint, little-big-city Boston, tucked into the corners of our apartment's back "office" while Dan and I went to gradu-ate school, lived off school loans and coupons, window-shopped for date nights, and learned to smash ourselves (East Coaster–style) onto any smidgen of space available on the public transportation system. There they witnessed our first Nor'easter—while winds whipped through the red-brick and gas lamp–lined streets, and we struggled through the front door like sheared lambs lost in a blizzard.

After graduation, these boxes dutifully traveled across the length of Interstate 80 from the East Coast to California, cramped in a U-Haul without any complaint, even amid the turbulent near-miss of multiple Midwest tornadoes. And then, to top it off, they suffered the slow, ardu-ous climb through the winding canyon roads of Cool, California, as we inched up the final incline to the Craigslist seller's address—all to claim our foolhardy mattress purchase. If you ask me, these faithful friends deserve a Girl Scout badge of service and a box of thin mint cookies.

And just when I thought we had settled down, these same boxes get called to arms. Isn't life always like that? Full of surprises, I mean—and full of change. This time, we'll move an hour and a half south (to Cupertino) for a year, for Dan's training. As we prepare for the move, our house is in shambles, piles of books and breakables line our dining room table, and my eyes are misting up over every TV diaper commercial.

Though I'm sure I should just suck it up and keep packing, I can't help but think—*not again*. We just did this!

We all have our *not agains*. And our questions and *what ifs* when faced with the unknown. Although some days, I do okay at shoving aside the worry, today it's not going so well. Pregnancy is making me *so* weepy, sensitive, and easily overwhelmed. I can't help but wonder: What will this year look like? Is this the new me?

After much deliberation, I've decided to keep my part-time job in Petaluma. I love it there, and at least it will be one familiar thing—one bit of solid ground amid the uncertainty. Most of the time, I think my plan is quite manageable. If all goes well, the time should fly by with a blink (and a birth).

I'll only be working two consecutive days a week, see? I'll leave Cupertino in the predawn chill, anticipating the morning's sunrise . . . As I envision it, the sun will still be backstage, batting her eyelashes and powdering her face while I drive past all the hardcore Bay Area commuters lining the Dutch Bros drive-through. Before she appears, I'll crank up the radio and the AC and peek at the horizon to see what vision awaits. As the golden light slides across the shadowed land, I'll wind through San Francisco, wrap around the endless span of bay, and cross the Golden Gate Bridge while, of course, belting out "California Here I Come" in a nostalgic, road-trip style.

For the last part of my drive, I'll enjoy the rolling stretches of sun-kissed hills that welcome me into Petaluma. My work will last until five-thirty, when I'll drive to my friend's house nearby to crash for the night and get some much-needed rest for the next day. The second day will be like a reversed version of the first. *And voilà!* I'll be back home in Cupertino for dinner.

Easy peasy, right?

Sure.

I stare around the room at the heaps of boxes, packing tissue, and fragile dishes ready to be packed away. I try to laugh, but I just can't seem to fool myself. Tears seem way more appropriate. I feel vulnerable again, like I'm struggling against a big, bad Nor'easter. But the storms in Boston were at least tangible, with snow careening from the sky. Here the gale is inward, unseen—yet no less real. My plan seems workable on paper, but only time will tell if it works in reality.

In the meantime, could someone please gift me with a monthly subscription of Kleenex?

⊰⊰⊰ LET'S TALK ABOUT IT ⊱⊱⊱

Adjusting to All the Changes?

You've been pregnant now for almost 12 weeks. What an accomplishment! Give yourself a pat on your belly, which probably isn't showing yet, because this early part of pregnancy is often the hardest. Yes, millions of women around the world are pregnant together with you, but that doesn't mean it's easy. Even if deep down inside you're thrilled to be pregnant—okay, maybe *very* deep down—you may still sometimes feel irritable, overwhelmed, sad, yucky, stressed, or even anxious. Yes, that's perfectly common.

It's okay if you just don't feel like you're glowing—you're not a firefly!

Since pregnancy is filled with change, it naturally fosters a whole range of emotions. In fact, you may even have multiple conflicting emotions in a single hour! Read on to get a better sense of common pregnancy experiences, and maybe even grab your partner or support person to join you.

Give yourself some grace if you don't feel your best in this first trimester. It may seem that your new hobby is puking, or perhaps stress—about taking care of kids, keeping your job, or having enough money—is overwhelming. After all, logistics for living are significant, right? Worries or anxiety can also creep in if you have previously experienced the sorrow of a miscarriage, are going through pregnancy alone, or were not planning on this pregnancy in the first place. Last, if we think of all the pregnant women with medical conditions or mental health problems (like depression or anxiety), and those who have had a complicated pregnancy in the past or are experiencing complications now, it is clear pregnancy is not quite as simple and perfect as we may have originally thought.

So, use this time to check in with yourself. How have you been feeling? Happy and content overall? If so, that's awesome! Cherish this time. If not, and you more commonly experience times of stress, sadness, anxiety, regret, irritability, guilt, or feeling you don't enjoy the things you used to, take a moment to reflect. Are these feelings short-lived, or do they persistently keep you from functioning or living to the full? Are you relying on cigarettes, marijuana, or other drugs to cope and feel better? Regardless of how you're feeling, it's important to remember you are not alone, and if you are seeking wholeness, there is help to be had.

Looking to give your baby the best present ever? It's *you*, being fully present—the best version of yourself. After all, when your little one arrives, you'll need wholeness to love, nurture, guide, and discipline your cute little bundle of energy. To be best prepared for this, *and* to have a healthier, more enjoyable pregnancy, take some time to invest in your mental wellness. It may take some work, but it's worth it.

Digging Deeper

Whew! Mental and emotional well-being is a big topic. If you're currently in a good space—hooray! If, however, it's something you want to learn more about, feel free to take a peek at B-4 which includes answers to questions like:

» How do I know if I need extra help or if this is just normal? (B-4b)

» In what ways can I be proactive about my mental health? (B-4b)

» Is it true that my mental health problems affect my baby and pregnancy? (B-4a)

WEEK 12

Baby

- Is about 2 inches long.
- Weighs about 2 ounces.
- Begins growing fingernails and developing fingerprints.
- Has some bones that start hardening.
- Has distinguishable external genitals.

Mama

- To help your baby grow, your body is now absorbing nutrients more efficiently.
- The uterus is the size of a grapefruit, which may start giving you a subtle yet cute little baby bump.

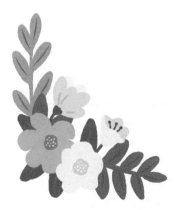

She and I, Worlds Apart

Sometimes, as an NP, I feel like a gameshow host—a serendipitous side-perk of the job I already love. I especially feel like the camera should be rolling when I make my theatrical entrance. I knock, open the door a sliver, ask the woman if she's ready for me to come in, and, upon hearing yes, emerge from behind the privacy drapes veiling the entry. Behind curtain number one is—me!

Another serendipity is the element of surprise. When entering the exam room, I never really know what I might find. Sometimes a woman brings her whole family to the visit, which makes me feel like I'm joining a party and should grab a karaoke machine. Other times it feels like a day care. A weary mother bounces a drooling baby, while she feeds a stroller-strapped toddler and tries to corral the child whose squirmy legs peek out from underneath the corner chair. And when, despite the "all clear," I enter to find a woman dry shaving her bikini area, the exam room feels like a spa.

Though it may be chaotic or surprising, I love how every woman's world fills the room. Before I enter, I read a medical chart and get a glimpse of what sort of story I may be entering—at least, as it's presented on paper. But as years of nursing practice have shown me, chart notes, diagnoses, lab values, and medications can only capture a tiny fragment of a life. They may describe part of her reality, but they certainly can't define *her*. So, I'm left to learn about each woman's world on the fly.

Sometimes, this process impacts me in profound and unexpected ways—like on this particular summer afternoon.

A twenty-one-year-old arrived for her first well-woman visit and pap smear, a routine screening for cervical cancer. As I began my questions, she started to share her concern over how different her digestion has been since "eating a lot of cheese" on her pizza about four months ago. But strangely, it hadn't let up since. She's also noticed nausea, bloating, and only a lighter than normal period.

Piecing together the clues, I asked the one routine question we maternity care providers are obsessed with—when did her last period start? This college student told me it had been a few months.

I proceeded with her physical exam and found her abdomen strangely *full* of something. I was pretty certain it was her fundus, the top of her uterus, which typically can't be felt. She had either an abnormal mass growing in her uterus, or a quite normal one—a baby.

Hmm.

Due to her symptoms and physical exam, I knew I needed to ask.

"May I listen for a moment?" I nodded toward the Doppler machine.

When she said yes, I smoothed the gel on her abdomen, and within moments of the Doppler's wand touching it, we heard another's heartbeat. Around 155 beats per minute—perfectly babyish. My guess is she was somewhere around 18 weeks pregnant.

When I verbally confirmed what she now knew, her tears streamed in the silence. The fetus had fully formed organs, and we would probably be able to determine the sex by ultrasound. In fact, she would soon feel her little one's kicks. We discussed her options, and within a few moments, she was certain.

"I just can't continue this pregnancy . . . I have only one more year of school. I have things to do. I've been planning—waiting—to try my luck on the big screen. I can't carry this baby and give it up for adoption either."

She wanted a referral to a clinic where she could get an abortion within a few days. As I connected her with the nurse to help coordinate this, it struck me. We were in such different places, she and I. I had finished my schooling and had a (relatively) planned pregnancy with my husband, whom I love. She was young, single, and just about to start her career. I could hardly wait to meet my baby and couldn't stop devouring books to see what my little munchkin was doing or how he or she was growing. This young woman, on the other hand, was overwhelmed by the thought of pregnancy. It was just too much.

I wish amniotic fluid could mysteriously swallow up women's woes and somehow transform unwanted pregnancies into desired ones. The difficult realities of life—that punctuate sentiments like: *I can't. I'm scared. I'm alone. I'm not ready. You weren't supposed to be*—these would vanish in a breath. *Puff.*

She and I, though hand in hand, our stories overlapping, were living worlds apart. If only I were as far along in my pregnancy as she was—I'd be happy to be just a few weeks closer to meeting my little one.

Am I an Imposter?

Lately, I feel as heavy as an elephant. I try to wisely remind myself a few extra pounds hanging from me does *not* mean this is the case. However, that concept is hard to grasp when my fun, turquoise pencil skirt only fits comfortably when I stop breathing, and every time I bend over, fat cascades from my waistline. *This is unsustainable.*

So, how large do I need to get before I can freely peruse the maternity racks and make a shameless purchase? Sure, I've managed to Mac-Gyver a solution—a rubber band I loop around the buttonhole on my jeans to afford another precious inch—but dealing with that extra hassle is getting old. Yes, I suppose now is as good a time as ever.

Determined, I set off on a scavenger hunt, searching for nearby maternity departments, which was *definitely* harder than it should be. *Because of course, that's what every pregnant woman needs—more work.* By the time I finally managed to spot one, I was ecstatic. The faceless mannequin with a pronounced belly felt like a prized trophy. *I made it!*

A flood of accomplishment washed over me, and I could picture a hero's welcome—fanfare echoing while the announcer calls, "Welcome lone wanderer, you did it!" But instead of jubilation, I was hit with a tidal wave of self-consciousness. A row of wall-mounted mannequin bellies seemed to mock me as I roamed past.

As I nudged my way farther into the department, it seemed that amid the clothing racks, I found myself in an unexpected proving ground—a terrain of unspoken competition among us pregnant women. Other shoppers' glances seem to ask: *Who here has the biggest belly? What are you doing here? If you're not showing enough, you're not one of us.* Are they really thinking these things? Or am I just imagining it because I only have love handles to show for my pregnancy?

Maybe I'm not the only self-conscious one, but I couldn't shake the feeling that I didn't belong—that I'm an imposter in this maternal world. *That's absurd*, I tell myself. *I have pregnancy rights, damn it.* Yes, shopping in the maternity section has now become a right in my eyes. Fact is, my clothes have been getting too tight and I need options. Sure, I can hang out in Dan's sweatpants at home, but I can't exactly show up to work in them.

That's right. *Hold your head high, mama.*

Unfortunately, the inner pep talk wore off moments later, like the fragrance of cheap perfume. And so there I was, back to timidly touching the myriad of fabrics intended to drape a blossoming mother's belly. There was certainly something for every approach to pregnancy—with options to either accentuate or conceal the reality of a growing babe. If you want to hide it so your friends don't notice, just hop inside this parachute and soar off to modest, prepregnancy land. If you want to show it off—finally—here's some Saran wrap, I mean, *tube tops* for you.

In the end, after all that, I left with only *one* shirt.

What a letdown!

The items I tried on were still too large for my unassuming bud of a belly and made me look like I was wearing curtains. Resembling household décor was not what I had in mind. However, the shirt that did go home with me had fabulous potential—it could cover the moon if I asked it to.

⟫⟫ LET'S TALK ABOUT IT ⟪⟪

Loving Your Body

Let's give credit where credit is due. Your body is amazing! Your organs and body systems have revved up and are working 24/7 to grow your little baby. What was once a mere speck will soon be a new person you'll cuddle, love, and care for. Even if you have health problems or are experiencing medical complications during pregnancy, your body is doing the best it can, day in and day out. How incredible is that?

While growing a little person, you've probably noticed how rapidly your body has started to change or feel different. You may even find yourself wondering things like: Is my body doing what it should be? Will I like my pregnant body? How will my body change? Will I get my prepregnancy body back after my baby's born?

Great questions!

Pregnancy can certainly change the way you think about your body. Some women love watching their bodies adapt to pregnancy and think it is the best thing that ever happened to them. They love how it makes them feel (probably except the first trimester) and can hardly wait to flaunt that figure.[1-3]

But other women struggle with the changes.[1-3] Pregnancy symptoms and changes are out of their control and make them feel miserable and uncomfortable.

And of course, it's totally normal to find yourself in both camps during various parts of pregnancy—or even on the same day.

Body image

Body image refers to how you think about, view, and experience your body.[3,4] Many things can influence it, like your physical and mental health, weight, and physical capabilities or disabilities; racial, ethnic, cultural, media and religious views; self-derogatory body talk ("fat talk"); as well as how your family, friends, and community talk about bodies, either in general, or more specifically—yours.[5-12] Of course, mainstream American culture's obsession with attractiveness and thinness is hard to ignore, too.

When you have a positive body image, you love, celebrate, and appreciate your body for its uniqueness and functionality and feel comfortable in it.[4,13,14] However, plenty of women have negative (distorted) body images, which means they don't like what they see in the mirror or in photographs, and they view their bodies differently than they really are.[4] Those who experience this tend to feel

> **WISE MAMA**
>
> Limit your exposure to media that doesn't help you appreciate your amazing body!

anxious, ashamed, and self-conscious, and may even feel awkward in their bodies.[4]

Those who have or have had unhealthy ways of relating to food or their body, or those with a past eating disorder (like anorexia nervosa or bulimia), can go either way with body image during pregnancy.[6,‡] Some women healed years ago and are pleasantly surprised when they aren't impacted by pregnancy's body changes or simply decide pregnancy is a great time to excuse themselves from cultural expectations. Alternatively, some women find pregnancy triggering.[15] It may bring up perfectionism, feelings of loss of control, or difficult thoughts about their bodies and their past, even thoughts they've dealt with already.[15]

> ## BE PROACTIVE!
>
> To learn more about your pelvic floor health and how to prevent or treat urinary incontinence, check out "Your Pelvic Floor" (week 31) and A-3c.

So, which body image group are you in? If it's negative, don't get discouraged. There's hope! The pain and suffering you're going through don't need to continue for the rest of your life, or even the rest of your pregnancy.

If you want it to be, pregnancy can be a wonderfully exciting time to learn or practice a new way of relating to your body. The little person growing inside of you could already be helping to launch you into being a better, healthier, and happy version of yourself. What's more, you'll be able to create a legacy, passing on a healthy body image to your child. You go, mama!

---

‡ Michele Minero, MFT, personal communication, July 18, 2015

Digging Deeper

It takes time to do something radical and completely countercultural—that is, viewing yourself as a woman with a special and useful body. Sometimes we forget our bodies are coverings for our souls and they deserve respect and love. This may especially be true if we feel a little chunky around the waist and our cute bumps haven't appeared yet. (It'll come—usually around the fourth month, though if you're a plus-size mama, it may take longer.) To help you in this process, feel free to check out B-4g for answers to some common questions like:

» What are some practical ways I can nurture a healthy body image?
» Do you have any tips for practicing daily thankfulness for my body?
» What are tip-offs that I may need a new, healthier relationship with my body?

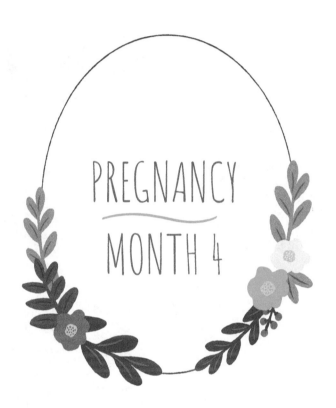

PREGNANCY

MONTH 4

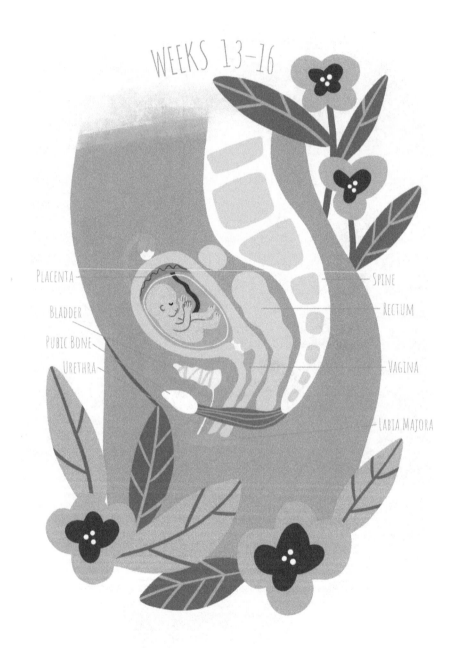

WEEKS 13–16

Placenta

Bladder

Pubic Bone

Urethra

Spine

Rectum

Vagina

Labia Majora

WEEK 13

Baby

- Is about 2 ¾ inches long.
- Weighs about 2 ½ ounces.
- Can now make facial expressions.
- Has fully formed lips and nose.
- Forms joints.
- Can now make and break down blood clots.

Mama

- May have gained or lost weight from pregnancy symptoms.
- Nausea may be improving.

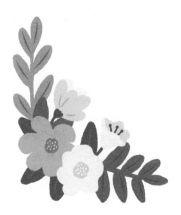

Parts Unknown

It's easy to underestimate the impact a growing, peapod-sized babe can have on not just a woman's life but also on her various body parts. Personally, I've been shocked (and semi-intrigued) by how my breasts appear to have taken on a life of their own without even bothering to ask my permission. They are now a full cup size larger than before, and my cleavage feels like a curvier rendition of the Grand Canyon. *Mind the gap, please.* I'm pretty sure only a turtleneck or a hazmat suit could cover it.

Getting used to such ever-evolving b(r)easts is not as simple and straightforward as an unsuspecting, nonpregnant woman might think. Take the other day, for example, when Dan and I were at home watching an English Premier League football game.

"*Ooowww*, you elbowed my breast!" I yelped, giving Dan a playful smack on the shoulder.

"Well," he defended, "how was I supposed to know it was way down there?"

I suppose he had a valid point. Here I was—marooned on the couch like a beached seal—with breasts that had no recourse but to wander off into uncharted territories. How could he have known where they'd be when I can't even seem to keep track of them? They constantly cascade

THE "SEASONS" OF A MILK FACTORY[7]

Lactation consultants Diana Marasco and Diana West liken milk production to seasons.
- Prior to pregnancy, you have a basic factory of milk-producing cells, dormant in *winter*.
- When pregnant, you're in *spring*! Milk-producing cells grow and develop, preparing the factory for production, causing breast tenderness and enlargement, and eventually colostrum production.
- Childbirth means *summer*—milk production comes into full bloom.
- Just as trees drop leaves in *fall*, production slows when breastfeeding is completed, and the factory prepares again for winter by disassembling unnecessary parts.

out of my bra, as if hopelessly searching for more appropriate—and less confined—places to rest. It's nearly impossible for either of us to predict where they'll be at any one time. So it's no wonder that when he leans in for a kiss, he accidentally jostles one of these wayward wanderers.

Clearly the time has come to try some way of containing them. *Hmm . . .* Leash? Fence? Bunker? Seriously, though, will a stretchy nursing bra be able to accommodate their ever-changing whims?

The pregnancy books disappointingly offered no advice on this matter. The only thing they do is mention that my nipples might already start producing colostrum. Great. Who wouldn't be tempted to squeeze the hell out of them after hearing that?

Jack and the Beanstalk

I'm relaxing in bed with a coffee-colored quilt swaddling me like I'm an oversized baby. Through our open window, I can hear the marathon crying of our neighbor's child. Man, I hope we never have a baby like *that*. Is there anything I can do to make sure that never happens?

I ponder the question but am too tired to get up and close the pane. I just don't feel like budging—especially after our hike today, which consisted of me dragging my body throughout the redwood forest, despite just wanting to lie down in a prairie like a log and rest my eyes and my *everything*. Ah, to let the sun sing me to sleep.

Don't get me wrong, the hike through the damp paths was beautiful. The trees towered above us like nature's own skyscrapers, and every time we ducked into or under them, I felt like a child, an Ewok, or an aspiring fairy tale character. If only I could have sprouted wings like Tinker Bell. Flight just seems so effortless compared to trudging along on the ground. If I had the energy, I would have climbed up, higher and higher, like Jack scaling his beanstalk. I would slowly escape everything around—until I found a jolly green giant waiting for me, or better yet, God.

⇛⇛ LET'S TALK ABOUT IT ⇚⇚

Move That Beautiful Self

Wait, don't go! Before you decide to skip this section because you hate to exercise, let me just say it's not as terrible as you might think. We're not necessarily talking about wearing spandex or joining CrossFit (in fact, don't do CrossFit now unless you're already a regular). Instead, we're talking about moving your body, most days of the week, so that your heart rate goes up and you get *at least* a little warm and out of breath (think brisk walking). Now, that doesn't sound so scary, does it?

Recommended activity

This type of movement includes walking, dancing, swimming, and hiking, and is often referred to as **cardio**. Some ladies are fortunate enough to naturally get this type of movement during the workday because their job involves keeping active. But if you're one of the many whose lifestyle does not naturally afford much physical activity, don't worry—with some creativity, you can find ways to fit it into your schedule, at least a few days a week. It can be a nice change of pace and is certainly worth it.

Now, if you're concerned about how much activity or movement is safe in pregnancy, here's a general guide: moderate-intensity aerobic activity is considered safe in pregnancy unless you've been advised otherwise by your maternity care provider (due to medical conditions or pregnancy complications).[1,2] In fact, if you've been used to vigorous-intensity aerobic activity prior to pregnancy, you can actually continue that level of intensity during pregnancy as well.[2,3]

In general, expect to get out of breath sooner while moving, and as your belly grows, you'll probably feel like modifying certain activities to get more comfortable. But, unless your maternity care provider has specifically advised you to limit your physical activity, make it a point to keep moving.[2,3] Otherwise both you *and* your baby would be missing out on its benefits.[1,3]

Benefits of staying (or becoming) active

And what are these benefits, you might ask? First, regular physical activity (i.e., most days of the week) will lift your spirits, relieve stress, improve your sleep, control your weight gain, maintain your fitness, decrease your body discomforts (like leg cramps and back pain)—and get this, it decreases your Cesarean birth risk.[1,4] Also, it can help control your blood sugar and blood pressure.[2,3] Think about it: there's no single medicine that can give you all these benefits.

In addition to these awesome perks for you, studies have shown that when pregnant mothers exercise, it also benefits their babies in amazing ways; namely, it boosts their brain development, sets them up for a healthier life through a healthy body weight, and fosters heart health.[5,6] Basically, it's like finding a pot of gold at the end of a rainbow (*well, almost*).

Disclaimer

So, if all this sounds great except for the fact that you're completely exhausted (because most pregnant women are), you have my permission to give in and rest. Guilt-free. Spread the word to all those concerned about you letting yourself go. This is pregnancy, and that's ridiculous. But the good news is that in the weeks to come, you'll slowly start feeling more like yourself and will have way more energy than you do

> Unless your maternity care provider has specifically advised you to limit your physical activity, make it a point to keep moving.

now. When that time comes, remember there are resources in the back of this book waiting to encourage and support you in making movement a daily routine. Yes, it's possible!

Digging Deeper

Pregnancy is the perfect time to prioritize regular physical activity since it has so many benefits for you and your baby. And trust me, it will have a positive impact on how comfortable you'll feel throughout pregnancy and in the homestretch. In B-2b, you'll find practical tips on how to get started or keep going while pregnant, as well as answers to questions like:

» What specific physical activities are recommended in pregnancy, and which should I avoid?

» Is it okay to get out of breath while working out?

» Are there pregnancy-specific considerations for physical activity and exercise?

» My job can be physically demanding; how do I make sure my baby and I stay safe while at work?

» What warning signs do I need to watch for when exercising?

SECOND TRIMESTER

WEEKS 14–27

WEEK 14

Baby

- Is about 5 ¾ inches long, head to heel.
- Weighs about 3 ¼ ounces.
- Has taste buds.
- Makes many different hormones.
- Continues to develop the kidneys.

Mama

- Joints and ligaments in your pelvis and throughout your body relax, especially during the first half of pregnancy.
  - Pay attention since you may be more unstable during heavy lifting or high-impact workouts.
- The placenta grows so it can better connect with your uterus.

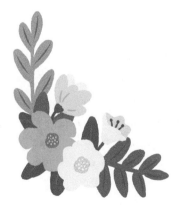

Bubbles

I have decided my baby will be a girl. She must be, since there simply aren't reasonable Hungarian boy names. *Zoltán* gives him thunder thighs, *Atilla* turns him into a bareback riding savage, and *Cseke* would likely be mispronounced "cheeky." And so, for a while now, I've been racking my brain for a Hungarian girl name that will suit my precious resident. It's as if, in searching, I might finally be able to register the fact that yes, indeed, I do have a baby within me. A person physically attached. In *me*.

Honestly, this process took a little longer than I expected, and I'm afraid it has been only partly successful. Sure, I know everyone's different, and the attachment process doesn't magically correspond to the baby's size. I've witnessed that bond form in some women right when they get a positive pregnancy test, and in others when they see that "blob" on an early ultrasound or feel their baby's movements around 20 weeks. But I've also met some mamas who don't feel connected until later in pregnancy, or even until after their baby's birth. There's a whole range out there, and now I've been wondering where I'd fall along the timeline.

Each week, I read about how much my baby has grown and wonder—is today the big day I'll feel connected? After all, she's the size of a pea pod. *Nope, not yet.* What about now that she's lemon-sized? She's quite a bit bigger than Thumbelina—which is a relief, considering I'd like to hug her one day and not just put her in my pocket or carry her along in my palm.

Thinking of names and the size of my little one has nudged me in the right direction, but it was not until today that the first bit of affection for my resident bubbled up within me like freshly uncorked Martinelli's—a surge like the cold fizz that cascades down the side of the bottle and the mist that sprays your cheeks—startling and strangely refreshing.

I love you, my inner voice whispered to my daughter. *I love you.*

Wait, what? Where did that come from? another, more familiar voice chimed in. *How can I love someone I've never met?* I don't even know anything about her personality or even basics like whether she has my dimples or Dan's eyes.

Is this just blind love? Or is this a glimpse of what a mother's love can be? Not blind, *unconditional*.

And why now? I'm in a cycling class, of all places! One minute I'm bobbing along in the row beside a gray-haired man I (mentally) refer to as Mr. Sweatband—who even wears those anymore?—and the next thing I know, there it is. A sudden, warm surge of feelings spontaneously flowing toward my little resident.

I love you. I love you.

I love you?

Yes, I love you. I wonder what it's like for you to be in there.

I remember early ultrasounds I've done for pregnant mamas around this stage, and I can't help but giggle. You must look so impish now, floating around and then bouncing up and down against the amniotic sac in uncoordinated jumping jacks. The image in my mind's eye makes me smile.

What's it like living in my waters? I wonder, willing her to hear my thoughts.

Are you soothed and rocked when I go about my day? Or does it feel like an earthquake?

As I bob and sway, each push of my feet against the pedals brings a new question.

Do you like it when I bike?

Do you get lonely? Or is mama's company and aquarium perfectly enough?

I wipe a bead of sweat from my furrowed brow (somewhat wishing that I, too, had the courage to wear a sweatband).

How dramatically will our lives change when you arrive?

Will we know how to take care of you? Will we do it well?

Family Reunion, *Where?*

If the United States Postal Service ever did go bankrupt, both my mother and mother-in-law would be in trouble. They're probably the last two to correspond by handwritten letters—you know, the floral *Thank You* and *Thinking of You* notes that get sealed in pink envelopes and once required sour-tasting stamps in the upper right corner? It's really too bad they live across state lines from each other. If they had it their way, I'm sure they'd much prefer to live in Green Gables' Avonlea, sipping raspberry cordials, strolling through seas of brilliantly colored wildflowers, and romping through muddy pastures as bosom friends.

Of late, my mother-in-law, Becky—who heard the news shortly before her Alaskan cruise—has been eager to talk with my mother about the announcement. I certainly can't blame her. After all, their kids are *finally* having a baby together! It's high time the two celebrated and analyzed this news from every insightful, grandmotherly angle.

PLANNING TO TRAVEL?

Start by checking with your maternity care provider. Second trimester is generally a lovely time—provided you focus on a relaxing destination and itinerary. Once you're 36 weeks along, you'll want to stick closer to home. After all, we don't know when you'll go into labor, right?

International travel has a few more considerations. Would your destination put you at risk for serious infections (from food, water, or mosquitoes)? Visit the Centers for Disease Control and Prevention "Traveler's Health" website to learn more. Would you need extra vaccinations and are they safe in pregnancy? Is there a good hospital with NICU nearby? What type of travel insurance would you need?

When traveling by car, tuck the lap belt under your belly, keep the shoulder strap over your shoulder, and keep the airbags on. As always, remember not to sit or stand in one place for too long. Keep that beautiful blood circulating to avoid blood clots. Stay hydrated, walk around every couple of hours, and point and flex those toes occasionally. You could even wear compression stockings for longer trips.

If traveling farther is not recommended for whatever reason, no worries! Work on having a blast at a local destination. It could still be truly special.

However, since we had not yet delivered the news to my parents before Becky and Tim set sail, her wait was prolonged. The trip must have seemed like a chasm of communication more vast than the span of turquoise-white icebergs on their voyage. I envision Becky peering through her porthole window, absorbing the sight of frosted mountain caps scoring the horizon. In some ways, this glorious trip would end too soon, but in another sense, it's way too long. After all, there's an important conversation waiting to set sail.

And sail it did once Becky returned home. In fact, the joyful news itself was no less extraordinary than the way she and my mother discussed it. Becky was so excited that she scratched all typical modes of handmade communication. There was no more time to waste. She picked up the phone, tapped the number, and just like that, they both landed in the 21st century.

Their phone conversation lived up to the expectations of both parties, my mother told me in our own phone conversation later. It was packed with excitement, laughter, and eager sharing about how the other found out about our secret.

I doubt raspberry cordials could have made it any more thrilling.

My mom confessed they pretty much lost it when they heard the news at my brother's graduation, which, of course, did not surprise even-keeled Becky. To conclude, my mother added, "I told her how much fun it will be when everyone is reunited in the hospital delivery room."

Reunited in the what?! I did a mental double take. *Did I catch that correctly?* You're planning to host the next family reunion while I—legs spread—am navigating the most transformational moment of my life? *Oh, and would you like one or two lumps of sugar with that?*

"Mom," I spluttered, "Dan and I haven't even thought that far ahead. We haven't decided who will or will not be at the delivery. Heck, I barely decided I would attend!"

In fact, I'd rather not, if that's okay with you.

Amid our laughter, my irritation softened. In her true graceful manner, my mother reassured me that our wishes would, of course, be respected once we knew what they were. My labor was not meant to be a show but a celebration.

It's amazing, though, how sneaky and prevalent expectations are. They're simply everywhere! We all bring our own thoughts and experiences of pregnancy and delivery with us, like unassuming companions on an adventure.

I try to hold on to this reality and not the tiny twinge of irritation that starts to rise once again in my mind. Whose pregnancy is this, anyway?

It's ours, yes. But, in a way, it's also theirs.

LET'S TALK ABOUT IT

Find Your Tribe

For all the expectations that people can bring into a pregnancy, it's really true—both pregnancy and parenting are things to be done in community. Why? Although both can be exciting and lovely, they will sometimes be so hard and exhausting that you'll just need a boost. Plain and simple. And yes, even strong, independent, self-sufficient women (and men) need community in this new season.

Community is what will give you a buffer for your soul, room to breathe, and an outlet when the world seems to cling to your back. It's vital for you, as well as for your partner or loved ones. You'll need your squad.

Not convinced? Take a look at other species. There's a reason most animals live in schools, flocks, prides, gaggles, and colonies. This way, they're never alone and are way stronger together. And think about all the free babysitting!

Taking stock of your community

Since community is so important in this season of pregnancy and on into parenthood, this is a great time to start reflecting on your own life and social support. Do you live in a herd or are you like a lone bear? Who is currently involved in your life and is both willing and able to provide support for you now and once you give birth? Also, who do you *want* to be around you and your baby?

You don't need an entire stadium full of people. Even a handful of committed, loving, trustworthy people will do. Think coworkers, neighbors, gym buddies, classmates, faith communities, mom groups (like MOPS), and of course, family. Or think parents like you, in the trenches—those who are pregnant or have youngsters. Finding people with these darling little poop-machines is a great way to see parenting up close, learn some survival tips, see what baby products work, and have people to talk, laugh, and cry with.

Also, consider older parents with grown kids (yay for experience!) and younger teens who would be great parent helpers once your baby arrives. Find people who live close enough to watch movies with, as well as those you can connect with from a distance via phone, video chats, email, social media, or text. A little reminder: to nurture your baby while also flourishing as a parent, you'll need more than just social media friends, even if you have hundreds.

Being intentional

Building your community may mean spending more time with certain friends or rekindling relationships with family members. Sometimes it may also mean making those hard decisions like moving to another town or parting ways with those who have toxic effects on you. These choices are never easy, but they can be the biggest gift you could ever give you and your baby. If this is you, find your courage and go for it! You're creating new, positive opportunities for you and your baby.

Now that you're hopefully starting to feel better, use these next two trimesters to build or strengthen your relationships and community. Sure, sometimes it may feel inconvenient, hard, or even awkward, but new things are like that. Embrace it. Trust me, you'll thank yourself later! It's an investment you'll be able to cash in on once your little one is here. You and your baby will need all the love and help you can get.

Digging Deeper

Living in community is an adventure in every sense of the word. While sometimes it can spice up our lives just right—offering us joy, meaning, friendships, and growth—other times, it can feel overpowering. In the latter case, it's tempting to give up and become a hermit. But hold on, there's hope! Effective communication is key and can strengthen and save relationships. It's all about practice. For more information on how to hone your skills—in addressing expectations, boundary-setting, listening, and honesty—flip to B-5, where we cover questions like:

» What are helpful tips to think about when I'm trying to have an important conversation? (B-5a)

» What expectations are worth exploring with my partner, family, and friends? (B-5b)

» How can I set boundaries when I've always felt that saying no is being unloving? (B-5c)

» I'm worried my friend may be in an unhealthy relationship. What are some tip-offs? (B-5f)

WEEK 15

Baby

- Is about 6 ½ inches long.
- Weighs about 4 ¼ ounces.
- Now has many body parts that are responsive to light touch.
- Starts forming teeth.

Mama

- Your blood volume continues to rapidly increase.
- Heartburn may persist from continued hormonal and structural changes.
  - Tums are safe in pregnancy, but if you're taking a lot, talk to your maternity care provider about better options.

Cute as a Button

It's strange how sentimentality strikes—sometimes wholly without warning. Such had been the case for me about a year ago, when I had the overwhelming impulse to sift through layers of disorganized family photos my parents had stashed underneath their bed. I lifted the bed skirt, peeked into that dusty forgotten space—once my perfect hide-and-seek haven—and reached an arm into a gap that seems to have shrunk dramatically over the years.

How did I ever manage to shimmy into that short crawl space all those years? When I close my eyes, I can picture it like yesterday—I dart past the dust ruffle, scooch forward until it drapes normally once more, slow my breath, and imagine myself as a still, wooden plank. The coarse fibers of the rug press into my cheek while giggles and footsteps zip past. Finally, what felt like an eternity later, an upside-down face pops into my view, and we'd shriek with glee. I was found. Even though it's supposed to be about remaining hidden, I now realize how my soul took comfort in being sought, and how relieved I was to be found—to be no longer alone.

I blinked back the memory, focusing on the pile of photographs before me—faded memories in color sprinkled amid those in black and white. I scooped up a random handful and let the images transport me back to distant moments—to my four-year-old sister, elated, flying over a snowbank by herself in a sled. To my mother and her sister posing together in the garden before an annual ball, wearing beaded, Hungarian headdresses and puffy, floor-length gowns. To a tattered, black-and-white portrait of my grandfather, who gazed into the camera with a gentle expression in his glasses-rimmed eyes—a snapshot of a time before he had any wrinkles or grandkids. And to fifth-grader me, dressed in neon shorts and shirt, with bangs hair-sprayed to the sky.

Wow. How time has passed! Definitely a good choice to let the bangs grow out.

Sifting through these images, I'm struck by how easily I forget about parts of my past, parts of me. While my mom gave birth to me in the physical sense, my family gave that birth a context—a history by which I understand and navigate my present. I sense that without this context, trying to understand myself would be like trying to grasp the whole picture by looking at one puzzle piece.

After tucking the photos back into their box like pieces of our family puzzle—bits of our heritage collected on paper—I slid it back under the bed into the place I used to hide, waiting to be found.

―⟨⟨⟨―

Now, a year later, this growing one within me has drawn me once more toward photographs, but this time, babies are the focal point of the images. I found myself wondering: What are babies *really* like? Or at least, what do they look like up close? A little investigation couldn't hurt. So, I scour the internet in this insatiable urge to see how my daughter might look when I finally hold her in my arms.

What I found was intriguing.

Little toes, petite yawns, and thumbs that have already found their home-sweet-homes. Babies swaddled in fuchsia blankets, propped up on fluffy, faux fur, or in little suits designed to look like dwarfs, bears, and ballerinas. Apparently, some are even elegantly displayed on trays like a mouthwatering Thanksgiving Turkey, Junior. Basted with love. Cute, creative—and a bit humiliating.

What compels grown adults to dress up their darling newborns like this? Am I going to feel this same urge for my little one? But even more importantly, how will she view her part as a piece of this family puzzle? Will she find in this family picture a nurturing place of belonging—one where she can be found and known in profound ways?

Pregnancy Is All Relative

Don't ask me what exactly I want my body to do. One moment, I want to be showing more so I look and feel more pregnant. The next instant, I wish I could feel normal again—my body topped with underwhelming breasts set above a smaller belly. But then back I go—I'd never want these things if it meant being *un*pregnant. I want to meet my little baby.

Maybe I just have to come to terms with the fact that pregnancy isn't as glamorous as it appeared when I was an outside observer. What do people really mean when they say they feel great in the second trimester?

I'll tell you. It's code for saying: It's as good as it gets. Enjoy it. Everything is relative.

The second trimester is way better than the first because that was when your body stabbed you in the back and decided to form baby organs at all costs. You never got off the couch or had the chance to move more than an arm's reach from the toilet or a trash can. It is also way better than the third trimester because you can still shave your legs and even your bikini area if you're especially motivated.

But it still doesn't mean you feel as comfortable as you did in your nice, old, prepregnancy body—a time when you didn't gag unexpectedly or suffer through rectal itching provoked by hemorrhoids. Luckily, this prepregnancy state feels so very long ago that pregnant ladies like me can hardly remember it. So, at times like these, you start to wonder. *Did prepregnancy really ever exist?*

And this is why, when you are asked, "How are you feeling?" there is only one logical response to give: The second trimester is great, amazing, awesome! It's the best time in pregnancy.

HANG IN THERE

If the fatigue, nausea, vomiting, or other common pregnancy symptoms are still too-faithful companions—good news is coming your way. You will likely start feeling better very soon if you haven't already. Any time now, you could wake up feeling more energetic or less nauseous. If your pregnancy symptoms are overwhelming, talk to your maternity care provider to explore other treatment options.

⇛ LET'S TALK ABOUT IT ⇚

Cultivating Gratitude

> *Joy is what happens to us when we allow ourselves to recognize*
> *how good things really are.*
> —MARIANNE WILLIAMSON

Authentic gratitude, or thankfulness, is wonderfully nourishing to our bodies and souls. It's pretty much like swallowing a spoonful of sunshine and letting it warm and energize our weary bodies. No, it doesn't mean our lives are perfect or problem-free (because when does that ever happen?), but rather, it means choosing to focus on and to embrace the blessings that are interwoven with the bits of life that aren't so perfect. It's a shift of mindset. A resolve to soak in whatever beauty and goodness we can, on a regular basis.

Benefits of gratitude

Amazingly, studies have found this sort of approach to living can have a profoundly positive impact on our overall well-being and health, as well as our ability to maintain relationships.[1] For example, studies have found gratitude leads to happier and more satisfying lives.[2] It can lead to better sleep, improved resilience to trauma, and maybe even less workplace burnout.[1] In fact, it can decrease stress levels, loneliness, depression, materialism, bitterness, envy, and possibly suppress the inflammatory markers linked with health problems.[3-5] Imagine, all this gained simply from the practice of cultivating and expressing gratitude.

Gratitude on the easy days

We all know, some days go so well gratitude feels effortless and natural. It's like we're just sprinkled with awesome. The blessings are big and right in front of us, almost impossible to miss. These are joyous moments— like landing a job or getting married. The best thing to do in times like these? Treasure them! In fact, if you're like most of us forgetful humans, you'll have some seasons when you wonder if these sorts of joyful days ever existed.

To prepare for these droughts, try writing down some of your favorite blessings as they occur—and save them in a special place to revisit when you're in a gratitude desert. You can practice this habit of collecting your blessings either individually or as a family. Who knows, you might create a fun tradition around it with your loved ones by regularly checking out what you wrote.

Gratitude on the hard days

First, if you've been writing down what you're grateful for, go back to that list or journal or blessings jar. Plunge through the memories and see if you can find a common thread. What have you been grateful for most often? Can you be grateful for it today?

Second, it's important to be persistent. A life of gratitude is often like being on an endless scavenger hunt. You may really need to rack your brain over this. That's okay. Slow down enough to find those blessings. It can be small as a ladybug, fleeting as a downpour, kind as a smile, refreshing as a cool breeze, glamorous as a full moon, powerful as the Colorado River, grand as the Himalayas, or as distant as the Milky Way. There are always gifts tucked in your day for you to find, designed to help you thrive.

Digging Deeper

Since the practice of gratitude has such tremendous benefits, it's no wonder that people have created all sorts of fun or artsy ways to savor it. To get in the habit of incorporating daily gratitude, or to inspire your quest on those harder days, try some of these activities.[6]

» List two or three things you're grateful for based on:
  • Your senses (like what you can see, hear, feel, taste, or smell)
  • What went well that day
  • Who you're grateful for

» Play gratitude ABCs. See if you can find something for every letter of the alphabet.

» Take on the gratitude challenge. Every day, identify something new you've not listed on the day before. See how long you can keep it up!

» Write what you appreciate on your mirror with a dry erase marker, on your shower wall with bathtub crayons, or on stones with paint.

» You can even use gratitude to spice up your relationships:

- Send a letter telling someone why you're grateful for them.

- Or fill out handmade or store-bought "appreciation" coupons for when they knock your socks off.

WEEK 16

Baby
- Is about 7 ¼ inches long.
- Weighs about 5 ¼ ounces.
- Begins regular breathing movements.
- Can make grasping motions.
- Has almost fully formed sex organs.
- Produces digestive enzymes.

Mama
- Nipples enlarge, while the color of your areolas deepens.
- Your "milk factory" is developing, increasing your breast size, likely making the veins on your chest more visible.
- You may have a more obvious baby bump. Plus-size mamas may take longer to show and may eventually have a lovely "B" instead of a classic "D" belly shape from the side.[1]

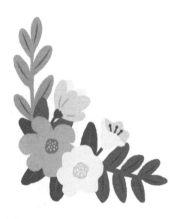

The World Sees!

I never really thought about how it would all go down the first time the rest of the world discovered the pregnant me. That it happened during one of my shifts at the Ob-Gyn clinic is perfectly fitting, though, now that I come to think of it. After all, here at the clinic, pregnancy is woven in our fibers—it runs in and through our thoughts and work, like the orange threads interlacing the sunset-hued, Ecuadorian tapestry Dan bought me as a wedding gift.

It had started as a normal patient visit.

Knock. Knock. I rapped gently on the door.

"Can I come in?"

"Yes," came the reply. "I'm ready."

"Wonderful," I said, entering to meet my new patient. After washing my hands (*now without gagging!*) I welcomed the young woman and introduced myself.

And then it happened. Before I even had a chance to say anything else, a wide smile stretched between her cheeks. Her eyes lit up, she leaned forward, and in a hushed, conspiratorial tone, she asked, "Are you pregnant?"

How did she know? Can she actually see something? I mean, I know I have love handles, and if Dan and I look hard enough at my belly's profile, we can see a little pooch. But it's pretty subtle—only a sliver of a half-moon, at best. I know some women start showing earlier, others later, but here, now, her question says it's finally happening for me. Someone else sees it, too! And she didn't even need a magnifying glass, prompting, or tip-off. At last!

Keep it together Meshi. You can't just jump around, flailing your arms in excitement, shouting, "Yes, I am! I am!" Keep your cool. You're not a high school cheerleader—you're a professional. A grown-up. Try as I might, I couldn't keep back the beginnings of a grin.

Yet amid the joy, I also felt vulnerable—exposed. My time with patients is about them, not me. Typically, the only hint about my personal life is my wedding ring. But now, I can't help it, my body is revealing what my words would not.

Striving for nonchalance, desperate to hide that it was my first time answering the question, I responded.

"Yes, I'm 16 weeks."

That's right, I thought, satisfied with the delivery. *I'm an old pro.*

She congratulated me, and we moved on with our visit while my soul nearly burst through my skin from excitement. I can't say for sure, but I *may* have leaned back a bit to show off my bump. *Just maybe.*

She had great timing, I thought after she had left. It was only last week that I finally decided to share the news with my employer and colleagues. While there's no formal etiquette for when I needed to tell them, and while I could have waited until the results of my twenty-week fetal anatomy ultrasound, I'd felt ready. I was tired of bottling up our joy and wearing looser fabrics to hide any evidence. It was time to let this new thread of our reality—pregnancy—visibly run throughout every part of my life.

Meeting Mother Atlas

On days when I don't work in Petaluma, I veg out. As far as I can tell, there's no real difference between how I lie around the house and how the giant zucchinis in our apartment's garden lounge on the soil of their beds. When I walk the meandering path to our backyard entrance, I stroll past the rows of thornless raspberry vines and the zucchinis' deep-green, shiny leaves topped by the floppy yellow, trumpet-like flowers from which they emerge. Each time I walk that way, I pluck a few plump berries, pop them in my mouth, and crouch down to admire the ever-growing vegetables. Yup, we have so much in common—we're both so skilled at resting.

While vegging recently, I've contemplated a few keepsakes to make for my little wonder so she knows she's special to me. I thought an animal mobile made of felt would be logical and as good a place as any to start. After all, don't all babies need something to look at when in their crib? As much as I want to lounge forever, I resisted the urge and started stitching together Lady Fish, Mr. Owl, and Baby Lion—my baby's future friends.

When not sewing, I've also started scouring the internet for a pre-owned baby carrier—a fabric marvel that, I've heard, keeps a baby close while also giving mommy a chance to go about her daily activities. *Sounds good to me.*

A listing on Craigslist caught my eye, so I dialed up the number in the ad.

"Hi," I said when a woman answered. "I was wondering if the baby carrier on Craigslist was still available."

"Yes, it is," she said, a bit flustered.

"Sold!" I replied, thrilled about the news. "I'll take it!" There was no time to waste. I needed to secure this hot commodity before it could be ripped out from under me.

Her response to my enthusiasm was cut off by a piercing wail. As I listened, I became certain there was with her, very close by—a monster. A miniature one, perhaps, but powerful, nonetheless. And loud. Her toddler screamed in the background, making it clear I had called directly into a war zone. How can this woman possibly be functioning right now? She sounded glad to sell the carrier—and would possibly add the toddler to the deal if only to get some rest.

Is this what I have to look forward to? A state of utter exhaustion? An existence of nothing beyond mere survival? She really sounded like she hadn't slept for decades. In fact, I felt so bad for her that I was highly tempted to ask her a few depression-screening questions over the phone. Just to make sure she's okay. My better sense got hold of me, and I held off, arranging to meet her the next day in the Starbucks parking lot.

While I was waiting in my car, watching people go in and out of the bustling coffee shop, I thought about the woman I was about to meet. Honestly, I wouldn't have been surprised if she never showed up. I don't think I would have if I felt the same way she must feel.

Much to my surprise, however, she came. On time, even. This woman was way tougher than I thought. *How do people like her do this?*

Motherhood has apparently blessed her with a complimentary backbone stronger than Atlas.

We exchanged hellos, and then she asked how far along I was, and if it was my first baby.

"Yes," I said, catching a glimpse of her tamed little creature strapped in his car seat. He looked cute. Even innocent. No one would ever suspect how capable his vocal cords were and how robust his lungs.

"Motherhood is incredibly difficult," she affirmed, "but worth it."

It was a familiar mantra. One I've heard many mothers reflexively chant. In a short conversation, they may say little else besides passing on this golden nugget of truth. And yet, as I placed my new purchase on the seat beside me and the harried mother drove away, I realized the mantra—familiar though it was—was all the more comforting coming from someone still living in the trenches of motherhood.

LET'S TALK ABOUT IT

When What-Ifs Overwhelm You

At this stage in pregnancy, you might finally be feeling well enough to think about gender reveal party ideas, or even to hunt for your baby bump, because, if you've been through all this, it sure would be courteous of your body to give you one already. You may even be wondering what it will be like to feel your baby's first movements. It's coming soon! If you've been pregnant before, you may sense your baby's movements in the next week or so, while if you're a rookie, it could be nearer 20 to 21 weeks.

Likely, having been pregnant this long, you've also realized that carrying a little one brings a bunch of interesting change and newness with it. There's always something to plan, prepare for, and think about. Even for those of you who've been pregnant before—each pregnancy, just like each child, is unique. In this, specialness saturates your body, even down to the microscopic level, as your baby's DNA courses through your veins.[2] Isn't that amazing?

If you're like most pregnant mamas, though, you may not only be thinking about the wonderful things but also those that are worrisome or even overwhelming. Some of you may be scared because of known pregnancy or medical problems while others of you have a lot of general concerns. Let's take a closer look at these types of experiences, shall we?

> Self-care activities include regular physical activity, adequate sleep, nutritious eating, meditation, cultivating spirituality, relaxation, hobbies, doing something you love, and connecting with loved ones.

Defining fear, anxiety, and worry

Fear, anxiety, and worry are related, but each is distinct. *Fear* is a reaction we get when faced with an immediate threat, as our bodies' survival instinct causes that famous *fight-or-flight response* to protect us. *Anxiety* is a bit more complex and consists of physical, emotional, and cognitive responses— having to do more with assuming danger or discomfort is headed our way. It may, for example, cause physical symptoms like tiredness, irritability, restlessness, nausea, and trouble sleeping or concentrating.

Sometimes when we're anxious, we don't realize it and refer to it as stress, freaking out, or panic. On the other hand, "*worry* is anxious thinking" which feels like an exhausting "mental workout." It's when we play out the possibilities of what could happen next by asking those tempting "what if" questions and ponder all the terrifying worst-case scenarios. Worry feeds into anxiety, which then feeds into worry, creating a feedback loop that can potentially interfere with our functioning.*

Of course, some degree of concern and worry is understandable during pregnancy. You're growing a baby, after all—an incredible thing and no small feat! Healthy (small) amounts of anxiety, stress, or worry can keep us attentive and motivated to identify and address problems. Unfortunately, though, unhealthy amounts of anxiety are easy to come by and are especially likely when we're tired, stressed, spending time with anxious people, or have let our self-care practices fall to the wayside.

---

* Julie Jorgenson, LMFT, personal communication, May 15, 2021

If anxious feelings or worrisome thoughts are forefront in your heart and mind or are impacting how you function in your daily activities, you may be suffering from an anxiety disorder. This is so common! Types of anxiety include generalized anxiety, panic disorder, phobias, and obsessive-compulsive disorder.[3]

Responding to anxiety

If you can relate to this realm of anxiety or have even been diagnosed with an anxiety disorder, be encouraged—there is help and freedom to be had. Although we can't control life and wipe out its uncertainties, anxiety doesn't have to write the narrative.[†]

To begin, ask yourself: What role do I want fear and anxiety to have in my life? Do I want to let them dictate my life and distract me from living fully? Or do I want to change my relationship with these so I can live richly and freely despite those uncomfortable feelings? For those of you dear mamas trying to cope by using substances like cigarettes, drugs, or alcohol, ask yourself: Do I want things to be different? What kind of mama do I want to be?

Sometimes medical problems can cause you to feel depressed or anxious. Ask your healthcare provider to order you labs—these often check thyroid levels, complete blood count, glucose, vitamin B12, folate, and vitamin D.

Thankfully, with the right support, we are capable of learning to recognize our fears and anxiety and developing healthy ways to respond. For those ready to take the next step, there are many options available such as therapy, lifestyle changes, and medication and supplements—or better yet, a combination of these.

Whatever your relationship with anxiety and worry, focus on clinging to your daily joys and soaking up the specialness in and around you. You only get this "today" once. Enjoy feeling your little one move and watching your bump grow. And when worries or anxiety try to crash

---

[†] Livia Perry, FPMHNP-BC, personal communication, April 1, 2021

your party, when they try to convince you to live in the past or the future, ground yourself in the present and remind yourself there is hope! With time, practice, and the right support, you can move closer to living your life according to your values instead of your fears. What a wonderful gift for your little one to experience and witness while growing up! You go, mama.

Digging Deeper

While early on in pregnancy everything can seem a little surreal, at this stage you may be finding you have more specific—more tangible—excitement, fears, or worries. This is a beautiful time to start integrating *daily* self-care activities into your routine to promote your well-being through whatever may come your way. Take time to explore the resources in B-3 & 4, meant just for you. You'll find more information on topics like:

» In what ways can I support my mental wellness and relaxation? (B-4f and B-3c)

» Help! I'm really struggling. How do I reach out for help and what can I expect? (B-4c & d)

» Are psychiatric medications safe in pregnancy? (B-4e)

» Is it okay if I use marijuana or an alcoholic drink to unwind? (B-4h)

Notes

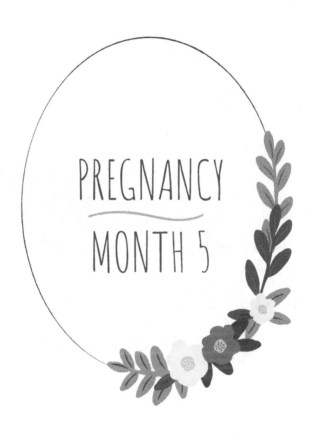

PREGNANCY

MONTH 5

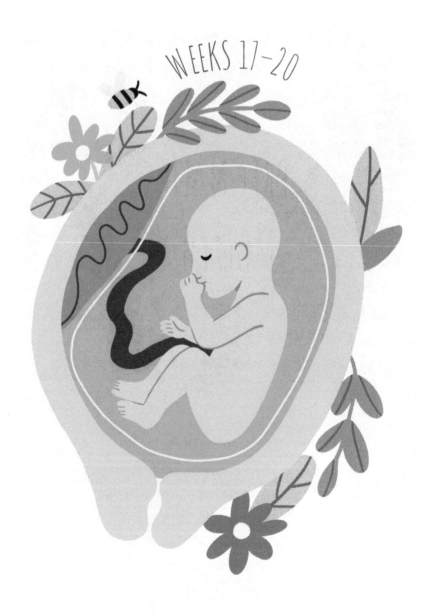

WEEKS 17–20

WEEK 17

Baby

- Is about 8 inches long.
- Weighs about 6 ¼ ounces.
- Starts storing fat.
- Has started producing blood cells in the bone marrow to support the immune system and carry oxygen.
- Forms bronchioles (breathing passages) in the lungs.

Mama

- Likely you need less sleep than in the first trimester.
- You may now experience occasional round ligament pain as your growing uterus causes these to stretch. Although not dangerous, these sharp, momentary pains on the sides of your belly can startle you while moving or twisting.

Hello, Pepper

It should have been easy, or at least, much *easier*. It always had been. Why should it be any different now? Sure, I chose a stretchy dress at the clothing store (I am pregnant, after all), but this—*thing*—had no shape. It had a floral pattern and style that by all rights should have been cute. And it *should* have worked. But as soon as I donned it in the dressing room, I was greeted with a sight that was both shocking and disheartening. For all the shape it had, I might have been wearing a pillowcase. I scrutinized the image in the mirror, not quite believing my eyes.

I have no waist.

Now when did that happen? And where on earth did it go?

I tore off that horrid nightmare of a dress and searched the mirror high and low, hoping to find my lost waist. *No sign.* I even scanned the tile floor around me, but I only spied ten little sausage-like toes peeking out from beneath my pregnant belly—pudgy appendages that I can now only *presume* are mine. It seems my ever-evolving body has managed to morph into the approximate shape of a Hungarian paprika pepper—long and ill-defined.

Sigh.

It used to be so much easier to find clothes that, firstly—fit—and secondly, fit *better*. But what now? Maybe it's time to try my luck again at the maternity shops. After all, more people *are* noticing I'm pregnant. Just the other day, in fact, when I was at the fabric store purchasing my stack of neatly folded cloth, the cashier randomly asked, "How much time do we have?"

Time for what? I'd wondered, looking around for a clue. Is this a literal or rhetorical question? No wait, this is a trick question—a riddle—right?

But by the grace of God, after a moment that felt like an eternity, it somehow clicked.

I have a belly. I am pregnant. This belly is getting bigger. The riddler must be seeing that I'm pregnant.

Oh, right! I've got this.

"I'm due February 5th," I answered.

Phew, I passed. Not with flying colors, but I passed.

Yes, I suppose it's time to revisit the maternity section. Leaving the beastly floral dress banished to the hanger, I shoulder my purse and give one last look in the dressing room mirror at pepper-like me.

There are worse things to look like, I supposed, as I envisioned the paprika-adorned merchant shops in Budapest's *Nagy Vásárcsarnok* (Great Market Hall). There, among the corridors of the old, beautifully patterned yellow-and-red structure, beside the Danube River, tourists and natives alike enjoy all sorts of savory aromas and goods—local produce, fresh pastries, aged wines, spicy salamis, smoked cheeses, pickled cabbage, and, of course, sweet paprika.

No, I decided, lingering in the memory of our visits to my home sweet (far away from) home. It might not be so bad to be like these peppers since, in the end, we'll get to greet our darling—who will surely be the spice of our lives.

Beyond the Saint Bernards

My favorite thing about going to prenatal appointments has caught me by complete surprise. Of course, I had no way of anticipating it when we made our initial selection of the small Ob-Gyn practice near Cupertino. The two midwives and the physician had years of experience, were well respected in the local medical community, delivered in a local hospital, and have a reputation for focusing on natural childbirth while minimizing unnecessary medical interventions. *Score!* Knowing all these were important to me, it seemed like a perfect fit.

And truly, from the moment I step into their office, a lovely and inviting cottage-style building, I feel welcome—ready to pull out my slippers and start lounging. This place is so relaxing, it could easily pass for a day spa, or the perfect venue for hosting a tea party—a far cry from the medicalized offices awash with uninspiring abstract art hung on sterile, white walls, and an almost-visible haze of disinfectant.

Each month I visit for my prenatal appointment, I check in at the secretary desk with the gooseneck-shaped legs, and then settle in the adjacent room on ornately carved mahogany furniture. All that's missing is my mother's home-cooked, layered potato dish, *rakott krumpli*.

While waiting to be called back for my visit, I'm content to let my gaze absorb the surroundings—the cushions patterned with a Middle Eastern–style needlepoint, the ornately woven Persian rugs, and the floral tapestries hanging on either side of the French windows. So thoughtfully decorated! Why can't all pregnant women receive prenatal care in such a rejuvenating and nurturing environment?

I wouldn't change one thing about this place. Not one! Okay, maybe two—those monstrous Saint Bernards lounging in the waiting room with me. While I'm fairly certain the clinicians wouldn't allow them to hang out if they were actually ferocious, and (for the moment, at least) they're not terribly interested in eating me, I still can't help but be a little uneasy around them. They're each literally the size of—me. Maybe I should consider bringing Dan in for my prenatal appointment as my bodyguard. These hounds are definitely capable of making any pregnant guest waddle back immediately from whence she came.

Although I'm thankful for all this mostly considerate planning (minus the dogs, of course), my personal favorite has to be—drumroll, please!—the toilet seat warmer. Unexpected, yes. And soothing? Very much so. An especially nice touch, indeed, since we pregnant women do spend quite a bit of time here collecting the urine samples our maternity care providers request.

Might as well let us sink into a warm, padded seat while we frantically try to accomplish the impossible: to somehow find that elusive stream dripping behind our mountain and get more pee in that barely visible specimen cup than on our fingers.

It's as if by providing this amenity, they are saying: We care about you. We believe you can—not just pee in a cup, but also push a giant bowling ball through your naive vagina, unmedicated even, if you so choose.

⇒⇒⇒ LET'S TALK ABOUT IT ⇐⇐⇐

Making the Most of Your Prenatal Appointments

By now, you've experienced a snapshot of what appointments are like with your maternity care provider. While there are many different settings, scenes, and types of maternity care providers themselves, at the core, they should all be oriented toward accomplishing the same thing: taking care of you and your little one. Since these meetings can have a profound impact on your pregnancy journey and the health of your baby, let's look at what you can expect from these appointments, how to prepare for them, and how to navigate your interactions with your provider. Ready?

Timing

In general, most women with healthy, uncomplicated pregnancies have a 10- to 20-minute prenatal checkup: each month until 28 weeks; every two to three weeks between weeks 28 and 36; and then weekly until the big day. Of course, there may be some variations on this theme based on where your maternity care provider works and your specific situation. You may need more frequent visits to your maternity care provider and specialist, and sometimes even extra monitoring of your baby (such as with ultrasounds or nonstress tests, which use an external monitor to track how your baby's heart rate responds when he or she moves).

Content

Think of your routine prenatal appointment as a huddle with your maternity care provider. It's a check-in, a chat about the game plan for the upcoming weeks, and a time to learn about select pregnancy topics. By now, you've probably figured out the general rhythm for your visits. To prepare you for your appointment, they collect some basic health information, such as your vital signs, weight, and maybe even a sample of your urine (to check for things like protein and bacteria).

During some visits, hopefully, someone is also checking into your safety and well-being by asking screening questions regarding mental health, substance use, and domestic violence.[1-5] Though these can feel a little awkward, please know that an honest answer helps your maternity care provider better understand how to support you.

The bulk of your visit with your maternity care provider will consist of checking on your little one (listening to the heart rate by Doppler and estimating growth with *fundal heights*, the number of centimeters between the top of the uterus and the pubic bone); following up on medical or mental health problems; addressing your questions and concerns (so bring them!); reviewing lab or other results and next steps; and covering relevant, educational pregnancy topics.

Phew! Yep, that's quite a list—is your head spinning? It can be a jam-packed session. This is also why it's nice to have grace for your maternity care provider. If they're running late, it's often because they're trying to cover a lot with mamas like you, or an emergency arose.

Preparation

There are a few things you can do to help set yourself up for a meaningful prenatal appointment. First, be proactive and take responsibility. Your active involvement can spark conversations that can lead to better understanding and ultimately better care. For starters, collect your thoughts before your appointment, and bring a list of questions or concerns you'd like to discuss. Start with your top two or three most pressing ones to help you prioritize.

And then, it's all about timing. Be sure to tell your maternity care provider *at the beginning* of your visit that you have questions or concerns to discuss. It will help them plan the visit so you have time to talk. If you had primed them for a question-and-answer time, but you find they are headed for the door and they completely forgot to get to your list, do remind them of your concerns. Though generally, if you wait that long, you probably won't get a very in-depth or satisfying answer. "Doorknob" questions are fitting for quick clarifying ones like: *So, should I be fasting for this test?* and *When will I get a call about . . . ?*

Follow-up

As you can imagine, it's not easy covering all these important elements of care in a single visit. Sometimes, your maternity care provider may be like a superhero, able to get to it all. However, there will undoubtedly be some appointments where you'll leave rushed, and maybe even a little disappointed.

So, then what?

The best thing to do is follow up and speak up. Express your questions and concerns. Otherwise, your provider may not have any idea how you feel or what's going on and therefore won't be able to get you the care you deserve. If you have something urgent that wasn't addressed, you can always call back with your question or leave a message with the front desk. If it's not urgent, bring your wonderful "leftovers" to your next visit.

That said, if the maternity care provider in question is repeatedly a poor communicator, dismissive, and gives the vibe that she or he is not interested in working with you, move on. You and your baby need better care. Switch to someone who shows that they respect you by making time for you and by being excited to collaborate.

Ultimately, both you and your child benefit when you are informed and involved in your healthcare and decision-making. Try it! Trust me, it's good practice and it's your right. Later you'll thank yourself, because if you cultivate them now, these mama-bear protective skills will benefit your little one through the years to come.

Digging Deeper

While being involved in your prenatal visits in these new ways is worth it and can be exciting, it can also be tricky. If you're not sure how to formulate your questions and concerns, check out some of the prompts below, based on content from the Childbirth Connection website.[6] Customize the ones that fit your situation best, and take them with you to your next prenatal appointments. Before you know it, you'll be bringing up your questions or concerns like a pro.

» "I don't understand _____ . Please explain this to me."
» "Can we review _____ today? I didn't catch everything you mentioned earlier."
» "I'm wondering where I can get more information about _____ ?"

» "I'm concerned about _____ . What are my other options? What if I take no action (*watchful waiting*)?"

» "You're recommending _____. What scientific evidence supports this as being the best?"

» "What could happen to me or my baby if I accept _____? What if I don't?"

» "I'm uncomfortable with what you're recommending. I'm thinking about getting a second opinion about _____ ."

WEEK 18

Baby

- Is about 8 ¾ inches long.
- Weighs about 7 ¾ ounces.
- Now has eyes and ears in their final position.
- Can make facial expressions and sucking motions.

Mama

- Your blood pressure will likely be lower in the second trimester.
  - To feel well and avoid dizziness, be sure to drink plenty of fluids—especially if it's hot outside.
- You may start feeling your baby's first movements (called *quickening*)! First-time mamas, or those who have an *anterior placenta* (one located in the front of the belly), may not feel this quite yet.

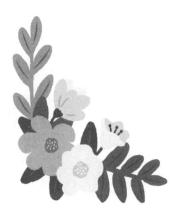

The Never-ending Question

It's amazing to me that I can have a little busy bee floating around inside me and yet feel nothing as she goes about her baby business. How's that possible? I've casually reassured pregnant mamas like me that it's normal to not feel their baby's movements until about 18 to 21 weeks, but now that I'm experiencing it myself, it seems quite shocking.

I can seriously have a five-inch person living smack dab in the middle of my core, and I'm completely oblivious? Come on now, really? If it were up to me, I would have felt something by now.

To make it worse, everyone around me is asking if I've felt my baby move yet. How do friends, family, and coworkers all know that it's time to inquire about this upcoming milestone? All day long, I hear myself giving the same two boring answers: *No* and *Nope*.

How disappointing.

I just keep wondering when I'll feel the first little flutter or nudge saying, "Hello, out there—Mommy, it's me." I look forward to this big day with the same expectant longing that grips children awaiting their first visit from the Tooth Fairy, or young teens looking for the signs of adolescence to begin. It's a big deal—and yet all we can do is wait. And then wait more.

I wish I could say that I've perfected the waiting game, but I'd be lying if I did. Honestly, it's just frustrating. I'm not sure which is worse—the inquisitive people or the situation I've found myself in. I just feel like snapping back like a fiery pregnant lady and saying, "Yes, I realize it will be a flutter, and I'll let you know when I finally feel something." *So quit bugging me about it.*

But, behind my inner defiance, a sneaking worry lingers. Will that day ever really come? Though the nausea has mostly faded, gas kneads my intestines so much that I'm sure, to catch my attention, my little one would have to drive a monster truck at full speed into the walls of my uterus.

I hope she can find one soon.

Biking Up Mount Everest

Naps are mysterious and magical. They can create multiple days out of one and refresh a tired pregnant body so brilliantly, it almost sparkles afterward. Yes, it might just be one of my favorites of God's inventions. To let my eyes close, my body sink into the softness below, and let my mind drift off into never-never land. *Perfectly glorious.*

I'm especially grateful for it today because Dan and I just returned from an exhausting road-biking date. We hadn't planned for such an intense trip, but life has a sense of humor.

We took a new route today, away from the popular Stevens Creek Reservoir, which was our typical favorite. It's such a beautiful trip but could also be quite risky due to all the semitrucks that use the same roads. Though we'd never had an issue before, I kept worrying that something would go wrong. While the scenario is unlikely, Dan took my concerns seriously and led us along a brand-new bike route today, just for me.

Isn't that sweet?

Happily, the road started out flat, stretching a few miles through rows of neighborhoods. But before I could get too comfortable, our leisurely path began inclining. And then, even more. It grew and grew, before my eyes, into a perfectly round hill, as if Mother Earth were reclining before me, showing off her sunny, pregnant belly cloaked in asphalt.

After making it up her hill, and in view of the next looming slope, I exhaled loudly—maybe even *really* loudly—hoping Dan would feel some remorse over what mess he'd gotten his pregnant wife into. If I thought that biking up hills before pregnancy was hard, I've found it was a breeze compared to navigating them while pregnant.

Pedaling round and round, slower and slower, I inched up the next hill. Mother Earth was reclining in a seemingly endless pile of voluminous curves.

"You're doing great, sweetie," came Dan's too-cheerful voice. "Keep up the good work."

Yeah, right! I thought, punctuating each word with the familiar, rhythmic squeaks of my leather clip-in shoes and the push of my ragged breath. *Dan's definitely* not *so sweet now.*

I looked up at the horizon, trying to see how much of the blessed belly of a hill is left, hoping it would help me muster the energy I needed to keep my screaming quads moving. Bad idea. The incline simply continued without even a whisper of an apology.

Okay, Dan's not at all sweet. Has he ever been? The accusations churned with my heaving breath.

I could see some walkers nearing our position, and I tried pushing forward with pride, hoping they might just be impressed to see a pregnant woman out there with them on Mount Everest. But I couldn't. I had to stop—*right* in front of them. How embarrassing!

It's all Dan's fault.

Yes, pregnant pride does come before a figurative pregnant fall. I walked my bike up the rest of the way, avoiding eye contact. Limitations seem to be my constant companion lately. There was a time when I could have pushed the whole way up the hill without stopping. But not today. Fighting back frustrated tears, I tried to let my breathing slow and focus on how far I *was* able to go—to accept my abilities as they were.

When we eventually made it to a flat road and wound along the creek, its calm, trickling sounds soothed my achy body. The cool breeze refreshed the scraps of my being. That nearly kicked my butt.

Nearly.

Though the excursion was tougher than either of us anticipated, I realized I was pretty proud to make it through despite having to stop. In fact, the endeavor seemed a fundamental step in reclaiming my place as a moving and active person in society. What's more, for the first time since being pregnant, I didn't burst into tears at my new body's limitations.

I guess I do have Dan to thank for that.

Could I possibly be getting used to the pregnant me? I wonder, as I curl up under my crisp bedsheet and indulge in yet another nap—ready to sparkle.

ᗥᗥᗥ LET'S TALK ABOUT IT ᗕᗕᗕ

Dad's Impact on Child Development

During and after pregnancy, mamas are center stage, receiving special attention, individualized care, and hopefully some pampering. While this makes perfect sense and is how it should be, sometimes dads are forgotten or overlooked. So, this section is designed to offset this trend and set the record straight.

Fathers—including biological, adoptive, and social fathers (father figures)—play a vital and unique role in a child's growth and development. Though a diverse group with a wide range of upbringings, personalities, interests, gender identities, and thoughts on fatherhood, men add (both individually and as a group) a depth of dimension to our lives.

If your life is complicated and your baby's biological father is uninvolved or not in a place to be a positive role model—take heart. This section is still for you, too. Other capable men can step in to help fill that void if you choose to live within a community and let them.

Though our understanding about the father's impact on his child's development is continuing to grow as more time is spent studying this valuable aspect of family, some of the elements we know already are astounding. For centuries, fathers have been skillfully adapting their roles so their children and families can survive all sorts of difficult situations and cultures; over the past few decades, this has meant dads jumping into more direct caregiving roles.[1] It turns out that this closer level of interaction can have many benefits that are now coming to light.

Dad's body changes too!

Incredibly, invested dads undergo biological changes to prepare them for fatherhood. Get this: his hormones will shift, and his brain will experience structural changes too! For example, his testosterone levels decrease to help him be more sensitive, empathetic, and focused on family.[2] The "love and bonding hormone," oxytocin, will increase whenever he plays with your baby and will also mirror your oxytocin levels throughout pregnancy if he lives with you.[3,4] Being around your hormones changes his. And as if all this wasn't enough to blow your socks off, certain brain regions will literally change size so he's better at bonding, nurturing, and interacting with your baby.[5] Now how amazing is that?

Dad's unique contributions

So, what are the benefits of a loving father's interactions with his child?

Studies have shown that a sensitive dad's interactions with his child (from day one) have a profoundly positive impact on his or her cognitive and language development,[6] executive functioning (the higher-level brain processes involved in behavior control),[7] and even mental health (like a decreased risk of depression and loneliness in older kids).[8] These benefits extend throughout the child's life.[1,9]

It doesn't stop there, though.

A dad's playtime with baby is another important way he can shape his child and their relationship. If you're pregnant with your first child, it won't take long after your baby arrives for you to realize Dad is *not* your clone, and he has his own way of doing most anything, including playtime. Not only is this okay, it's ideal! Mamas tend to be more affectionate during play while dads tend toward rough-and-tumble play. Come to find out, a dad's play style is more repetitively stimulating for your little one, which not only fosters bonding but also gives your baby the chance to safely explore and engage the unpredictable, full-of-surprises world around them.[10] So, when you see dad doing things differently than you, remember—his way, if done sensitively, benefits your little one. By allowing and encouraging this kind of play, you're expanding your baby's horizon.

Friend, as you journey through pregnancy and prepare for your darling's arrival, remember papas and papa figures are profoundly important. They can beautifully complement your interactions with your little one. If you have a partner, go ahead and share some of these awesome dad facts so he learns how pivotal his role will be in your baby's life. Let him talk to your belly so your baby can start getting to know daddy.

Oh, and when your little one does arrive, be sure to give dad the time and space he needs to figure out fatherhood. No need to swoop in at your baby's smallest whimper. This space and your encouragement will not only build your relationship and make him a better dad, but it will also likely teach you a trick or two.

Digging Deeper

After reading this, some of you mamas in a relationship may be looking for more ways to celebrate and support your partner in his unfolding role as dad. What a great idea! Check out the list below for ideas suggested by Dr. Anna Machin.[1] For those of you mamas who are not in a relationship with someone who could be a father figure, consider making a list of men in your life (uncles, grandfathers, friends, brothers) who you'd like to involve in your child's nurturing. The more the merrier!

» Check in: How is he doing during your pregnancy? After delivery?
» Involve him: Bring him to prenatal appointments and include him in conversations and decisions.
» Find dad-specific resources, like dad-only prenatal classes (in person or online), or schedule a guys' hangout where inexperienced dads ask questions of experienced dads.
» Throw him a "daddy-shower."
» Identify his unique role:
  • For during delivery: contraction timer, water boy, advocate, massage therapist, cheerleader, coach, cornerman, and communications specialist
  • For after the birth: lead diaper changer, baby burper, breast pump sanitizer, tea maker, cuddler, visitor manager, and take-out master

WEEK 19

Baby
- Is about 9 ½ inches long.
- Weighs about 9 ¾ ounces.
- Has already had more than 20 million heartbeats.
- Is already receiving immunity benefits from you.

Mama
- You may not notice it yet, but your body is now making colostrum, your baby's first milk.
- Because of greater blood flow in the pelvis, you may have increased sexual arousal and ability to orgasm.

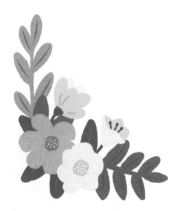

My Butterfly

"No," "Nope," and "No, I have *not* felt my baby's first movements yet."

It's taking forever.

Discouraged, I repeated the too-familiar mantra to my mother over the phone. Desperately wishing for any nudge of a new answer, I searched my mind for any minor changes within me that I might have possibly overlooked.

"Hmm . . . Well, there is one thing. I noticed an occasional, ever-so-slight, movement in my belly—like a small gas bubble bobbing along sideways." It was like something tracing an imaginary horizon line on my insides.

With a giggle, a very hopeful Nana-to-be exclaimed that this sounded very "suspicious," and I should pay closer attention to these feelings. "If you feel gas-like bubbles in your belly, in the same spot," she added, "and no gas comes out—you've got to wonder if it's really gas you're feeling."

I'm so proud to call this wise woman "Mother." Just like that, she put me at ease.

Once we ended our chat, I plopped down on our quilt-covered bed and gazed up at the ceiling fan, excited, but hardly daring to hope that today might be *the* day. Taking a deep breath, I focused on the fan—its blades spinning around and around above me like a mesmerizing carousel.

A little carnival music, crunchy kettle corn, or a petting zoo would sound delightful right about now. So would the cheerful dance of iridescent circus bubbles, emanating from the candy-striped booths where children run and gather to touch these magic spheres. I can picture it now—standing in awe like a child while God envelops me in a swath of shiny bubbles that soar up, hover, shimmer, and then glide back down again to kiss my cheek, perch on an outstretched palm, or balance on my big toe—the encore before their final bow. *Pop!* In so many ways, the path of pregnancy feels like that of a bubble's—it is unique, up-and-down, and filled with mystery and miracle.

Bathing in the image and letting my mom's words feed my hope, I quieted my soul and waited under the gentle breeze of the whirring fan.

Okay, let's see what exactly is going on with these inner bubbles. I held my breath and gaze, and then there it was. That strange little sensation. Like tiny little butterflies fluttering around in me.

Colorful ones—
gently beating their wings,
making ripples
as they swim through my waters.

Then they were gone.

I tried telepathically asking my little butterfly to move again. *Just to be sure.* And then it happened. This time, a movement in the pit of my stomach.

Hooray! I jumped up, grabbed the phone, and called my mother and sister to announce the arrival of this monumental day: Yes, yes, and *yes!*

I *finally* felt my baby move.

Squeals resounded so loudly over the phone that even my little one deep inside must have heard their excitement.

The Broken Record

I thought this day would never come. Last night was like the night before Christmas because we knew today we would see our baby by ultrasound. To prepare, I dutifully started chugging the 32 ounces of water during the hour before for our fetal anatomy ultrasound. The liquid rushed down my throat, splashing into a sea of who knows what, until my bladder screamed.

In the meantime, Dan and I soared down the highway to San Jose in our old gray Jetta, grinning at any driver who happened to make unexpected eye contact. While I've been perfectly content assuming this little one is a girl, and am therefore excited to find out officially, I remind myself the real purpose of this appointment extends far beyond this. The radiologist will check my baby's growth, look closely at her organs and body parts, and even explore her living accommodations, so to speak (noticing items like the location of the placenta, length of the cervix, and volume of amniotic fluid). I wonder if she'll cooperate during this exam, showing off all her little parts as needed, or if I'll need to come back in a few weeks for a recheck.

When we finally arrived and walked through the outpatient radiology waiting room, my heart sank. There were so many people ahead of me, waiting to be seen. Are they running behind . . . by a year? There's no way I'll be able to sit for an hour with a full bladder. I must have looked desperate enough because shortly thereafter, the door swung open, the technician paused, took a deep breath, and took a stab at my name.

"Em-ee-seeeee?"

It's an expected variation, and I applauded the attempt. (Come to find out, "EH-meh-sheh" isn't an intuitive pronunciation in the States.) Dan and I stood up, assuming it was my turn, but the ultrasound technician asked him to stay behind for a few minutes.

Okay, no problem.

Next thing I know, I'm lying on the table in the dark room and the technician is about to start the assessment. *Um, minor problem: Where is my husband?* When I asked when Dan could come in, she had the nerve to say, "After the evaluation is done."

Wait, what?!

"I would really like him to be in here with me."

"Preferably not," she responded while squirting warm gel all across my belly.

I kept insisting, saying that it would mean so much to us if he were here with me.

"He's actually also a physician," I added, "and very much enjoys looking at ultrasounds."

My pleas fell on deaf ears.

"Is there anything I can say or do to have him brought back?" I eventually asked.

"Preferably no," she parroted.

Unbelievable! This should be unheard of. Even a healthcare provider can't navigate this crazy healthcare system? How could we ever expect nonmedical people, let alone non-English speakers, to adequately advocate for themselves? At a loss for what else to do, I finally decided to stop bothering her so she could at least do her job.

About five minutes later, an intercom came on in the room.

"Do you have patient Parker?" asked a woman over the speaker. "Her husband would like to be brought back. He's a physician."

I proudly listened to the conversation. *Way to go, Dan. You pulled out the doctor card.* I later learned that he simply asked the front desk staff if there's a reason why he couldn't be with his wife. He told them he was a physician and really wanted to be back there. Within two minutes, there he was, standing by my feet—and seeing our little one before even I could.

Though I was glad to have Dan there, and the rest of the ultrasound exam went smoothly from a technical standpoint, the process was quite disappointing. The technician had the screen pointed *away* from me. Here they were, getting a peek inside at our little one, while I was left out in the cold. But I'm growing the darn thing, aren't I?

Working to let go of my frustration and get comfortable, I put my hands behind my head and focused on my husband instead. Intently studying our baby's black-and-white images, he didn't glance away even for a moment. The intensity of his gaze, and how he seized this chance to get to know our little wonder—from the inside out—both caught me by surprise and warmed my heart.

"Cute," says the technician. *Click.* We have a souvenir snapshot—our baby stretched out, with her arms behind her head, too, a mirror image of her mama.

What seemed ages later, the ultrasound tech granted me the grace to empty my bladder before showing me my own baby on-screen. Grateful, I hurried off. Once back in the exam room, I settled in to see what Dan and the technician had been enjoying this whole time.

There she was. The little dot with a beating heart had now grown into a little baby—a daughter. Her petite legs were crossed at the ankles, daintily.

All I could do was stare back at her face through the monitor, treasuring the sneak peek. This could very well be the last in-depth ultrasound for the rest of pregnancy. In fact, for many women, it is.

She's so cute. And yet looks so much like a little alien.

On the car ride home, I conference-called my family, sharing the sex of our cute little monster, to the sound of more delighted shrieks.

My dad calmly reminded me that she was not a little alien but really was never "meant" to be seen in this state when she was still assembling herself and growing. She will, he added, look very cute and normal when she appears in February.

LET'S TALK ABOUT IT

Knowing Your Healthcare Rights

The healthcare system can often seem like a whole different planet, with all sorts of unknowns. Staff often wear martian-like uniforms or white coats, can interact a little robotically like WALL-E, and even use strange words or phrases. Even something as simple as exiting a building, which you've done countless times in your life, can feel like an accomplishment by the time you make it through the labyrinth of hallways. No wonder things get confusing.

Since there is no official bus tour to guide you through this strange land of healthcare, let's see if we can make it easier for you by exploring your rights as a patient—a set of fundamentals designed to ensure you receive the proper care, tailored to you. We touched on aspects of this in "Making the Most of Your Prenatal Appointments" (week 17), but now we're going more in depth. After all, with this knowledge comes power, and power means better healthcare for you and your little person, remember? So, find your seat, make yourself comfortable, and hold on.

Before we take off, a word about the landscape of healthcare: unfortunately, the quality and access to resources in the U.S. vary greatly by location.[1] Although there's ongoing work being done to ensure *all* people—regardless of race, ethnicity, income, age, sex, or sexual orientation—receive equitable care everywhere, sadly, we haven't arrived at this vital destination.[1] This is even more reason to know your rights. As you navigate the healthcare system and go about your life, advocate for yourself and your sisters alike—speak up, ask questions, give feedback, fill out surveys about your healthcare experiences, and in turn, be part of the movement to improve the rights of childbearing women nationwide.

> ꙰ ❀ ❁ ❀ ꙰
>
> Finding respectful care congruent with your cultural or religious background is both a right and an important part of your experience.[2]

Privacy

Now, for every healthcare experience, you are entitled to receive care in privacy and to have your health information protected, both part of a law called ***Health Insurance Portability and Accountability Act of 1996 (HIPAA)***. It's your call who you'd like your information shared with, and you can always request to have a copy of your medical record, even if your bill isn't paid yet.

Preferences

Don't be hesitant to share specific cultural or religious preferences with your maternity care provider. For instance, some women may need a prescription for gelatin-free prenatal vitamins, others might prefer female providers, or need to bring a special meal to the hospital after birth. It may also include inviting friends or family to your visits or labor. Feel free to have them attend but check with your facility regarding how many people are allowed. You may need to prioritize, alternate, or have them draw straws.

Being informed

Also, it is your right to understand your care—so if your maternity care provider starts speaking in a way you don't understand, seek clarification.[2] It's vital for you two to be on the same page. Sometimes, this may even mean requesting an interpreter. If needed, please speak up. You not only need to understand what your maternity care provider is saying but also be able to express yourself. This is to be a dialogue, not a monologue. Healthcare facilities should have ways to access phone interpreters, which will typically provide more accurate translations than when family members or friends interpret.

Evidence-based care

When you're receiving care, it's your right to have care that is based on current scientific evidence.[2] I know, this sounds like a no-brainer, right? Still, any time you're offered a procedure, medication, test, or treatment, let that beautiful voice of yours ring out and ask for the rundown: What are the pros, cons, and risks? Trust me, this will help you decide to accept or decline what's offered, seek a second opinion, or perhaps even change your mind—which, by the way, is possible, even if you've signed a consent form.[2]

Labor considerations

And now, for that glorious day—birth. Did you know you can choose what type of birth setting you'd like to use? This may partly depend on your insurance, so be sure to find out in advance what options are covered.

Prior to labor, you're entitled to get information on comfort measures available to you. And guess what? The day of, you're free to go with the flow and change your mind as you labor! Labor loves to extend little surprises along the way, but generally, unless there are specific medical reasons not to, you can move around during labor

> **IS IT TOO LATE?**
>
> It's okay to change your mind about a medical procedure, even if you've signed a consent form.

in a way that feels right, and you can birth in a position of your choice. And when your baby and you are no longer one, but two, you have the right to uninterrupted time together, assuming neither of you requires immediate medical attention.[2]

For now, and for your future medical interactions, remember—your patient rights are designed to help you experience meaningful, ethical, up-to-date healthcare tailored for you. Hopefully, as you remember these elements, the world of healthcare will feel more familiar and less like a trip to a distant planet.

Digging Deeper

Did this whirlwind tour of your rights in healthcare inspire you to be involved in your care? I hope so! Next, skim the questions below and see if any of them apply to your current situation. If you answer yes to any of the following, it's a splendid idea to speak up at your next appointment.

» Is there something in your prenatal care that doesn't make sense?

» If you're receiving any treatments, procedures, or medications, are you unsure of the pros/cons/alternatives?

» Are there any important cultural, ethnic, or religious preferences for your prenatal care that you haven't yet shared with your maternity care provider?

» Do you need more information to decide on where you'd like to have your baby?

WEEK 20

Baby

- Is about 10 inches long.
- Weighs about 11 ¾ ounces.
- Has very fine hair, known as lanugo, all over the body.
- Is covered in a thick wax-like substance, called *vernix caseosa*, which hydrates and protects the delicate skin.

Mama

- The placenta is fully formed.
- You may have a harder time bending forward, since the top of your uterus is level with your belly button.
- The blood vessels attached to the placenta enlarge, and blood flow to the area continues to increase.

Oh, Hello!

"Wow, Meshi, your breasts are huge!"

My close friend's unusual greeting stunned me as she walked through our front door for our girls' night in. Well, that's a first.

How am I supposed to respond to a comment like that? Should I say, *Thank you?* or *You're telling me!* or *Pregnancy's transforming, what can I say?* The best I could do on a whim was announce I finally got around to buying a bra that fit these big girls.

As she settled in with a glass of water and I began to set the table for our dinner, I felt compelled to share the story of the bra-shopping escapade. Before I could stop them, the words spilled out, and I launched into a rambling recount of the events that led to my purchase.

"Up to this point," I shared, "I had been layering my clothes, wearing a tight tank top over my bra for extra security—a fabric fortress, if you will. But that only worked for a little while. Finally, I grew so tired of stuffing my breasts into thimbles (worrying every time I bent over that I'd become a human jack-in-the-box) that I had to make my purchases.

"I didn't anticipate bra buying would be such a conundrum," I told her, gathering momentum with each detail. "But I guess I should have known better, since nearly everything else in pregnancy has proven to be more difficult than it should. So, there I stood—frozen like an ice sculpture between the rows of hanging bras.

"Should I just buy a bigger regular bra that fits now, or transition to a nursing bra before I'm breastfeeding? Sure, pregnant women can do either, but there's one problem. Nursing bras can look so *blah*—so bland and neutral. Great if I'm looking for camouflage in the desert, but not so hot if I want to feel pretty any time soon."

My pause was met with an encouraging smile from my bosom buddy (*yes, pun intended*).

"All women," I plunged on, "those with blooming bellies included, should be able to feel beautiful and celebrated, don't you agree?"

She nodded.

"Exactly! So, I figure, purchasing a regular bra seems like a good idea. But then, is it wise to spend money on something that will soon become nothing more than a closet decoration? Still, if breastfeeding goes well, I'll end up practically living in my nursing bras for months or even years, so maybe I should pace myself and enjoy the days free of them for as long as I can."

Elbows resting on the table, her hands cupping her face, my friend sat with a glimmer of amusement in her eyes. I grabbed our plates, and— figuring I was much too far into the story to stop now—continued.

"So finally, I stopped waffling and put myself out of my misery. I gathered one of each type of bra—a sexy, yet affordable black nursing bra (a true find) and a regular, polka-dotted purple one. Armed with options, I advanced on the fitting rooms.

"The regular bra came first. Almost immediately, I heard my breasts exhaling a sigh of relief. They felt secure, comfortable, and welcome. They had finally made it 'home'—this one was a must-have.

"Next, I tried the nursing bra. As soon as I fixed it in place, I was lured into figuring out how this new contraption worked. I unclasped the hook above the cup, folded the fabric down, and—boo! There were me and my breasts, staring at each other under the fluorescent lights.

"They hung there sheepishly and so exposed," I admitted, waving a hand. "I can't blame them. This is all so new to me." The comment received a sympathetic chuckle, and I continued to the nearly breathless conclusion. "So, what could I do, but toss both bras into my shopping basket and head to the checkout line?"

Outside, our other friend pulled up in front of the house, and I moved toward the door, ready to welcome her in.

BUYING A BRA

In pregnancy, use regular or nursing bras.

- You may need to size up in pregnancy, since both your rib cage and your breasts are expanding.
- If breastfeeding, use nursing bras and tanks. Think easy access and accommodating cup size. Also, find a soft and ultra-comfy nursing bra for nighttime support. You'll love it!

"Thankfully, with both of them I can alternate," I said, wrapping up my surprise rant. "That should help avoid pain from one bra pushing into the same places all day long."

"True," my confidante agreed, as I turned to welcome the next guest.

Had our friend not arrived then, who knows, I may have shared the other questions that the nursing bra had prompted before I'd left the dressing room that day. I'd wondered, as I peered into the mirror: What ensemble of experiences will come from using the foreign collection of straps and clasps? Will I get all tangled in them? Am I going to be like those women whose breasts appear unabashed at the sound of their baby's every hungry peep? Or will I use a nursing cover, and if so, for which of the many reasons? For my own privacy? To keep my curious baby undistracted? Or because I felt the need to hide everything—as if breastfeeding were something unnatural?

The second and last guest made it past the white picket fence and up the path, and so I left these wonders unsaid. There will be time to discover the answers later, but for now . . . I opened the door with a greeting, forgot about my breasts and their intrigue, and settled into the evening.

You Can't Buy Back Time

Wow, I am now halfway through pregnancy. Finally! This remarkable landmark signals that the end is no longer an eternity away, which means—yikes! What am I going to do about my job, my career?

I've always thought when it came time, I'd focus fully on mother-hood, but I'm not so sure anymore. After all, I've worked toward my degree and certification for so many years—and I love what I do. Am I ready to give it all up for good, or at least, take a long and indefinite pause? Is it selfish to still think about establishing a strategic trajectory for my professional life? Can work and family life even exist in harmony, or is the concept merely a figment of my hopeful imagination?

As I wrestle between the pull of motherhood and career, my mind is drawn once again to those women who have been most influential in my life. At the top of the list (aside from my own mother) are my grand-mother and her mother. Both embodied dedication, resourcefulness, patience, and long-suffering. Yet what stands out the most is their love.

War had already separated them from kin and country, and they were not going to let the measly 600 miles between us do it again. My childhood home in Oregon was far from theirs in California, but—that's right—not too far for the determined. They made up for it with long phone calls, surprise packages, and slumber parties when we visited for a month each summer.

To get down to Mountain View where they lived, sometimes we overnighted it in an Amtrak coach—watching trees, rivers, and dirt blur by as we crunched on travel-size boxes of Corn Pops and Fruit Loops. Other times, we made the excruciating drive in our non-air-conditioned 1976 Ford station wagon, the three of us children smashed together in the back seat with our parakeet, *Csiri's*, cage. We watched my mom slice apples and green peppers while our bird's yellow feathers fluttered, and her birdseed spilled into our sweaty laps with the road's every turn.

While the drive could be rough, it was always worth it. At the other end, we enjoyed nonstop, silent Marco Polo games in my great-grand-mother's swimming pool; oodles of her warm, Transylvanian corn-bread pudding with jam, called *puliszka*; classic American musicals and long-forgotten Marilyn Monroe; and rollaway beds in my grandmother's living room. During these months, these matriarchs created a rich world of transplanted Hungarian tradition steeped with old American heri-tage—and we loved it. Sure, this hybrid world was peculiar, as outdated as it was out of sync with most everyone around us, but it's all we knew.

And it was lovely.

Thinking back on these memories now brings up more than just heartwarming days of my odd childhood. It inspires me to think about what I'm to do with what these role models have laid behind—and, in a way, *before*—me. Did they mean to carve out a motherhood roadmap for my life, or did they simply try to bless me with the full measure of their resourceful, creative, and boundless love?

As these memories mingled with my desire to cultivate my career, I happened on a nugget of wisdom. At the clinic, a patient came in for her appointment and on her intake questionnaire, she had jotted down her professional occupation as "mother and wife." With great excitement, she explained she had just quit her former job because of a change in her priorities.

"I missed out on the first two years of my oldest child's life," she lamented. "I didn't want to make that same mistake again."

Man, what timing.

"You can *never* buy that back," she added.

I nodded, tucking that bit of wisdom in my heart and letting it simmer with my childhood memories. It struck me that there are as many types of mothers as there are cuisines, and with all their differences, the single most important feature is their love.

So, what sort of mother do *I* want to be? I hope my love for our baby will be so entirely captivating that it will guide my career decisions and illuminate my path going forward.

Perhaps I would be content doing a little work on the side, while I figure out what mothering is all about. Though I might not get a chance to make *puliszka* every day with a part-time job, I should be around enough to help create our own little eclectic Hungarian American–hybrid world, Parker style.

⋙ LET'S TALK ABOUT IT ⋘

Supporting the Working Mother

Many pregnant mamas in the workforce begin to wonder at this time what their work future will look like. As your curiosity rises and the mental wheels start turning, remember that as a mommy, your ultimate job will be to love your child(ren)—in your own special way.

Motherhood goals, realities, and options

Your mothering style—whether like or unlike other moms'—will be unique, both shaped by who you are and who you are becoming. In this, there is beauty and magic. For your baby's entire life, you'll be his biggest fan, assessing what he needs to survive, develop, thrive, and navigate society, whether you're earning kisses, messy diapers, and minute-memories or you're among the larger percentage of American women earning money.[1]

Regardless of where they're slaving away, mamas are busy multitaskers living complicated lives. Only some women have the luxury to choose whether to be home 24/7 with their baby. Get this: 72% of mamas with children younger than 18 years old are in the workforce, and of these, 55% work full time.[2-4] It's no wonder mothering looks different for every family.

> For a refresher on tips for physical activity while pregnant, check out "Move That Beautiful Self" (week 13) and "Move That Pregnant Bod" (B-2b).

So, how will this little bundle impact your career or work goals? If you're still figuring all this out, that's okay! You've got time. In the coming months, consider your finances and standard of living, reflect on your motherhood dreams and life goals, and talk with your loved ones and employer. This is also a great time to start asking coworkers, friends, and families about child-care recommendations and options. These may include a family member, partner, in-home day care, nanny, or even a friend with young children.

Work considerations

In the meantime, let's help you protect yourself and your job while working during pregnancy, since in work, as in life, it's important to prioritize your well-being. If you're safe and feeling well, your baby is more likely to be also.

In the working world, this means it's vital to get adequate rest and breaks to pee, eat regular snacks and meals, avoid chemicals like cleaning detergents and secondhand smoke, have time off for prenatal appointments, be able to sit down when you need to, and protect yourself from frequent bending, heavy lifting, or standing all day. By the way, this list also applies to all you stay-at-home mommies. Tap into extra babysitting help to make this type of self-care possible. If you don't have family around and can't afford to hire a babysitter, consider starting a babysitting swap with friends or join a parenting group.

If you are part of the workforce, it's good to remember every employer is different. Some are ready to spoil you to make sure you're well taken care of during pregnancy, while for others, it's near the end of their priority list. If you find yourself in the second (stressful) situation, please know you have options. For one, consider asking your maternity care provider to write you a *work accommodations* letter, which lists temporary and reasonable work modifications designed to keep you working and providing for your family.[5,6] There is also the option of going on *leave,* but this is often time-limited and may have other implications for your job security and how long you can stay home postpartum. Be sure to think through your leave options before jumping into them.

Yes, working moms have a lot to consider, but as you go about exploring your current work environment and what mothering may look like in your future, remember—there are so many creative solutions to every problem. Look around you and ask for help. Your brilliant mommy mind is designed for this.

Digging Deeper

We often hear terminology like *work accommodations* and *leave,* but don't quite know what to keep in mind when considering them. For more information on these two, including answers to the questions below, check out A-3g.

» How can I find out if I'm entitled to work accommodations?

» Do I ask my maternity care provider to write a work accommodations letter, or do I wait until they offer?

» Should I go out on leave?

» What is FMLA? Is paid leave available for all pregnant women?

» My boss fired me because I am pregnant. Is that legal? Where can I turn to for help?

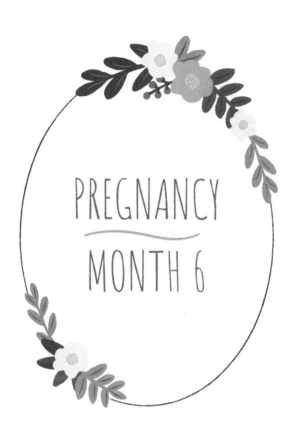

PREGNANCY

MONTH 6

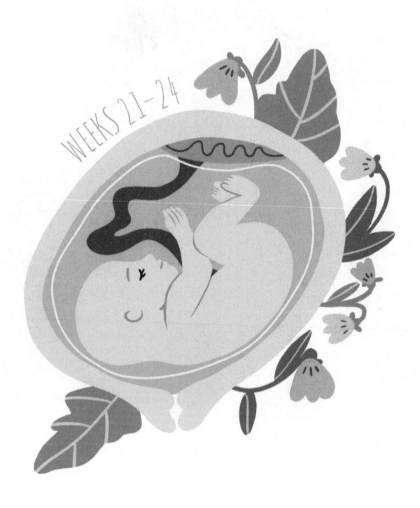

WEEK 21

Baby

- Is about 10 ¾ inches long.
- Weighs about 14 ounces.
- Now has opaquer skin.
- Builds a thin layer of fat under the skin.

Mama

- The uterus continues to expand up toward your diaphragm by about one centimeter per week until delivery.
- Higher estrogen levels and increased blood flow cause vaginal discharge. If it's white, odorless, and non-itchy, it's normal— even if it warrants wearing a panty liner.

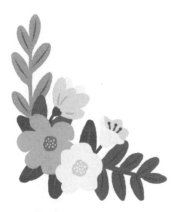

Baby, Are You Still There?

As far as I can tell over the past two weeks, my little girl has been quite enjoying her accommodations. Although it's still too early for us to see the wave of movement wash across my belly, or for Dan's hand to feel anything other than my bowels, her flutters and shifting motions have punctuated my days. I wouldn't be surprised if she were trying to hurl herself through the eye of my belly button. For this reason, I've taken to giving her a gentle talking-to whenever her motions pick up significantly.

"Baby," I say, "the world I live in is vast and spectacular, but it's also saturated with imperfection. Take your time. Get strong and sassy. There's no need to catch a glimpse of the bigger world encircling your own before your time."

And it appears she has taken the words to heart—quite impressively for a twenty-one-week-old. She still hasn't cannonballed out of me, which I'm grateful for. However, I fear she may have misunderstood me. I didn't tell her to stop playing or to stop having fun, did I? *Some* movement is not so bad. Just don't be trying the Great Escape.

I've just been so exhausted over the past couple of days at work, so now I'm not sure. Has she been moving, and I missed it? I was completely distracted and forgot all about her. Better to have this kind of memory lapse now, instead of after she's arrived, but still. Is she okay? I haven't had any cramping, pain, or bleeding, or anything abnormal, but you know—a pregnant mother's imagination can be as much a strength as a weakness.

Little one, please give me a little nudge and kick so I know you're alive and well.

Nothing.

It's quite common to not feel my baby move all the time around this gestational age, I try reassuring myself. In fact, some women are just barely starting to feel their babies move. Plus, feeling a baby's movements takes getting used to, and when they're this size, they're still small enough to slip under the radar.

My pep talk worked somewhat—for about two minutes.

Shoot, my fears interjected a moment later. *I wish I would have purchased a home Doppler so I could listen to her heartbeat.*

On the other hand, I've probably just been too busy to notice, and she's perfectly fine. It's not like my thoughts are what sustain her little body.

Logic wasn't winning.

What if there really were something wrong with her? What are the chances that something would suddenly go wrong in a healthy pregnancy? *So very rare*, says Meshi the NP. But Meshi the mother has some other ideas. I did wake up lying on my back the other day. Could it be that my large vena cava vein didn't return enough blood to support my baby?

I finally decided to follow the advice I tell all my pregnant mamas: drink some juice or eat something to raise the blood sugar a bit and sit or lie down on your side to do a little investigative work. No, don't worry about starting kick counts yet (those usually start around 27–28 weeks) but just pay attention and see what's up. So, I took a swig of orange juice and plopped down on the familiar old green couch, the one I practically lived on the first trimester.

Move around, baby, reassure me. *Please.*

I waited. And waited some more.

Aha! There it is—a flutter! And another one. Phew! Thank you, God! That had me worried. I guess I much prefer my baby practically hurling herself through my belly than her being a nice, obedient, well-behaved girl. After all, nice and well-behaved girls are not what our world needs.

A Mother's Pictures for Her Daughter

Today was my lucky day. When I came home from work, there was a big manila envelope waiting for me on the kitchen counter. My name was written on it in my mom's familiar handwriting beside a few tiny, red Hungarian folk-art tulips and hearts.

What a nice surprise!

I must admit, whenever I get mail, excitement takes hold. In the frenzy, I become voracious—almost tiger-like—ready to consume and absorb every element of my find. Although it's tempting to sink my teeth into it and give it a good, savage shake, so far, I've contented myself with shoving my pointer finger under any crack in the seal. No, I've never had the patience for peeling an envelope millimeter by millimeter along the seam, nor have I reached sufficient sophistication to own a letter opener.

With unbridled anticipation, I soon had the envelope open. Reaching inside, I pulled out a stiff sheet of paper bearing copies of three color photos of my mom—a younger and pregnant version of the woman for whom pregnancy was the height of joy. I stood there, holding her in my hand, gazing at her belly's profile, studying each of the three instances when she was pregnant with us kids. She looked radiant and so happy. Is that how I'm going to feel and look one day in pregnancy?

I then read her simple comments underneath: *See how big I got? Don't worry about getting larger.*

Wow. Wait a minute, I didn't even realize how uneasy I felt about growing bigger until now. But I guess it had made me a little nervous. My mother's right. So right. This is exactly what's supposed to happen. Babies grow and so bellies bloom. Wasn't I the one who said I'd prefer a life-size baby to a pocket-size Thumbelina? Well, this is part of it.

I placed my mother's reminder of a healthy pregnancy on my nightstand and noticed I had changed. Just from one thoughtful letter, my spirit had lightened. Drinking in each detail of those photos, I had felt a sense of freedom—as if in some way I was being blessed with the calm, peaceful joy infusing each image. With my mother's gentle prompting, I loosened my grip on things out of my control, more comfortable with what body transformations might lie before me on this adventure.

⫸ LET'S TALK ABOUT IT ⫷

Pregnancy and Baby Keepsakes

What do you say we have a little fun? You're over halfway through pregnancy, so let's get this party started! Before you know it, your little one will be bouncing on your lap, licking your face, and begging to catch a glimpse of life as it was when he or she was yet unveiled. "Mommy, what were things like when I was inside?" she'll ask while climbing on you like you're a tree. And you know what? At some point, you'll wonder that, too, and in the moment of nostalgia, you'll miss the closeness you two share now.

Yes, really.

So, join me as we explore how you can commemorate this special pregnancy to share with your child. Turn on your favorite music, grab a pencil and some paper, get comfy, and let's get those creative juices flowing. Feel free to jot down ideas or circle those you might like to try.

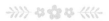

If planning a maternity photoshoot, aim for around 35 weeks, when your belly is in full bloom. If you wait much longer, it may turn into a newborn and family session—surprise!

Pregnancy mementos

For starters, let's think about what you may wish to record for (1) yourself, (2) your partner or loved ones, or (3) your baby. Are there certain activities you've been involved in during pregnancy? Trips you've taken or are planning to take? Crazy food cravings? A list of top baby name contenders? Think of what details you might want to capture, and through which different types of media—perhaps pictures, notes, mementos, collages, music, art, sewing, or even scrapbooking.

Let your personality shape this activity and guide your path toward saving and *savoring* key moments during pregnancy—ones that capture some of its special, funny, and surprising snippets. No, we're not talking about how many days you vomited or how many times you had meltdowns but rather, things you want to remember.

Pick one or a few ideas that sound fun, meaningful, and rejuvenating. It's up to you if you'd like to go for quick and simple ideas (like buying a postcard, jotting down a few thoughts or facts, or smash-booking) or more elaborate and time-intensive ones (like writing a poem or song, belly casting, making a memory book, coloring a coloring book, scrapbooking, blogging, collecting something, or making a pregnancy playlist).

Consider taking weekly or monthly belly profile shots. It's quick and simple, and you can pore over these shots for years to come. Toddlers and children love seeing and hearing where they came from (though not in the "birds and the bees" sense), and I have yet to meet a mama who regrets taking these. You can even go all out and have maternity pictures taken by a friend or a professional. Maybe even get your sexy on with pregnancy boudoir photos.

Baby keepsakes

Remember, the fun doesn't have to stop here. Try planning for baby keepsakes during pregnancy to make life simpler when your little one arrives. These can be special items you'd like to give your baby or objects used to capture the early months of your baby's life.

Not sure where to start? Check out the following options or surf the web for DIY items or ones available for sale. If you're feeling industrious and would like to make your keepsakes yourself, you go girl! If not, allow yourself to be guilt free. This is meant to be a fun commemoration, not a chore, and one thoughtfully purchased item can be such a treasure. Consider it a job well done even if you land on a single small but manageable keepsake. Remember, as the American naturalist John Burroughs said, "The smallest deed is better than the greatest intention."

Now, before we leave you with an awesome starter list of options, here's a quick word on one traditional memento: a baby blanket. Unfortunately, while these are often soft and snuggly, great care should be taken around blankets since they pose a suffocation risk for your baby. If you have a special blanket or are planning to make one, consider hanging it on the wall for decoration rather than wrapping your snuggle bunny in it, or *only* use it while you are directly with your little one, watching closely to ensure your child stays safe. It can also make a great floor cover for when your baby's doing supervised play- or tummy-time.

So, whatever you end up choosing to do for a keepsake, remember this process is meant to be fun and refreshing, like mint lemonade. These activities are not only great for when you've got the itch to do something special for you or your baby but also perfect if you need a creative outlet, an emotional pick-me-up, or if you feel like your pregnancy is dragging on. This is your time!

Digging Deeper

As you think about how to treasure and capture specialness around you during this season, relish the freedom of this activity. Tap into *you*, your personality, style, and what you love, considering what fits your life. When you do this, in a sense you're also passing along parts of you. Your goal is not to select the most costly, involved, or social-media-worthy activity but rather to preserve some valuable part of your story to share with your little love. There are many more ideas out in the virtual world, but here are a few to get you started:

» Create or purchase a memento with your baby's name (such as artwork or a wooden toy).

» Write a letter to your baby with your hopes for his or her life.

» Ask your family and friends to write letters or notes of hope, blessings, or wisdom to your child and compile them for your child to read once grown.

» Frame a favorite quote, scripture, or holy text. (Tip: use acrylic instead of glass, so if it falls off the wall, it doesn't shatter.)

» Create baby handprint/footprint keepsakes made from a purchased kit or homemade salt dough.

» Compile a baby keepsake or pregnancy shadow box to display pictures and mementos.

» Track your baby's development with a milestone marker (such as monthly photoshoot props or clothing stickers).

WEEK 22

Baby

- Is about 11 ½ inches long.
- Weighs about 15 ounces.
- Can hear.
- Continues to develop unique fingerprints and toe prints.

Mama

- It is common to wake up more during the night, which impacts your well-being, concentration, memory, and mood.[1]
  - If snoring, apnea, or restless leg syndrome affect you, ask your maternity care provider for help.
- Skin changes are occurring, such as a pregnancy "glow" from increased blood flow and hormones. Other common changes include skin darkening on your cheeks, old scars becoming more visible, or the development of an exotic, temporary, dark line on your belly (*linea nigra*).
  - Limit your sun exposure.

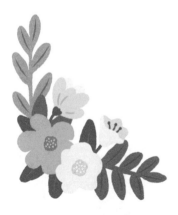

What's in a Dream?

Like many other pregnant mamas, I, too, have become a dream weaver. It's incredible—even without lifting a finger, we women can concoct the strangest, most vibrant, and elaborate nighttime experiences. It's as if each of our little brewing dumplings ignites a spark of inspiration within, often with newness every evening. And, given how rarely we sleep through a night nowadays (peeing, peeing, and then peeing again, for starters), it's much easier to remember our dreamland's terrain.

Dreams are curious things, full of surprises. While some seem poignant and prophetic, others can have an entirely different vibe—ranging from bizarre nonsense to disturbing nightmares. Yes, a dream catcher could come in quite handy! When faced with the theater of dreams, a mama's mind can easily take the raw collections of images and occurrences and stitch together all sorts of wild stories related to her life—finding in them evidence of her thoughts, fears, and feelings, as well as her hopes for her changing body, her baby, the birth, or even mothering. So, really, I'm not sure why I was so surprised the other night when, in my dream, I accidentally left my baby on the closet shelf.

In keeping with the theme, I had another memorable—and quite strange—dream the following night. To begin, I was panning for gold in a stream, which, given the surroundings, I supposed was a typical day for me in this dreamscape. *Why ever not?* While the refreshing ripples tickled my toes, I spotted a lazy town close by, like those in Old West movies—complete with a hot and dusty main street, lined with clapboard façades and widely swinging tavern doors. There was even a sheriff wandering the streets, with his gold star badge glinting in the sunlight below his perfectly curled moustache.

Yep, definitely the Wild West.

It seems, though, while I was casually minding my own business, a large and speedy horse appeared as if from nowhere and had the nerve to select me as a target for a good chase. Desperate, I threw my pan down and ran to my own horse, certain I'd be much safer if I could just escape to another town nearby. Trouble was, after much sidestepping and shuffling, I found I had no idea how to even hop onto my own damn horse. *Great.* Worse still, I had this unsettling realization that I was also responsible for getting two toddler girls (whom I can't recall ever meeting before) to safer territory—and they were nowhere to be found. And how will I even recognize them when I see them?

Where are you? I called, frantic. *Where are yooouuuuu?* I yelled louder, hollering through my cupped hands. No reply. I could hear nothing except the sound of charging hoofbeats. Surely, I should have been trampled by now.

Yet the landscape shifted from the water bubbling over the rocks to slanted shadows cast along the dirt road, and then to—a darkened stairwell? It rose before me, receding upward to a landing where, much to my surprise, I saw the girls I'd been searching for—waiting for my arrival. Each wore a bright yellow, puffy snowsuit.

Of course.

Falling toward me like autumn leaves, they leapt down to meet me on my horse, which I had apparently figured out how to mount. I caught one of the girls, settling her in front of me before I made a quick swoop to collect the other as she attempted to drop past me.

But before we could get away and seek a haven in the great unknown, there was one last thing to do. We stopped by the nearest mercantile to grab some necessary provisions. You know—beef jerky, porridge, and a corset. *The usual.*

Finishing up the purchase, I was told that if I just waited a moment, someone would kindly escort us to safer territory. This is unexpected but seems to be good news, so I guess we'll wait. We left the shop and stood outside. We waited and waited. Nothing. In the stillness, the second hand on the town hall's clock ticked loudly. *Too loudly.* In the once-empty streets, there appeared a silent group of onlookers.

Is this a trap?

Heartbeat pounding in my ears, breath held in worry, I surveyed the scene, looking for the source of my dread. My gaze scanned the faces in the crowd. Before I could even exhale, I spotted my answer: that same beast of a wild horse appeared and started pushing its way through those gathered—its muscles rippling with the movement.

Pulse racing, I leapt onto my horse, grabbed the girls by their hands, and swung them up and around me. Off we galloped, and the wild horse slowly faded into the distance.

Phew. We made it, but just barely.

I woke not long after.

What on earth does all this mean? I lay there, puzzling over the events that had trotted through my dream.

Am I trying to learn how to save someone entrusted to me, but feel unprepared?

Yes.

Do I feel like I'm embarking on an unknown adventure but don't even have directions?

Definitely.

Are yellow snowsuits a must in every lost child's wardrobe?

Maybe.

Should I be wary of wild horses?

Always.

Pregomania

"It's so hard to know what a baby really needs," I sighed, as Dan and I folded laundry.

He continued, silent.

"How am I supposed to figure this out?" I added. "People keep asking if I'm going to have a baby registry, and I have no clue. It's easier said than done and depends on if I can ever figure out what to put on the stupid thing."

"It's really not a big deal," he said softly. "A baby doesn't need much."

Dan continued sorting and folding clothes, apparently unfazed and content to listen to the lively beats of Bacilos from our stereo.

So annoying! He's not taking this seriously. At all.

Throwing a wrinkled tee shirt onto the bed, I stormed out.

Sitting down at the computer, I started surfing the web in haste, hoping that by some miracle, I'd get some clarity. The internet is *always* such a dependable resource for information, so what could possibly go wrong?

Oh yeah, *everything*.

My heart sank. The baby industry is so expansive and robust. It's utterly overwhelming. Between business strategy, marketing, and consumer reviews, I am thoroughly confused. Rather than answer the few questions I had, the search brought even more knocking—hounding me for attention about cribs, diapering, bottles, and pumps. Do I need a bouncer, a swing, *and* a playpen? Drop-side or stationary crib? Solid or pressed wood? Regular, biodegradable, or cloth diapers? Glass or plastic bottles? Manual or electric pump?

Will the questions dissolve if I just ignore them?

I could feel myself turning into the hardcore American consumer, thinking she needs to buy every item with a baby picture. Everything's a *must*. I'm thrown to and fro by the product promises, reviews, and recalls. Could someone please give me a life jacket?

I slammed the laptop closed with a huff. I'd gotten nowhere. How is it that Dan is not the slightest upset by our empty (and not to mention completely nonexistent) registry?

In my misery, I called my friend Ann, a seasoned mother, begging her to rescue grumpy little old me from this nasty mess. *SOS!* Patiently, she listened to me rattle off my frantic questions and then proceeded to give me a response only an experienced mother could give.

"You don't need much. You'll need diapers, wipes, and clothes in the beginning. However, the most important thing will be for Dan, you, and the baby to have time together."

What? That's it? Just a handful of items and special time as a family?

With just a few simple statements, she saved me from myself and in turn rescued us Parkers. She threw me the life jacket I so desperately needed and inspired me to play this consumer game with an entirely new strategy. I can outsmart this clever and unrelenting opponent by seeing: What is the *least* amount I can buy while still having everything I need? Yes, that seems much more enjoyable.

Hmm. I wonder if maybe Dan has been onto something all along. After all, if it were up to him, the baby would sleep in a drawer, get washed in a mixing bowl, and play with cardboard boxes.

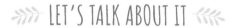

LET'S TALK ABOUT IT

Creating Your Nest

Simplicity is the ultimate sophistication.
—Leonardo da Vinci

Getting your nest ready for your little darling is a fun and exciting process but also a little overwhelming. If you're wondering where to start and what general concepts to consider as you begin, you've come to the right place! Of course, some of you may not be ready for this and would rather wait. No worries, this section will be here for you when your time comes.

Keeping it simple

First, taking a minimalist approach to buying is a wise way to go. Although at this point you may be tempted to have your entire living space be transformed into all things baby, eventually, you'll get sick of it. At some point, you—yes, you, my dear pregnant one—will be pacing up and down your house like a voracious lioness, ready to toss every baby item into a trash or donation bag. Save yourself the trouble now by avoiding purchases that don't have a clear functional or sentimental purpose. In fact, this may be a good time to start going through your living space and storage to donate unnecessary items before you bring new ones in your home.

Your evolving nest

Since babies grow quickly and their developmental needs change constantly, your baby won't always need teething toys and rattles and will soon become more interested in textured balls, stacking toys, board books, and eating specs of dirt off your floor. Consider your nest a nurturing environment that will keep evolving as you go. Pace yourself and remember, the less stuff you have, the less mess there will be to stress you out later.

To help cut out the extras, think of using items that grow with your baby. For example, some car seats have a broader weight range, some cribs convert to toddler beds, and some high chairs can be used with older kids. Look around your home carefully to see what you can work with. For example, if you have a recliner that rocks, you don't necessarily need a separate rocking chair. You just need a comfy place to sit with your bambino when you need to hold, feed, or comfort her—and soothe yourself, too.

>>> ❁ ✿ ❁ <<<

For safety reasons, car seats, cribs, mattresses, and breast pumps are best purchased in new condition.

Another example is a diaper bag. Sure, if you've always dreamed of having one with a cute, baby-themed print—go for it. Find one you like! Just remember, a backpack or tote can also work just fine. The more hands-free, the better. In fact, at some point you'll probably find yourself tempted to chuck the diaper bag anyway, especially when you're longing for your pre-baby days. When that day comes, a standard bag or your current purse will help you feel more womanly and less motherly.

The bottom line? You may already be more prepared for your baby than you think. Isn't that an amazing thought?

Staying safe

Finally, before purchasing, using, or adding that must-have item to your registry, do your research. Not everything is safe for your baby just because it's out on the market. While shocking, it's true. Always do a little investigative work, even if you received it as a gift. Eventually, you'll find brands you trust and get in your groove, but early on, it will require some work.

When researching, check for any recalls or bans on the item (for example, drop-side cribs are now a no-no). Safety standards for items in which babies can sleep, lie, stand, or sit can get updated every few years, and they do often get recalled. So, check online or call the manufacturer to find out, especially if you're buying used or pulling something out of storage.

In addition to checking recalls or bans, determine if the item has any potential environmental toxins. This is a biggy that many of us forget about. While not everyone can go toxin-free, do so whenever you are able. Since young children have a more vulnerable immune system—more susceptible to germs and illness, and less efficient at clearing out potential hazards compared to older kids and adults—it's important to minimize your child's exposure to these chemicals. Also, health problems from such toxins can be serious and may take years to develop.

Unfortunately, these toxins are present in many items around us—like in plastics (bottles, toys, dolls, dishware), mattresses, flame retardants, canned foods, nonstick cookware, certain diapers, engineered wood products, lead-based paint, and even in soaps and sunscreens. Unbelievable, right? For this reason, it's not always wise to buy something just because it's on sale or cheap.

As you start preparing for your little one's arrival, researching and cultivating the list of must-haves, remember — less is more. Spend your money on a few nice, good-quality items that are safe and will last. All we need to do is look around the world at many cultures and peoples to see you don't need many *things* to raise your child in riches.

CAR SEATS

If you need help installing your car seat, find an inspection station near you. Hospitals, firehouses, or police departments usually offer these for free. Look up local options by visiting the National Highway Traffic Safety Administration's website (www.nhtsa.dot.gov) or find a national Child Passenger Safety (CPS) Technician through Safe Kids (www.safekids.org), which lists professionals worldwide.

Digging Deeper

If you're ready to dive into the baby registry list and start compiling ideas on the most essential items, check out the appendix for details and categories designed to help springboard you into preparing your nest. Also, remember to pace yourself and take breaks to stretch that beautiful body of yours and mentally refresh. This list can't be done well in a day. In fact, you might enjoy looking around to see what coworkers, friends, and family members are using for possible ideas. In A-3i, you'll find answers to questions like:

» Can you ever have too many burp cloths?

» How many diapers will I need each week?

» What medical supplies should I have on hand for my baby?

» Which chemicals on an ingredient list should I avoid?

» What types of materials are good for my munchkin and the environment?

WEEK 23

Baby

- Is about a foot long.
- Weighs about a pound!
- Now has fully developed eyelids.
- Has more visible nails.

Mama

- More clotting factors mean a greater chance for developing blood clots during pregnancy.
  - Yep, this is one more reason to stay active. If you have a desk job or are traveling, get up and move regularly.
- You may start experiencing normal, painless hardening and tightening of your belly (Braxton Hicks contractions).
  - It is normal to feel these toning contractions occasionally throughout pregnancy—or not. Stress and dehydration often increase these, so rest up and stay hydrated.

Sugar and Spice

> *I'm not afraid of storms, for I'm learning how to sail my ship.*
> —LOUISA MAY ALCOTT

When a woman starts attending a well-designed prenatal class, parts of her are bound to change. I suppose that's the point, isn't it? To not just prepare for that grand day by learning about the stages of labor and the available comfort measures, but also to better understand how a woman's body is intricately designed for this transformational event. It's a place for asking the pressing questions, receiving special homework activities, and learning about possible labor decisions—so that, in the end, you can leave the class as a more confident woman or couple. For each woman, it's meant to prompt the realization—my body is made for this.

Having only had two prenatal classes, I'm still in the process of realizing a beautiful labor experience is not some fairy tale but rather a definite possibility. These sorts of thoughts come to mind at the most random times, like in spin class, for instance. There I was, staring at myself in the mirror like the other fifteen women cycling. We focused straight ahead without a smile, sizing up all sorts of things like whether we were satisfied with our own athletic performance, our instructor, and our bodies from this angle or that.

This time, though, the persistent questions in my mind were: Who is this person staring back at me? What am I made of? Am I more than sugar and spice and everything nice? How tough am I, really? Can I handle what is typically considered the most profound and intense experience a woman may go through?

In my last two husband-coached Bradley Method childbirth classes, we reviewed the stages of labor by watching the seemingly impossible—natural labor—unfold before our virgin eyes. As these women endured excruciating pain, they more easily resembled well-oiled machines than fragile members of humanity. Remarkably, they had found the balance between the instinct to fight and surrender. What focus and determination! Of course, not everyone takes that route, but—wow, it was inspiring.

The more I think about labor, the more I find myself teeter-tottering back and forth between (1) wanting to go through the challenge of labor to meet my baby, and (2) trying to postpone it for as long as possible. This is the only time she will be small enough to fit inside of me, where I'll feel her from the inside out! Plus, labor is undeniably a significant process, changing a woman and everything else in her life. *Yup, I can wait, thank you very much.* I mean, what if something goes wrong?

The image of my bobbing figure in the mirror faded as fear mounted in my mind. Then, by some miracle, those doubts were replaced with a certainty—God is in control. And He has a plan for both our lives. No matter how helpful worrying seems, it accomplishes nothing other than to rob me of any potential bliss today. It's as if I'm saying, "Here thief, take everything I have."

Why should I let that happen?

And so, climbing off my bike at the end of class, I basked in the knowledge that I had already started changing a bit. *Just a tad.* Sure, the person staring back at me in the then-foggy mirror was still scared but also open. Someone taking a measure of comfort in her own balance between the *fight* (trying her hardest during labor) and the *surrender*— knowing that come what may, God will be near.

My Mother Tongue

As I continue counting down my pregnancy days and watching my belly inflate, there's one question that's been weighing on my mind: Am I going to use Hungarian or English (or both) to connect with my little baby once she's born? Sure, from inside, she's already hearing both languages, but which will I use to sing her a sweet lullaby, talk to her, or encourage her during tummy time?

Ever since I can remember, I've planned on passing on to my children my family's language and culture. It must have been hearing all those random adults telling me how lucky I was to have parents committed to teaching me their mother tongue, and how sad they were that their parents didn't make that same choice. It was a missed opportunity, they'd said. Those words sunk down deep within me and nurtured my resolve like a hot ember. I didn't want to make a choice that would gnaw at my heart later or disappoint my children.

Of course, over the years, I have learned more about the nuances involved in parents' decisions about whether to pass on their native culture and heritage—a decision usually rooted in love, regardless of which option they choose.

Sometimes, when emigrant families move abroad, they cling to their lost world like a precious treasure to be transported and preserved wherever they go. If possible, they may pack a special vase or tablecloth, a bag of spices, some photos, or even a musical instrument—anything to remember and recreate the sounds, smells, tastes, and images of their homeland.

Other families try to absorb as much as they can of their new world in an effort to fit in, make a living, and start a new life—hopefully, a better one. These families focus on learning and teaching their children the ways of their new world.

Neither is easy, and either choice can make sense for a family.

So, what will I do?

Every time I look in the mirror and study my face, I see evidence of the family roots that span the ocean between me and my father's and grandparents' home country. My high cheekbones are like so many others' in Hungary, and my nose, well, it's a reflection of the one gracing my father's bearded face. Although it's taken some getting used to, these characteristics are a reminder of my ancestry—from my carburetor-inventing great-grandfather to the special tastes and scents of traditional dishes shared at family meals.

As one who has experienced the blessing of knowing how my life is part of a larger story, I wonder: Could I really change my mind now about raising my child bilingual and bicultural?

Sure, I have experienced some of the inconveniences of growing up between cultures as a Hungarian American—like when people never know how to pronounce my name, or how I mixed up the meaning of *tuxedo* and *straitjacket* in a college game of Taboo, or the time I envisioned the cartoon moose, Bullwinkle, when Dan referred to the famous boxing movie, *Rocky*. Embarrassing moments like these are ever a reminder that I grew up in two overlapping spheres of culture.

But, even so, if I don't try to pass on my Hungarian heritage as I know it, it's as if I'd be passing along only a small bit of myself instead of all of me—neglecting to share a core part of the Emese my parents raised.

Still, the thought of teaching the Hungarian language to my baby makes me the most nervous. While I know there are benefits to learning more than one language at a young age, doubts fill my mind about how I am to accomplish this. Sure, I speak the language fluently, but what if I don't know enough? After all, I grew up in the States, and while my family once used to communicate solely in Hungarian, this is not the case anymore. Plenty of English words get peppered in, slowly diluting both the spoken sentence and the distinctness of our culture. So, am I versed in our language enough to express my love fully and freely, or will it make mothering awkward?

And then how will I teach her my language and culture here when there is no real Hungarian community around me? I suppose there is an entire country full of Hungarians a mere fourteen-hour flight away, but my parents live in another state and Dan doesn't speak Hungarian. How can my little baby possibly get as much language exposure as I did?

The unanswered questions seem to pile up before me like a big mountain I must either pass over or push through. While I don't yet know what things will look like for us Parkers, one thing's for sure— my Hungarian heritage is a beautiful gift passed on by my parents and extended family, a gift embedded within me that cannot be forgotten.

⇶ LET'S TALK ABOUT IT ⇚

Sharing and Creating Your Family Story

> *Preserve your memories, keep them well,*
> *what you forget, you can never retell.*
> —LOUISA MAY ALCOTT

A few weeks ago, we touched on pregnancy and baby keepsake ideas and how they could be a fun way to commemorate special moments. Hopefully, you've found a couple feasible ideas that excite you. Today, we're delving into another creative topic—commemorating aspects of your family story (or infusing it with newness). While this can certainly be about your biological or adoptive family's heritage, it can also be broader. Think recording family history or reshaping future traditions, or both.

So, for those of you who may not know your family story (or would rather forget it), this section is still for you! It's your opportunity to consider how you'd like to shape your own family culture—to create and share the thread of meaning that runs through your story line and world.

Savoring your heritage

This is an opportunity to consider what parts of your family and spiritual heritage you may like to capture for your little one. Maybe a family tree? A favorite family recipe? A photo? A language? A prayer? A spiritual practice or religion? As you think about how to share this story, jot down your ideas.

While you contemplate this topic, you may also want to start this conversation with your partner, loved ones, and family members. A little caveat: These subjects may create a lively discussion. Enjoy it, embrace it, learn from it, and let it grow you. And don't be surprised if you and your partner (and even family members) have different ideas on what's important to pass on. Also, know that there may be some topics you'll just have to figure out as your baby gets older, and that's okay.

Although you can't determine everything now, it is possible to capture some special elements of your past. To do so, look through family albums, watch family videos, and even arrange meetings with family members. Not all of the story may be pretty, but are there parts you wish to remember and pass on? If so, there are many creative ways to record this history, and you can always include some of the physically tangible items in a cute keepsake box or baby book.

Creating your own story

So, what about creating a family story and heritage of your own? Well, part of this process happens organically as you get to know your little one and you grow together as a family. The other part you develop intentionally. This last category includes certain elements of life or values you find important enough to commemorate or honor.

The goal of these family traditions, whatever they may be, is to help ground your family and reinforce your core values. Some people even find it helpful to write a family charter (highlighting these values), revisiting it from time to time to ensure their life decisions are consistent with their ideals.[1] If this sounds like something you'd like to do, a helpful first step is to pick words to define your little community. Some examples include *honesty, forgiveness, fun, exploration, adventure, deep, spiritual, inclusive*, and *inquisitive*. You could even get fancy and mount keywords on your wall for a little decorative reminding.

For a simpler option, find books with meaningful themes and set aside time to read them to your baby and older children. Before you know it, this tradition may morph into your baby reading to you!

Being realistic

Now for a little reality check: When your baby first comes, your world will be a little messy and chaotic, full of unexpected moments of joy and

ACTIVITY IDEA

Take a trip to your favorite local bookstore and find some special reads. Even older kids can have a blast with this type of outing.

challenges. This may be a tricky time to launch or continue traditions with any gusto. Remember, within a few months, there will be more rhythm to your day, and you'll be able to think a little more about your family life. During such transitional seasons, give yourself grace and keep things simple.

Hopefully, these pages sparked ideas for new and meaningful ways to prepare for your little darling while he or she is incubating away. Enjoy this opportunity to carve your own path—to share or create your family story, your own way.

Digging Deeper

Collecting family keepsakes and preparing your own family story can take as little or as much time as you'd like. Allow yourself to continue adapting and exploring over the years to come. Consider it artwork in progress. When you're ready, pick one or two items off the list below (or something else you're thinking of) to get you started.

Family Keepsake Ideas

» Family tree

» Favorite family recipe

» Photo

» Language

» Prayer

» Spiritual practice or religion

» Ceremonies, special events, traditions

» Stories

WEEK 24

Baby

- Is about 12 ¾ inches long.
- Weighs about 1 ¼ pounds.
- Is now considered viable, meaning that if born early, there's a good chance for survival.
- Develops a layer of brown fat uniquely designed to protect against hypothermia after birth.

Mama

- The kidneys enlarge and now filter about 50% more blood than before pregnancy.
- You may notice bleeding gums when you brush your teeth.
  - To prevent cavities and periodontal disease, brush your teeth and floss daily, and keep up with your dental cleanings at least every six months.

Claustrophobia

Sometimes, I wonder what job I could enjoy if I weren't in nursing.

When I was in elementary school, I thought being a secretary could be quite fulfilling. I remember trying out press-on nails and then sitting down at the piano or my hand-drawn typewriter, tap-tapping away. My fingers would blur with methodical clicks, which, of course, made me feel quite accomplished. I had letters to type, phone calls to answer, and file cabinets to open and close with my long, beautiful, shiny pink nails. Each time, though, my grand aspirations deflated once one snapped off or pivoted sideways. How *unprofessional.*

During this inner exploration, I've also discovered what jobs I should avoid. A tour guide and businessperson are most certainly on that list somewhere, but the role at the very top is—a team mascot. I can't imagine how terrible it would be to wear a hot, dark, cramped suit, even if it did mean running around the bleachers dressed as a leprechaun. I'm sure that instead of bolstering the crowds or posing with fans, I'd find my heart start to pound with the fear of getting stuck in that stifling, inescapable space—overcome by that panicked sensation of breathlessness I get sometimes when on a plane, in a drive-through car wash, or while standing in an elevator.

Surprisingly, I now experience elements of this panic with pregnancy. Yet in this it's somehow reversed—like claustrophobia inside out. My tight belly has made me feel like there is not possibly enough room to accommodate my little one. I'm only 24 weeks along, but my belly is taut, my stomach squished, and my lungs already grieve for the golden days of freedom.

I just want to be more spacious and expansive, like the bright open vistas around me. How lovely it would be to let my baby stretch out within me like a towering tree, her limbs rustling in the breeze and swaying my insides with a rhythm of glorious serenity.

Is there any magic trick for this? I'd sure be happy to hear of it.

Whenever the unsettling moments of claustrophobia hit, I practice some guided imagery—picturing the morning fog lift from the shimmery surface of a lake—and then take a few deep breaths. It's amazing how much of our reality can be changed simply by adjusting our thoughts and our focus.

So, what's the big deal? There's plenty of room in here. I pinch the skin around my belly, give it a little tug, and watch it stretch like taffy at the state fair. See, my belly has potential. It has capacity. It will have no trouble blossoming in due time. I'll panic another day, but not today.

I hope.

Shifting Pelvis and Perspectives

Today is an odd sort of day. It's the first time I've felt like a ship on stilts, or at least a ship at sea—like the ones we saw resting in the water off the breathtaking coast of Cape Town while visiting our South African friends. Except this time, there is no World Cup 2010, no towering flat-topped Table Mountain behind me, no endless span of ocean ahead, or the spectacular, cultural richness of Africa everywhere I turn. Seeing any of these would make me feel better now that I've carted my suitcase up a flight of stairs and found my pelvis popping and shifting around like JELL-O.

Seriously? Sure, I always tell my pregnant patients to be careful when lifting heavier objects, because their bodies are making relaxin hormone to loosen the joints and prepare for childbirth. But really? I didn't expect to get injured so easily.

Discouraged, I turned to memories of the trip to boost my spirits. As I paused on the stair, visions of the stay danced through my mind—painting our faces with stars and stripes, blowing into the plastic vuvuzela horns at the Cup games, witnessing the traditional African dances, and cramming into a local's living room so we could enjoy authentic, sticky flavors with our fingers as light filtered through the small windows set in the asbestos walls.

Ah, and then there's the time when we almost got trampled by an elephant on a safari. Actually, let's skip past that memory and instead remember when we peeked in on the postpartum unit to satisfy my professional curiosity.

Mothers with colorful headwraps sat in their white-sheeted beds, cupping their naked, premature babies against their beautiful, dark-skinned chests—effectively keeping their babies warm through *kangaroo care*, and eliminating the need for incubators. See, here's another great example of how mommies are amazing.

Why, yes, I do believe I'm feeling better already.

Tucking away the images of this African journey, I turn my thoughts toward something else that may help: focusing on the conveniences of pregnancy. Perspective, it's said, can make quite a difference. So, why not test this out?

What can I be grateful for?

First, by having my little one tucked inside of me, she's with me always. This is quite relieving for a newbie like me because I'm still getting used to the idea that I'm responsible for someone other than myself. For now, I don't have to race around the house to find her. She's not playing in the toilet—she's in me, safe and sound.

Second, feeding this little munchkin is a cinch. Whenever I feed myself, she gets what she needs. I eat, and just like that, she grows. Ta-da! No need to figure out breastfeeding, warm a bottle, spend time on burping, change diapers, or even consider what fussy foods might bother her little tummy. Yes, it would be wise to enjoy this while I can. I heard newborns feed nearly nonstop—almost every one-and-a-half to two hours initially, for 30–45 minutes at a time. *That's intense.*

And last, my baby doesn't cry at all right now. That's so lovely. My ragamuffin may kick, turn, twist, and punch me, but that's it. She's silent. I don't have to do the detective work to figure out why she's crying.

Yes, in many ways, things are much simpler now than what's to come. So, can I, Mrs. Boat-on-stilts, stop fixating on myself and instead find a way to still enjoy this unique time? Just maybe—with some focus and a prayer.

⇛ LET'S TALK ABOUT IT ⇚

On Becoming a Mommy

Dear pregnant mama, as you continue growing from the inside out, you may have started noticing much more than physical changes in yourself. Beyond getting tearful at the sight of any baby commercial, you may even be getting philosophical, wondering: When do I begin becoming a mama?

Great question! Certainly, this change happens when your baby's born. Every time a new little life enters the world—voilà!—a new mommy is made.[1] On a deeper level, however, you may start sensing that transition to motherhood way before you meet your baby face to face. Pregnancy is a wild time of metamorphosis, remember? Though it may not sink in until your baby is in your arms, at any time after that positive pregnancy test, you may start feeling different about yourself and your life's purpose—begin feeling a tad bit "mommyish."

In this way, pregnancy is like a chrysalis that gives you a chance to start taking on butterfly-like (mommy-like) qualities. Day by day, tiny, itsy-bitsy changes can happen in your sentiments—when your perspective shifts and you start imagining your baby's cute ringlets and find him and your dachshund matching plaid vests, or you envision the long walks you'll have together, the homemade applesauce you're sure he's going to love, and the sweet scent of his soft skin as you hold him close. The convenient thing is that pregnancy can give you a chance to role-play motherhood in your thoughts and daydreams and see what fits your style.[1]

Now, as you can imagine, being smooshed inside a chrysalis (or having someone smooshed inside of you) isn't a breeze. It can get cramped as you navigate the challenges brought with change. Becoming and being mama is a major transformation that looks different for everyone.[2] This time of reshaping your identity can be exciting but also hard, complicated, and confusing.[2] Don't give up, though; in time, you'll learn how to fly.

In many ways, the process of transformation describes not only the journey of pregnancy but also motherhood itself—it is beautiful, messy, and full of unpredictability. One minute you feel happy and content and then the next moment, you may feel like a sobbing crazy lady because your coworker joked you had pregnancy brain, or because you missed your baby's subtle hunger cues and now he's hysterical.

Amid the changes, let pregnancy expand your horizons. This is a gift, especially for us perfectionists. You may be competitive, have trouble asking for help, or want things to be "just right," but if you're not careful, these tendencies can make motherhood more challenging than it needs to be.[3,4] Instead, let this journey encourage you to loosen your grip on life and practice the art of going with the flow—it's an indispensable outlook for the coming days of motherhood.

For more thoughts on choosing a name for your love bug, check out "Baby Naming" in A-3h.

Digging Deeper

For those of you looking for an opportunity to get your creative juices flowing, here's your chance! Please grab:

» Paper (white or colored)

» Old magazines and newspapers

» Glue

» Colored pencils or markers

Once you've assembled your goods, make a collage representing this process of transformation. Choose, cut out, and glue onto a paper the images and words that resonate with you. The beautiful thing is—there's no right or wrong way to do this. Turn on some inspiring music and see where your creativity takes you. You can even shape items into a butterfly. You may wish to add to this over the coming weeks of pregnancy. Enjoy!

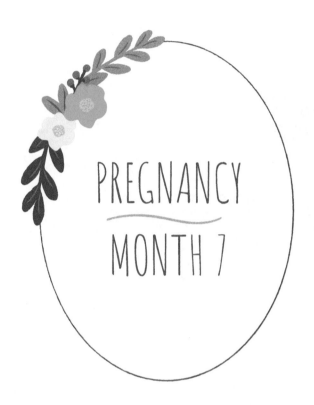

PREGNANCY

MONTH 7

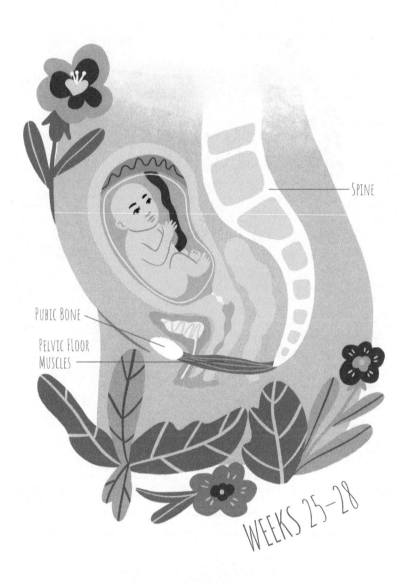

Spine

Pubic Bone

Pelvic Floor
Muscles

WEEKS 25-28

WEEK 25

Baby
- Is about 13 ¼ inches long.
- Weighs about 1 ½ pounds.
- Continues to develop the brain.
- May have up to 44 breathing motions per minute.
- Releases steroid hormones through the adrenal gland to help prepare for birth.

Mama
- Your nose may be stuffy more often, since blood flow and swelling in the area increase throughout pregnancy.
- Lighter- or darker-colored stretch marks may be appearing. Although there's no magic potion to prevent them, good news: they usually improve postpartum.
  - In the meantime, feel free to flaunt them proudly—like a motherhood tattoo.

"Momsters"

"Taqueria El Favorito" is an appropriate name for the nearby Mexican drive-through, since it's our favorite authentic Mexican restaurant from which to grab burritos, and a perfect place to practice the little Spanish I can barely claim to know. Having extra time on my hands today, I stopped in, rested my elbows on the sticky plastic table, and people-watched while dipping my burrito in fresh salsa, savoring the flavors.

There was nothing too interesting to spy on until a group of four sat down nearby—two mothers with two trailing little girls. A year ago, I didn't care too much about observing mothers with their daughters, but now I'd have to admit pregnancy has changed me. Curiosity fills me, and I can hardly help myself.

Since it's only a few days before Halloween, I probably should have expected to see something unusual. After all, cotton spiderwebs stretch across neighborhood windows, "Boo" signs stand by front doors, and neon skeletons and ghosts dangle from trees. In just a few days, our Santa Rosa neighbors will be corralling their kids through the streets for the annual Halloween parade.

Despite the seasonal décor, I was still not at all prepared to see these two, thirty-something-year-old women dressed in black, their makeup creating pale faces overlaid with thick black scars. I was equally unprepared to see their two little girls dressed in fishnet stockings and dog collars, with skirts too short to offer any warmth. It was spooky—though to be fair, I still have nightmares from watching *Ghostbusters* at a childhood slumber party. Could it be these elaborate costumes are for the famous Mexican Day of the Dead celebration to honor passed loved ones?

I'd like to say it was just the costumes that unnerved me, but sadly, it was also the adults' interactions with the kids. As they settled in and had their lunch, I could hear their conversation peppered with expletives and saturated with impatient commands.

"Stop moving around!" growled the woman with matted hair and vibrant, painted flowers amid the scars.

"I said, BE QUIET!" the other one snapped.

What exactly, I wonder, prompted these mothers to interact so harshly with their children? Could it have been a lost job? Single parenting? Financial hardship, losing a loved one, or bad news? Although I'll never know, I knew I'd never forget the sadness and confusion in the little girls' eyes.

Eventually, with an ache in my stomach, I got up and made my way back to my faded gray Jetta.

For a moment before leaving, I just stared straight ahead at the grooves on my steering wheel.

Motherhood sure isn't always pretty. There will be days without relaxing stroller walks; calm nighttime cuddles; tasty, pureed baby food; or the agreeable toddler. The thought is overwhelming. Especially since mommies don't get a breather just because things aren't going well. Their job is nonstop—like the traffic I hear from our apartment window—and sometimes, its ever-present nature pushes mommies past their limits. Apparently, it can make "momsters" of us all.

I am hopeful, though, when I think about the profound impact mommies and daddies (and really, everyone) can have on children's well-being. All every child needs to flourish is at least *one* loving, dependable, and invested adult in their lives. Surely that's doable, right?

Happier still, children's souls were created with a buffer system—they don't need a perfect parent but a loving one. God must have known that raising children is a beautiful, yet messy human endeavor—full of blemished moments of impatience, tiredness, overwhelmingness, and sometimes overarching growliness. Thankfully, all is not lost when our babies have a raging diaper rash, our work stress carries over to home, or we lose our tempers. While all these are good to avoid, it is reassuring to remember children can do well when their mommies are simply "good enough" less than half of the time. What a relief for all of us with a perfectionist streak, we who are experts at feeling guilty.

Will someone make note of my scary mothering while I'm in a vulnerable state someday? I sure hope not. But in reality, very likely yes. If or when it happens, may I have the grace to forgive myself, wisdom to remember the nature of motherhood, and the resolve to help mommies in need, like me.

What If I Don't Like to Play Ball?

Before the birth of my first child I worried and worried that I wouldn't be a natural mother, that I wouldn't be able to get it right. I realized eventually that there is no such thing. All of us learn from page one starting on day one— there is no shortcut to learning how to bring up a child, and I don't think you ever stop learning.
—Rowan Coleman

Truthfully, I'm a little concerned. Okay, maybe a lot concerned. With my maternity leave plans looming in my mind, I'm forced to confront the reality that at some point, I'll need to start interacting with my daughter in the flesh—like actually feed, clothe, and diaper her. No big deal, right? That's kind of the point of pregnancy even, to eventually have a baby to cherish and raise.

Yes, but still, I'm just not like one of *those* women—the "natural mothers," I call them. The ones who relate to children effortlessly and spend countless hours causing eruptions of uncontrolled laughter and giggles. They make funny noises, weird faces, and silly gestures. They roll the same ball back and forth, over and over, there and back again, even though they just finished doing that a second ago. Children flock to them as to bubbles or balloons.

I don't get it. How is all that any fun?

And what's more, if I don't like it, what does that mean about me? Yes, I partly blame having the hand-eye coordination of a worm. But despite this handicap, can I still be a good mother?

Faced with these worries, I sat down outside our apartment home underneath the towering evergreens and called my mother for a little wisdom. I could sure use some reassurance.

"Each mother has her own parenting style," she encouraged, "and individual ways to show her child they are loved. At the right moment, and not a second early, you'll come up with your own unique ways to express who you are and to show your baby you love her."

Really? Is that how it works?

Come to find out, my mother didn't really enjoy playing ball with us either, and in fact, she didn't do it very often. But here's the clincher: When she did and when others do, it is not the ball rolling specifically that makes the experience so exciting. It's the playtime with the little love, the interactions, the eye contact, the silly faces, and the making of funny and sweet noises together. Truly, it's about forming a deep and trusting relationship—the sense of security and attachment that becomes the foundation on which your child will develop close relationships throughout her life.

In these times spent doing the same thing over and over, you discover things about your child's personality. What does she do in response to that darn ball? Does she like it, go for it, or hate it? Does she get scared? Is she oblivious? It's amazing how such a simple, spherical object can become a tool through which a mother can get to know her little dumpling.

And *that*, I realized, is how a parent is transformed into a helpless robot, rolling the ball back and forth. I guess all this time, I had it all wrong.

⋙ LET'S TALK ABOUT IT ⋘

Planning Your Maternity Leave

Thinking about maternity leave can be both exciting and a little daunting. You may not yet know how close to your due date you'd like to work, how long you'd like to be on leave, or even what your options are. So, no wonder! In "Supporting the Working Mother" (week 20), we covered *work accommodations*, so you can work safely while pregnant, and *leave*, a limited time off from work. Well, today my friend, we're moving on to bigger and better things—maternity leave. After all, who wants to give birth at work?

Planning ahead

Research has shown that paid maternity leave improves mamas' and babies' health.[1] And yet, as of 2022, the U.S. is still the *only* developed country that doesn't have a national, paid parental leave, which means 84% of its private sector workforce is without access to paid family leave through their employers.[1-4] Crazy, right? No wonder pregnant mamas like you are left scrambling, trying to piece together time with their new little loves using federal and state maternity leave laws and vacation time.

Depending on the circumstances, women eligible for partially paid leave can stop working a few weeks before their due dates and remain off until six to eight weeks after delivery. After birth, mamas may also use saved-up vacation time, bonus baby bonding time (a state- or employer-based benefit), and federal Family Medical Leave Act time (up to twelve weeks unpaid).[2,5] If they're lucky, this buys them the option of three to six months of maternity leave. But in this far-from-ideal world, about 25% of women go back to work as early as two weeks after delivery![1,2,6]

> **DID YOU KNOW?**
>
> About 50% of women would stay home longer if they could, and most would prefer an average of six to seven months of maternity leave.[9,10]

If you're planning on expressing milk (pumping) at work or at school when you get back, consider mentioning this to your employer or student support services before starting maternity leave. They may need time to prepare and establish a designated space for this. Did you know that **Break Time for Nursing Mothers** is a federal law under the Fair Labor Standards Act (FLSA) that requires some employers to give you reasonable break times for expressing milk, as well as access to a private (non-bathroom) space for your baby's first year of life?[7,8] Breaks taken in excess of standard, compensated breaks, unfortunately, are not required to be paid.[7] This law applies to those women who are entitled to over-time pay and work at a business employing at least 50 people.[7]

Other federal laws (like *Title VII*, *Title IX*, and the *Pregnancy Discrimination Act*) and some state laws can also legally protect you while expressing milk at work or school.[2,8] There are wonderful, creative solutions for finding spaces for those of you who don't have desk jobs, so start dreaming and don't give up.

Check with your employer, maternity care provider, or social worker to find out what state maternity leave and lactation accommodation laws are available to you. Other great resources (also noted in appendix C) are Center for WorkLife Law, Pregnant@Work, and A Better Balance.

The early days

The first three months after birth will be a sweet blur, filled with precious surprises, smiles, tears, fears, extreme tiredness, and adjustments to your roles, schedule, and expectations. You'll thank yourself if you keep things extra simple during this time and limit responsibilities outside of mothering. In the first few months after birth, save yourself and don't plan on accomplishing anything monumental while your little wonder naps erratically. You'll need time for sleeping, eating, and for taking your own naps. *Really.*

Don't be hard on yourself if you're less productive, your house is a mess, you aren't performing great at your job, and you notice your ingenious thoughts are as rare as a hot date. This time is not meant for that—you're helping your baby adjust to this new world, in your arms, one breath at a time. This time is about slowing down—for once. Remember, by three months, you should feel a little better (and even more so at six months!) as you start having more time to sleep, are able to shower for longer than a minute, and can once again think in complete sentences.

Returning to work

When it comes to returning to work, having flexibility is a rare and lucky thing. An understanding boss is worth a million, and sometimes the only way to find out is to make a request. It's worth asking if there are creative return-to-work options like working remotely, part time, job sharing, or even possible job function changes (such as with better hours, lower stress, or less travel).

Last, it's okay to take some time to decide how you feel about returning to work when you do. While you likely have your guesses now, you may surprise yourself! Some women realize they miss their baby more than they thought when back at work, while others are shocked to realize how much they miss work when at home. Some mamas find they'd rather work full time while their partner, family member, or a nanny does the daily caregiving. Give yourself grace to find out what's comfortable and works for you and your family. If you're not sold on your return-to-work plan, don't sweat it. Sometimes you just have to start somewhere and then readjust as needed.

Digging Deeper

If you're working, planning for your baby's arrival takes some thinking through. This is a wonderful time to start developing a postpartum care plan (see A-5a) and to think more about what's next in terms of maternity leave. Below you'll find a list of questions to consider and help you get organized. For the answers, ask your employer and maternity care provider, search online for your state's maternity or family leave laws, and call the resources noted here and in appendix C.

» What are your leave options? Are they paid or unpaid?

» When can you use them? How long can they last?

» Is your partner eligible for parental or paternity leave?

» Do you have any flexible or creative return-to-work options?

» If planning on expressing milk, is there a designated space at work?

» If there is no space for expressing milk, does your job qualify you to get break times and a space for pumping under the Break Time for Nursing Mothers federal law?

» What child-care options exist for when you go back to work?

WEEK 26

Baby

- Is about 13 ¾ inches long.
- Weighs about 1 ¾ pounds.
- Can now react to loud noises with a blink-startle reflex.

Mama

- You may experience breathlessness as your uterus pushes up against your lungs.
- If it hadn't before, constipation may develop due to (you guessed it) your uterus pressing on your digestive tract.

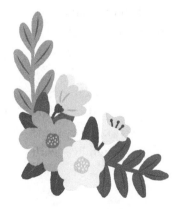

The Not-So-Blank Canvas

Pregnancy infuses the ordinary woman with something extraordinary. In pregnancy, the former wallflower is now noticed. Sure, there are plenty of pregnant women roaming the streets, but each one catches the eye of the women passing by. It's quite an odd experience, to be scanned wherever you go.

The pregnant belly is a beautiful thing, full of baby, and thus—mystery. With the pregnant bump greeting the gaze, women of all walks of life encounter a rush of unexpected emotions.

To biological mothers, the belly is a reminder of times past, when grown or growing children were once so close, when their babies could think of nothing better than to be by their sides, and when days were packed with unbounded delight and complete exhaustion.

To those who have tried to have children, though, the round belly is an assault, a jury challenging her core. It's a reminder of longings unfulfilled and of repeatedly dashed hopes as monthly cycles march on. Questions resurface: Why me? Doesn't it matter to God, or anyone, how my soul aches for a child as yet unformed? Will I really never experience the luxurious inconveniences of pregnancy?

Sometimes, I feel self-conscious and even guilty when I'm out of the house, since I don't know what emotions my pregnancy elicits in the people around me. I don't know what whirlwind of thoughts will wash over her, whether it will offer colorful and sweetly refreshing daydreams, feelings of in-the-trenches comradery, or an afternoon haunted by disappointment and sorrow.

It's been especially difficult during clinical work when I meet with women who have been waiting to conceive. I am no longer a blank canvas—just another person who may or may not be going through what they are. Instead, I am in the group of "other" women—those who already have what they want.

At this point, all I can think to do is suck in my belly to shave off a few extra inches, care for women in every way I can, and hope my budding bump will not feel like an offense. Who knows, maybe by some miracle, they won't even notice that I'm—quietly and gratefully—with child.

I Wish It Wasn't a Night to Remember

Just for the night, can I detach my belly? I promise I'll reattach it tomorrow. I just want one good night of sleep. Instead, each one gets worse. I'm finally starting to understand why my pregnant patients are always so tired. *I get it.*

Last night I tossed and turned, the same way I've always imagined the leading character in "The Princess and the Pea" would as she tries to sleep atop a pile of mattresses. No single sleeping position felt adequate or remotely comfortable, and I don't think I even had a pea wedged underneath me.

On my side, I tucked my legs in as if trying to cannonball into dreamland. Splash! Immersive reprieve would have been most welcome. How nice it would be to swim among fancy dreams or even plain ones. But no such luck.

Position change.

I laid on my back with legs bent, then butterflied out as if trying to flutter my way into a deep sleep. How I would have liked to beat my wings—to softly land and rest my weary body. But no luck. My wings must be too weak or my body too bulky for flight.

Dramatic position change.

Maybe better luck with my other side?

Nope.

I elevated my annoyingly heavy head at various heights. Stupid idea. I then elevated my legs with pillows in all sorts of hopeful positions.

No can do.

Not even a body pillow could save me now.

If I just could have somehow expanded my pelvis, given it a little more room, and stretched my back. But might as well ask for the impossible.

Instead of complaining about the pregnancy-induced earthquake, Dan leaned over, plopped his tired arms around me, and even tried to raise my spirits with a back rub. His half-asleep efforts were unimpressive, but sweet. We even had our first 3:00 a.m. chuckle together, which then made me want to press close to him. I shimmied and scooched myself over inch by inch only to find an unexpectedly massive, round obstacle between us.

What in the—? Oh, yeah.

I sniffled. This baby is already separating my husband and me. Though right beside me, he feels so far away.

⫸⫸⫸ LET'S TALK ABOUT IT ⫷⫷⫷

Getting Rest

At some point, you'll be willing to empty your piggy bank or maybe sell your partner just for a few glorious minutes of sleep. The culprit? Insomnia—which is defined as a difficulty falling or staying asleep, waking from sleep too early, or having nonrestorative sleep.[1-3] But how can it be so difficult to sleep when you're so tired? Well, remember you have a cute belly, an active baby, peeing is your new nighttime hobby, and you may also have heartburn, back pain, excitement, worry, weird dreams, obstructive sleep apnea, restless legs, or leg cramps. And then, as if that weren't enough, we're asking you to sleep on your side and no longer flat on your back. It's a conspiracy. (*Just kidding!*)

Sleep goals and benefits

So, you've probably heard sleep experts recommending nonpregnant, healthy adults (ages 18–64) get between seven to nine hours per day (in contrast, your newborn baby will be getting an average of 16 hours!).[4-6] Since the perfect amount of sleep during pregnancy is still a mystery, the main thing is to listen to your body. Sleep when you're tired. If you can't sleep, then rest. Why? When you sleep or rest enough, you feel better, your body is happier, and a better *you* interacts with the world. This is especially important if you struggle with your mental health.

Did you know sleep positively affects your immune system, mood, heart health, blood pressure, growth, stress hormones, and risk for obesity and diabetes?[6-9] *Wow, what a list!* It restores every part of you. And in pregnancy, the gift of sleep just keeps on giving: it decreases your risk of gestational diabetes, preeclampsia, depression, Cesarean birth, and preterm delivery (which is when you give birth before 37 weeks).[10-12] Adequate sleep can even shorten your labor and may even help reduce your labor pains.[13,14] Yep, it's pretty much a miracle.

If not sleep, then rest

It may come as no surprise that as we approach the finish line, most pregnant women sleep fewer hours and experience more sleep problems.[3,11-16] Most of the time, the culprit is all those terrible night-wakings, though about a third of your pregnant friends will find it hard to sleep in, and some will have trouble falling asleep.[11] And sleeping parties (when pets and children sleep with you) don't help.[17]

So, when you're lying awake that blessed night, remember you aren't the only lady flip-flopping like a flounder. Instead of getting frustrated that you aren't having that deeply restorative sleep, realize dozing can give you some beautiful benefits, too. If you really can't sleep, don't torture yourself by staring at the clock's second hand. Get up and do something enjoyable and relaxing. The secret, though, is to avoid TV, computers, smartphones, and e-readers because they emit a light that will, in fact, wake you up more.

On another note, all this trouble sleeping is almost as if nature is slowly training pregnant mommies to become night owls—which can certainly help prepare us for taking care of our little munchkins when they arrive. However, if you're waking up unrested in the morning, make it a point to take a nap instead of just loading up on extra caffeine. Get creative if you need to—your body needs it. At work, use a bathroom stall to pause for a few minutes, if you must.

Digging Deeper

Rest, relaxation, and sleep are beautiful things we all deserve to enjoy, wouldn't you agree? For practical tips on making this happen during pregnancy, check out B-3. There you'll find answers to questions pregnant mamas often wonder about, like:

» Help! How can I get more comfortable in bed? (B-3a)

» Are there any safe, natural things I can try to help me sleep? (B-3a)

» Even if I can't sleep well at night, what are other ways I can rest and relax? (B-3c)

WEEK 27

Baby

- Is about 14 ½ inches long.
- Weighs about 2 pounds.
- Starts becoming light-sensitive as eyelids open.
- Grows longer hair on head, eyebrows, and eyelashes.

Mama

- Your body continues to blossom and gain weight, affecting your baby's childhood and adult weight.
- For one baby, if you started pregnancy at a healthy weight, expect to gain about a pound a week until delivery.[1]
- For twins, if you started pregnancy at a healthy weight, expect to gain about 1–1.5 pounds a week until delivery.[1,2]

Note: If you started pregnancy overweight or plus-size, your weight goal is less, and if you started underweight, it's more.

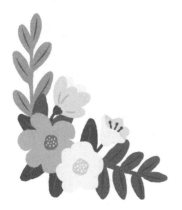

Symphony

Ah, a nice hot bowl of chili with a salad sounds perfect after my evening commute back to Santa Rosa. There's nothing like the warmth of comfort foods—like mac 'n' cheese, casseroles, or stews—to nurture us, even when our loved ones are hundreds of miles away. Stirring the pot, I watched the colors swim about—the red and black beans, purple carrots, red peppers, and white corn kernels. It's quite amazing that these individual items, all with different textures, properties, and tastes, are able to create such a symphony of flavors.

While the soup simmers on the stove, I crack open the kitchen window to let in a stream of cool air. Condensation streaks down the panes, each cleared swath revealing the evergreens in the yard, dripping from the afternoon rain. *Drip. Drip. Drop. Drip. Drip. Drop.* Onto the bushes and the pinecones below, they fall. I stand transfixed by their meditative rhythm—a pregnant statue, staring at the beauty my soul so desperately needs.

Lately, the glamor and excitement of pregnancy have dissipated, only to be replaced by its weariness. My belly grows tighter and bigger every day, and my emotions carry me up and down on a whim. The miracle of pregnancy has taken on a new twist in my mind, that is—it's a miracle that so many women survive this state and forget so easily all its trials. I've gone so far as to think that if I ever did write a pregnancy book, I'd have to call it something like *The Joy of Pregnancy: The Biggest Lie Ever Told.* Or perhaps this one: *Growing, Growing, Growing, but Never Glowing.*

Sitting down to enjoy my dinner, though, with the steam curling up from my bowl, I had a thought. Maybe, in the end, a woman's pregnancy story could become something like this soup. After all, time is on our side. In time, these highs and lows, the light and rich textures, could intermingle—simmering together into a rich medley of memory. As I breathed in the rising aroma of the soup below, hope also rose within me. Perhaps, I dared to imagine, I will emerge on the other side of this journey, savoring the mélange of experience—that colorful symphony bursting with a flavor I'll never forget.

Sex: What Happened?

"You make this like an obstacle course," Dan laughingly confessed earlier today.

I can't blame the guy. While sex used to be effortless and simple, it certainly has become more complicated and, well, interesting. Sure, this is expected especially as women get toward the end of pregnancy, but I'm still caught off guard. *This is what it's like, really?* Perhaps a pregnancy roadmap could spread the word to my circle of pregnant mamas. Sex would be nicely marked as one of the many possible destinations and would have a starred disclaimer about the terrain: NOT FOR THE FAINT OF HEART.

Especially today, I couldn't seem to get comfortable. Carrying on with business as usual, I got sandwiched—between the mattress, my belly, and Dan, like a multi-layered human sub sandwich. *I'd like extra aioli sauce with that, please.* No wonder I felt consumed more than savored.

Now, if only he could hover above me or grow wings and levitate, that could change things entirely. Or maybe he and I could put our medical and nursing minds together and invent a one-of-a-kind contraption from which he could swing in like Tarzan or hang from a trapeze at home. *Hmm, yes, that might actually work.* I'd love to see Dan swing around our room. It might be hard to catch him, but we could work out the flaws.

Since our trapeze wasn't an option yet, my mind drifted to those many other fun, pregnancy-compatible sex positions. Surely one of these will be better! Hands and knees do help a pregnant woman feel much less like a sandwich. Why yes, this is splendid. *Glorious.* Perfectly doable—until my breasts caught wind of the position change. *Ting-a-ling!* My Hungarian bells went so wild that if they really could have rung, any church bell choir would have been put to shame. So, I did what any reasonable woman would do—I stuffed a pillow under them to mute their performance. *There we go, so much better.* Finally.

But no sooner had that been taken care of than my little bladder called for attention. *Help!* it cried. It needed attending to—and fast. In fact, I couldn't do anything else but fixate on relieving that pressure. I quickly updated Dan on the desperate state of affairs, which, as you can imagine, very effectively killed any potential last flicker of passion. Fizzle, and then—*puff!*

Well, sex is certainly not for the faint of heart, I remind myself. Perhaps we'll have better luck next time when we adventure to that wild corner of the map.

⋙ LET'S TALK ABOUT IT ⋘

Getting It On, or Not, While Pregnant

Okay you sex goddess, you. The answer is, yes! If you're having a healthy pregnancy, sex and orgasms are perfectly safe throughout your *entire* pregnancy (no matter how well-endowed he is).[3,4] There are a few instances where your maternity care provider will recommend holding off from penetrative sex or doing anything that arouses you to orgasm (like if you are high risk for preterm birth, your bag of water breaks, or you have a *placenta previa*, meaning the placenta covers all or part of the cervix).[3,4] So, if you don't get the word to refrain, go for it. *No, you will not traumatize your baby.*[5,6] He or she is tucked safely inside, surrounded by uterine and abdominal muscles, amniotic fluid, and the mucus plug in your cervix.

Staying safe

Before we journey further into this mysterious topic of sex in pregnancy, let's start off with a few important reminders on how to keep yourself safe. First off, this entire discussion about sex is built on the assumption that you and your partner have a positive and caring relationship: you feel safe, respected, honored, and you are not coerced, discriminated against, or experiencing any manipulation or violence.[7] If this is *not* the case, please talk with your healthcare provider or check out www.thehotline.org, taking care to do so in a safe time and place, where you can clear your internet's browsing history, or where it would not be misused. You may be scared but take heart—there is a way out. You deserve to be respected and safe.

Now for all you ladies who are starting a new relationship while pregnant, have multiple partners, or have a partner who *may* have a sexually transmitted infection (STI), remember: It's vital for you to protect yourself against STIs and to get tested.[8] Everyone, even the person who makes your heart swoon, can harbor nasty STIs. Seriously. Many people don't know they have an STI, and if you contract it and aren't treated, it can cause serious problems for you and your baby (like premature birth, organ problems, or stillbirth).[8]

So, unless you and your partner are exclusive, *always* use condoms, don't share sex toys, and have your partner tested for the works (including gonorrhea, chlamydia, syphilis, HIV, and hepatitis C). Be sure to find out about their genital herpes history, too, since it's not part of a routine STI panel and acquiring it could have significant implications for childbirth. Check in with your maternity care provider about how often to get retested for STIs during your pregnancy.

Adapting to changes

Now, on to the juicy details about sex in pregnancy. It's totally normal for you to see changes in your body, sexual desire, satisfaction, and relationship with your partner.[3,9,10] Sexual desire and experiences can change from moment to moment as your body blossoms and adapts to all this upheaval. Some women turn into prowling cougars while others want to smack anyone who mentions the "s" word. Usually, by the third trimester, most couples have briefer and less sex because, *man*, it's a lot of effort.[9-11] Have grace for yourself wherever you find yourself and communicate with your partner.

When (or if) you do have sex, you may notice your body feeling and acting differently, especially in the third trimester. Your breasts may leak colostrum, making you feel like a beautiful Italian fountain, or you may notice increased breast sensitivity, which may turn you on or make you head for the hills. The sensations in your vagina and clitoris may decrease, and you might notice more vaginal dryness or decreased libido.[9,12] Everyone's different. You may not even feel like having sex.[6,10,13] Also, certain antidepressants can decrease libido or make it harder to have an orgasm.[14]

On the flip side, women are usually happy to find it easier to climax. Any associated abdominal cramping should resolve within 5–10 minutes. If, by the third trimester, orgasms feel weaker or are harder to have, don't stress; things should normalize by about three to six months postpartum.[9,13] And of course, don't be surprised if you spot a little after sex or leak urine (more on this in "Your Pelvic Floor," week 31). If you are more than spotting after intercourse, check in with your maternity care provider to confirm all is well.

Focusing on intimacy

This is also a perfect time to remember that although sex is a gift, it's only one avenue for being intimate with your partner. This is especially important for those of you who have been advised to not have sex while pregnant to avoid certain pregnancy complications.

CIRCUMCISION

While we're on the topic of intimacy and sexual organs, let's consider for a moment this common yet controversial surgery. Circumcision is an irreversible procedure that removes from the glans penis the sensitive tissue called the foreskin (or prepuce), which is designed to protect the glans and urinary opening. At birth, the foreskin is fused to the glans, though later in maturity it is retractable.

Parents often choose circumcision for religious reasons, but nonreligious factors include potential health and sexual benefits, and social or family norms.[15] Though pretty common in the U.S., the worldwide rate of circumcision is only 30%, and data indicates the trend is declining in the States.[15,16]

If you're having a baby boy, take time to get the facts and weigh the pros and cons. While surgery may be presented to you as a no-brainer, the choice has its own ethical considerations and potential health impacts. To delve further into this topic, check out Evidence Based Birth's "Evidence and Ethics on: Circumcision."[17]

So, if you're not having penetrative sex for whatever reason, indulge in all the other glorious ways of physical affection: kiss, hug, hold hands, cuddle, stroke, massage, and lick away. Or just spend some time together doing what you love. This may be exactly what your soul needs, especially if you already have little ones hanging from you all day long like Christmas ornaments.

The bottom line? Pregnancy and having a baby can profoundly change aspects of sex and relationships. However, it doesn't mean it can't be fun or special. Be proactive. Resolve with your partner to work on intimacy as you traverse the road of (and *to*) parenthood. A connected mommy and partner will mean a happier and healthier baby and family.

Digging Deeper

Many of you pregnant mamas or moms-to-be are interested in sex and are eager to hear some practical tips for making it possible with a blooming belly. Remember, a little imagination, guts, and a sense of humor go a long way. Try new things and make memories in as many ways as you can. To get you started, check out B-5 where you'll find answers to questions like:

» How can I spice up my sex life? (B-5d)

» What do I need to think about when purchasing sex toys? (B-5d)

» Are all lubricants created equal? (B-5d)

» Are there positions that make sex easier while pregnant? (B-5d)

» Is oral or anal sex okay in pregnancy? (B-5d)

» What if I don't feel comfortable with how my partner wants me to have sex? (B-5h)

THIRD TRIMESTER

WEEKS 28–40

WEEK 28

Baby

- Is about 15 ¾ inches.
- Weighs about 2 ¼ pounds.
- Has the sense of smell.
- Has working tear ducts.

Mama

- To prepare for labor, your body widens the pubic symphysis, the joint connecting the right and left pubic bones.
  - Try a maternity belt or pelvic floor physical therapy if you're having pain, popping, or instability.
- Continued increase in blood volume may lead to anemia or can cause psychiatric medications to be less effective.
  - Reach out to your provider if you think you may need an adjusted prescription. Your third trimester labs will reveal whether you are anemic and need to increase your iron intake.

Extreme Nesting

Strange how sometimes a casual comment can stick in our minds like it was glued there. Dan made one such remark, which has been bugging me ever since. He says I'm starting to nest.

What exactly does he mean by that?

Mulling it over, I find an odd picture comes to mind: it makes me feel like a pregnant bird. I'd like to say a swan, but in all honesty, I feel and probably *look* more like a turkey. Since I don't have a beak or any feathers, I now also feel strangely bare, almost wishing I could grow wings and tack on the missing pieces. Then I could soar around outside and really look the part—collecting twigs, grasses, and leafy things for my nest.

Both the picture and the statement are surprising, though, for as far as I know, I've been preparing for months now. Case in point? The square patches for my darling's citrus-colored quilt are now mostly connected, the felt animal mobile is dangling above her crib, and the pile of baby items in the corner of our bedroom is slowly growing.

So why would he say I'm starting now? Well, I suppose I have gained a new sense of focus over the past few days—an intense drive to purge our tiny mousehole of all things unnecessary. Let's sell it or put it in storage, *ASAP!* The extra chair, the legless table propped against the wall, the folded-up shelf, and the unused desk. All of it must go!

> ⟫⟫ ❀✿❀ ⟪⟪
>
> For ideas on what to gather for your labor, check out A-4h.

But who could blame me? Wouldn't anyone, even non-nesters, do the same? I just can't imagine fitting one more person in our apartment, even if she will only take up twenty inches of space.

It's time to simplify and then maybe purchase a few key items for labor—like aromatherapy, flameless candles, and music. With such a list, I realize it sounds like I'm packing for a romantic getaway. But in a way I suppose it's true—I'll be meeting my little love for the very first time.

Cloudy with a Chance of Sunshine

I reached into the carefully arranged cardboard box and pulled out a slightly padded, white . . . *something*. It didn't look like any of the other washed-and-folded-with-love baby items my mom had gathered and brought with her on her visit—the soft overalls with an elephant patch sewn on the chest, the terry cloth pajamas, and pastel-toned, elastic-bottomed newborn nightgowns—now stacked in tidy towers nearby.

Could this be another cute pregnancy shirt that once draped my mom's belly when I was inside?

I grabbed both ends of this mysterious object and stretched it out and out (and out), like a festive, accordioned garland. There, suspended between my hands, was the biggest, baddest, hugest, largest, most enormous bra I'd ever seen. The cups were so big I think it probably could have doubled as a boat or been repurposed as beanies.

"You can have my old bra," my mom enthused, as the expanse of the thing flopped in front of my face. "It will be perfect for breastfeeding."

Um, what?

The piles of my old baby clothes blurred as my wide eyes pooled up with tears. My little bells will one day fit into these monsters?

"How can I possibly fit into that bra?" I blurted out, throwing it down in shock and horror. The stress of the thought tipped the scales—the first domino to fall in a long line of worries that tumbled out of me.

"I feel so unprepared to have a baby and I don't have a beautifully decorated baby room and I can't remember how to change a diaper—" my ragged words fought with my tears to be heard. "Besides, I don't even know how often to bathe her!"

I sobbed and sniffled.

So, other people will mother alone, don't know where they'll live, or how they'll support their baby, and I'm worried about my breast size and decorating a room? I guess so.

It may seem trivial later, but right then the issue was monumental. In the onslaught, my mother and Dan mobilized—and fast. Both tried to comfort me as I sobbed on the couch, tears streaming down my face, soul like a heavy cloud primed to give the world a good downpour.

Eventually, when my shirt had apparently been watered well enough, the storm subsided. The clouds parted, a ray of sunshine peeked through, and I found myself laughing over how ridiculous it was to cry over all of this.

But of course, that didn't last.

With a shift in the winds of my worries, in rolled the thunderheads, ready to take center stage. Folks, looks like you're in for torrential summer downpours today. Dry and then wet. Don't go anywhere without your umbrella.

Up and down my emotions climbed and plummeted like a barometer, leaving me—and my family—an exhausted, harried mess. This pattern continued until, eventually, there were no more tears to cry.

As I reclined on the couch, feeling lighter, wetter, and infinitely more drained, Dan and my mom thought it appropriate to speak some truth into my soul. *Thank God!* Although I do feel unprepared, they reminded me, we are lucky enough to have the most important things in order: health, food, shelter, and clean water.

Plus, when our little one arrives, she'll have what she really needs: my body to keep her warm, milk for food, our attention to meet her needs, and our love for comfort. Everything else—except for diapers—is secondary and (likely) superfluous.

I just desperately hope that mega-bra falls into the last category.

⇶ LET'S TALK ABOUT IT ⇷

Feeding Your Milk Monster

Congratulations! You've made it to the third trimester. You barely see your toes, are more tired, and you can no longer squeeze through tiny spaces. All these changes do a fabulous job reminding you—your baby is coming and it's time to prepare. So exciting!

It's easy to think that preparing means buying tons of objects. Although it's fun to find bedsheets and cute onesies, let's not forget what your baby is really going to need is milk (lots of it) and your love.

So, breastfeeding or formula?

Getting up to speed on feeding your baby will help decrease the after-birth cluelessness factor. Will you opt for breastmilk, formula, or both? As a reminder, we're not talking about rice cereal or applesauce at this point. Babies only require milk or formula for about the first six months of life (sometimes with additional vitamin D).[1] They don't even need water!

In a perfect world, everyone would be able to exclusively breastfeed for about the first six months of life, and then continue breastfeeding until desired, even up to age two or beyond (for reasons we'll cover shortly).[1-3] However, since we know life is rarely perfect, this is a great time to ask your maternity care provider and care team for information you need to decide how you'll feed your baby. This is especially true if you have medical problems (like diabetes, lupus, or HIV), use illicit drugs or marijuana, are enrolled in a substance use treatment program, smoke cigarettes, drink alcohol regularly, or if you will be restarting medications after birth.[4,5] Certain medications aren't compatible with breastfeeding, but many are, including many of the psychiatric medications.[6]

> ## BREASTFEEDING LINGO
>
> Did you know you've got options when it comes to breastfeeding terminology? You may hear *chestfeeding* or *lactating* as alternatives to *breastfeeding*; *expressing milk* (by a machine) as an alternative to *pumping*; or *human milk* or *mother's milk* as alternatives to *breastmilk*.[10] Use what you prefer, and if the distinction is important to you, be sure to let your maternity care provider know.

Breastfeeding hesitations

While some women can hardly wait to breastfeed, others are hesitant or uninterested. Hesitations can happen for many reasons. Maybe you've struggled with breastfeeding in the past with a baby who didn't latch, had a tongue-tie, or was a preemie. Or perhaps you felt you didn't make enough milk. Be encouraged—if you're open to it, you could still become a breastfeeding guru. Every baby's different, and you've changed since then. You're older and wiser, more experienced, may have more support, and may even be more motivated to make things work.

Also, for those of you who feel like breastfeeding just sounds yucky—it's okay to feel that way. This may be especially true if you've never breastfed or you have a history of sexual trauma. Take heart, breastfeeding may seem way different than you expect when you're in the moment. Some women even decide to express milk via pumping and then give their breastmilk in a bottle. It's hard work but a viable option for the dedicated.

So, breastfeeding or formula? Let's consider the facts to help you make an informed decision, shall we?

Breastfeeding benefits

Breastfeeding comforts your baby and boosts his immunity (like against cancer, colds, ear infections, obesity, and heart disease).[1,7-9] It even decreases his risk of sudden infant death syndrome (SIDS).[1,7-9]

As if that list doesn't make you want to stand in awe of this wonderful design, listen to this: our bodies even change their ingredients and quantity to exactly match our babies' nutritional needs as they grow.

LACTATION CONSULTANTS

A fantastic resource during and after pregnancy, these professionals can help address topics such as prior breastfeeding problems, breastfeeding after breast surgery, feeding twins, breast pain, milk supply, baby's weight gain, baby's latching, and weaning.

For example, when your baby's born, he'll be a virgin eater. So far, your little one's received all his nutrients through the umbilical cord. Now, your baby's got to learn how to suck, swallow, and breathe in a coordinated manner. Solution? Your body makes a concentrated, sticky milk called *colostrum*. By drinking this first, it makes it easier for your milk monster to learn to feed while also getting tons of immune cells needed to promote gut health. *It's food with brains!*

Many haven't heard that breastfeeding has amazing benefits for mommies, too. For example, it decreases your risk of cancers (breast, ovarian, and endometrial), depression, high blood pressure, and diabetes (especially if you had gestational diabetes).[1,7-9] It can even decrease your postpartum bleeding and stress, help you get more sleep, strengthen your immune system, and may help you get back to your prepregnancy weight quicker. *Yes, that's a gorgeous list.*

Formula factors

Formula, on the other hand, gives your baby vital nutrients and calories, but since it's void of live cells, it can't give you both those same glorious immune-boosting benefits. While it can be a lifesaver for certain babies, it may take some trial and error to find a formula your baby tolerates. Part of the challenge is that formula, made from cow or soybean sources, does not contain the enzymes (found in breastmilk) that aid digestion. Also, the cost of formula can add up. Count on spending an average of about $1,500 for formula annually if you go this route.[8]

Parting considerations

As you try to decide where to go from here, it's important to step back and catch a glimpse of the big picture: regardless of which feeding options you choose, the most important things are to love that little milk monster of yours and to feed your darling when he or she is hungry! Whether you decide on human milk, formula, or a combo—release yourself from any judgment over the choice. Every family and situation is different.

Digging Deeper

Deciding how to feed your baby can sure be a process, right? Yes, there are many considerations, and sometimes we can even have a game plan, but then life brings unexpected twists and turns. *The nerve.* For fun, try your luck with the following true/false questions. Hopefully, you'll learn some useful and surprising facts about breastmilk and formula feeding.*

1. Breastfeeding is the best option for everyone. T/F

2. Breastfeeding decreases my chance of diabetes, and breast and ovarian cancer. T/F

3. It's possible to bond with my baby through formula feeding. T/F

4. Formula and breastmilk both offer my baby the same immune benefits. T/F

5. I can breastfeed even if I smoke cigarettes. T/F

6. Some breastfeeding is better than none. T/F

7. Breastfeeding is supposed to hurt. T/F

8. In a perfect world, a baby gets only breastmilk for about the first six months of life. T/F

9. When I go back to work, I have to stop breastfeeding. T/F

10. Feeding a baby with either breastmilk or formula is a huge accomplishment. T/F

* Answers: (1) F, (2) T, (3) T, (4) F, (5) T, (6) T, (7) F, (8) T, (9) F, (10) T

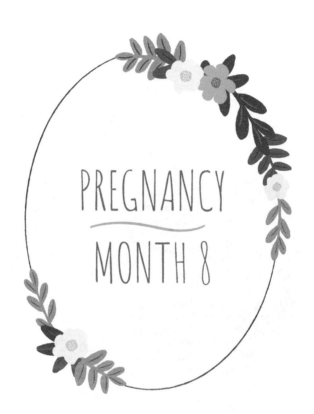

PREGNANCY

MONTH 8

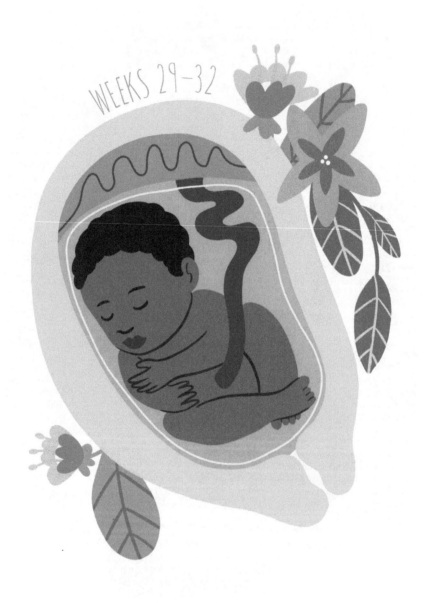

WEEKS 29-32

WEEK 29

Baby

- Is about 15 ½ inches long.
- Weighs about 2 ½ pounds.
- Continues to develop and mature the brain.

Mama

- Because your enlarging uterus pulls your lower spine forward, you may be experiencing back pain.
  - Back exercises and a maternity belt can help.
- Currently and into postpartum, parts of your brain are being restructured to enhance social, caregiving, and baby-bonding skills![1-5] Talk about an upgrade!
  - Be patient with yourself and jot down reminders if you notice temporary changes in your short-term memory.

Gratitude and Grace

There's nothing like the Thanksgiving holiday to knock some sense into a pregnant lady and give her a dose of perspective—possibly with a side of culture shock.

This year, we'd been invited to a gathering in California's Central Valley. When we reached this agricultural hub—after three hours and several much-needed pit stops—we parked in the lined drive of a ranch-style home nestled in the heart of a rural neighborhood. People were gathered in the yard amid bubblegum-pink lantana and trees heavy with ripening oranges.

Of those milling about, many appeared to be farmers, wearing the traditional cowboy boots and jeans—though often with an unexpected urban twist: a punk variation of hairdos with a rainbow assortment of bobs, curls, and spikes. Wow. Mere hours from home may as well have been another world. The main solace here is that black seems to be a popular clothing color for this crowd, and I happened to choose a black dress. *Score.* I smoothed out a wrinkle, hoping it might prove to be a type of camouflage, allowing me—and my expansive belly—to blend in.

Still self-conscious, I walked with Dan up the front path, where we rang the bell and stepped inside. Soon, we struck up a conversation with a few guests nearby. Getting my bearings amid the small talk, I idly watched a toddler weave through the room, picking her way between legs and chairs, all while sucking on a pink skull pacifier. It seems pacifiers come in all sorts of shapes I'd never expected.

As the afternoon continued, though, it quickly became apparent that while our backgrounds and choice in pacifiers may be a bit different, in fundamental ways, we were all the same—hungry, and excited to spend time with old friends and new acquaintances. We could hardly wait to savor the flavors of the traditional turkey dinner—soft slices of meat dripping with gravy next to piles of stuffing, cranberry sauce, and green bean salad. And, of course, the dessert table.

Ah, the dessert table. It's not so easy being a pregnant woman during the holidays, when there is no shortage of delicacies to please the cravings. So, I'd mentally prepped for this. *That's right.* My plan was both easy and brilliant. I'd trick myself into feeling I'm eating dessert to my heart's content simply by nibbling on multiple small helpings throughout the evening. When I got full, I'd stop. Distract myself. Think of anything *but* the creamy pumpkin pie, the fluffy whipping cream, the caramelized pecans on top of the rich sugary slices, and the flaky apple pie à la mode. That's right, I'd think of anything else. Anything but.

Anything else.

Let's see, what else is there to think about? New plan—run. If all else fails, just run.

Unfortunately for me, my strategy quickly proved not only tricky, but surprisingly awkward. Every time I went to the dessert table, the same stocky man was also returning for more. I was there according to plan, and there he was, shoveling slices of pumpkin and pecan onto his plate.

I tried not to make eye contact, hoping he wouldn't notice thanks to my black-dress camouflage. But he did, and eventually he tried to strike up conversation.

"Eating for two?" he asked with a chuckle.

Ha ha, very funny. Why do so many people assume pregnancy is either an excuse for women to eat anything or for others to make remarks? Also, why is this stranger looking at what I'm eating anyway? What I really wanted to say was, "Well, we apparently know why I'm at the table, but why are you?"

Instead, I just smiled and walked away, leaving my snippy remarks unsaid. It's Thanksgiving, after all. Might as well focus on all the blessings—like yummy food, good company, and my growing baby.

Ode to the Female Body

Sometimes, the ordinary can become extraordinary. This time, in a typical Sunday church service, I saw something that prompted a reminder and revelation. There, one pew in front of me, a petite woman hoisted up her son—a comparatively monstrous first grader—while belting out the words of a praise song.

I became so intrigued by the extraordinary sight before me, I'm afraid I lost all track of time and the matters at hand. I glued my gaze on the fascinating scene, and while I continued to sing along with the familiar melody, I did so on autopilot, my mind humming with questions.

For one, how was her son not deaf by now? And two, would she crumble before me? When was she going to drop the kid? After all, she didn't look particularly strong and nor was he small. It seemed just a matter of time.

Ah, I know! It must be her hips allowing her to accomplish this surprising feat. All she'd had to do was stick one out, prop him on her makeshift shelf, and—ta-da!—he was securely suspended, singing beside her, cheek to cheek.

Up to this point, women's hips have just fallen into my mental category labeled *curves*. They're the things guys like and women criticize—the place where stretch marks appear, where jeans never fit quite right. But I realize now that's so superficial. Hips are about functionality. They support, hide, accentuate, and are a vital tool for activity and adventure. Even now, in my case, they cradle my baby before her debut.

And what other body parts might be taken for granted? The vagina, perhaps, unassumingly tucked in between the labia and cervix. This poor, forgotten little soul has got to be one of our most underappreciated anatomical parts, and women often don't even know how to refer to it without blushing. It has more nicknames than you could rattle off in a breath—hoo-ha, downstairs, vajayjay, penis flytrap—and yet, it has the capacity to allow women to explore their sexuality and express love. In ways, it serves as a secret sanctuary: a sacred space for connection and intimacy. And in many cases, it also serves as a passageway—the avenue by which a baby is introduced to his mother and her world.

I surfaced from this reverie long enough to note that though the modern Madonna and her boy in front of me swayed in time with the music, her boy hadn't wobbled even the slightest. It truly is a wonder, and, I must admit, a bit disappointing.

Hoping a little more time would do the trick, my thoughts continued. How incredible that during and after pregnancy, a woman's breasts can undergo such a gutsy transformation, not just in size or shape, but also in the mind's eye. Our breasts—which we pad, push up, or secure down, which we measure in cups and obsessively wish were bigger, smaller, higher, or fuller—can, in motherhood, become an accepted ally. For in motherhood, the focus becomes less on their form and more on their function. They are the comforting softness upon which our little darling rests over our hearts, secured by our embrace, and, if we wish, the nourishing source of sustenance for our baby's growing body.

As we took our seats, the last guitar chord ringing through our midst, I found my awe over the female body—incredible, functional, and uniquely designed to live and love—drifted into curiosity. How's a mother supposed to have her body to herself while filling so many needs and functions? How does a mother thrive and not get burned out being at her family's core? What's the secret to being as sturdy as this woman one pew over?

I sure don't know. Still, as I sat there, attempting to realign my focus, I knew I was resolved to find out.

⇶ LET'S TALK ABOUT IT ⇷

Nurturing Your Spiritual Self

People are like stained-glass windows. They sparkle and shine when the sun is out, but when the darkness sets in, their beauty is revealed only if there is a light from within.
—Elisabeth Kübler-Ross

During this incredible journey of transformation, we mamas experience a lot, right? Amid the changes, tapping into your spiritual self can be a wonderful way to help adjust. So, what is this spiritual self? It's that precious, unseen part of you, deeply yearning for meaning. We all have a drive to distill meaning from the whirlwind world around us, and we embrace different methods for doing so.

Defining spirituality

Now, when it comes to spirituality, we're not necessarily talking about religion. Spirituality crosses all cultures and societies and relates to that which affects your spirit—anything that offers you meaning, hope, and purpose in life.[6,7] This can include people you love, a sacred deity you worship, nature that awes you, music that moves you, and art or even a sport that captivates you.

To live in touch with the spirit has tremendous benefits. For example, it can improve your quality of life and ability to cope, decrease stress and pain levels, slow disease progression, and even bring emotional and physical healing.[6-10] Many religious or spiritual people have been found to experience less anxiety, depression, suicidality, and substance abuse, and, get this—they even live longer despite serious health problems—when they regularly attended religious services.[7,11-13] In essence, even amid monotony, stress, difficulties, illness, and suffering, spirituality allows you to look beyond the superficial and find hope, comfort, and peace. We all can benefit from this—in pregnancy and beyond. Yes, even when blowout poops hit the fan, you can look beyond and cope!

Tending your spirit

There are all sorts of lovely ways to tend and care for your spirit. Ultimately, it all relates to what you find meaningful and what you long for. In which direction(s) do you feel pulled? Some mamas make it a point to get out in nature more, spend time with family, develop a meditation practice, pray more, play an instrument, learn Pilates or yoga, or listen to spiritual podcasts or music. Others of you may find yourself drawn to getting involved in a faith community or exploring your family's religion.

Whichever route you find for spiritual practice, as you invest in your spiritual self and cultivate this important aspect of self-care, remember this

Share with your maternity care provider if you have any spiritual or religious beliefs that influence your healthcare wishes (such as blood transfusion, birth control, labor, or postpartum practices).

amazing fact—doing so not only rewards you but also your family and friends. The benefits of being spiritually centered can pour out and overflow to those around you, especially your little one(s). Before you know it, your precious babe will get to learn from you firsthand how to approach, experience, and navigate life with meaning and purpose.

Digging Deeper

Let's take a moment and ponder your spiritual self and how you can nurture this beautiful part of you. Go ahead and grab a refreshing cup of hot or iced tea and find a quiet spot to sit and pause. *Breathe.* Isn't it so nice to sit for a moment in stillness? Now, consider your answers to the questions below. If applicable, feel free to explore these with a partner or loved one for added richness.

» What brings your life meaning?

» What core values do you live by?

» Are there any spiritual beliefs that help you cope?

» What spiritual needs do you have now?

» How might you start incorporating activities into your life to bolster your spirit?

» Do you believe there is a higher power?

» Do you have any core values or faith beliefs you'd like to pass on to your baby? If so, what are they?

WEEK 30

Baby

- Is about 16 inches long.
- Weighs about 3 pounds.
- Sleeps often.
- Makes blood cells in the bone marrow.

Mama

- Protective immune cells are now efficiently transferred to your baby through the umbilical cord.
  - Ask your maternity care provider about the recommended Tdap vaccine offering protection against pertussis (whooping cough) and more.[1-4]

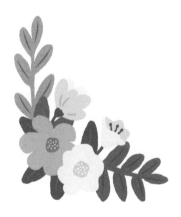

When Are You Due?

I'm starting to realize pregnancy is much too welcoming an invitation to connect with womankind. Is it the round belly that has a special allure? Or the waddle that puts others at ease? While I'm sure they mean well, and at times I don't mind, I do hope I can soon figure out a graceful exit for those moments when I just don't feel like chatting; for an introvert like me, constant conversations get exhausting.

Part of the trouble is an unexpected conversation can come from anywhere—at the gas station, the frozen food aisle, or the crosswalk. In the strangest or most ordinary of times, women materialize and make their approach. They strike up conversation, carefully opening with a line of questions to break the ice—questions women seem to run through as though marking them off a mental checklist.

"When are you due?" asks the bank teller, opening with the typical line.

"February fifth," I respond, too weary of these conversations to add a smile.

"Is this your first?"

"Why yes, it is." I pass along my ID, willing her to not inquire further. She does.

"Do you know what you are having?"

"A girl," I answer, glancing down at the plastic card in her hands. How does everyone know how to do this inquisition? I must have missed the memo.

"Oh that's wonderful," she exclaimed. "A little girl, and your due date's around the corner. That reminds me when my little Suzie was born. Boy, did she hardly sleep for the first three years. But those were the days . . ."

She trailed off, staring into the air behind me. When she transitioned from reminiscence to reality, she added, "Do you have a name picked out?" It's the last of the main questions, the grand finale of the pregnancy conversation that seems to always start with the due date.

"Still playing around with names," I muttered. Because—who knows?—maybe we'll change our minds.

"I see," she said, with a conspiratorial grin. "You still have time."

She handed back my ID, unchecked.

And that was just one in a long line of impromptu discussions that often end with me becoming privy to all sorts of personal details of someone else's pregnancy. It's as if simply by being pregnant, I've signed up to become a keeper of stories at all odd hours of the day.

Due to this completely involuntary sleuthing, I now know the checkout lady's baby just turned thirty-one, the dental hygienist had a surprisingly easy labor, and, according to the woman at the crosswalk, I should definitely sleep with my baby once she's born.

And they all start with the same questions.

It's not that the question list is exhaustive, nor is the heart behind them anything other than genuine excitement and celebration—it's just that sometimes I don't feel like interacting with people or talking about pregnancy. It isn't my sole identity, you know. I do have other things to talk about.

I haven't yet figured out how to stop the scenario entirely, but I have discovered a sort of bypass. If I'm really feeling antisocial at the first question, I cleverly give a hurried synopsis, like: "I'm due in February with my first child—a little girl."

There, take that!

The sweet lady then beams as if she's been let in on a big secret, and I'm perfectly thrilled. She completely forgot about that last, unanswered question. Before she realizes I've pulled a fast one on her, I end the exchange with as much grace as I can manage and make a beeline for the door.

Am I in There, Somewhere?

I've been pregnant for 30 weeks now. That's quite a long time, especially if I think of it as 210 days, or even 5,040 hours. As I glance at my Humpty-Dumpty shadow skimming the sidewalk, I realize I sometimes can't even remember who I was those 302,400 minutes ago.

I study an old picture of myself from last year, holding up a chocolate pie with a big smile—a snapshot of a time when things were simpler, more carefree. I could go from event to event and not get completely exhausted. I could tie my shoes, flop onto the bed facedown, and hug Dan without feeling like a muffin. I could exercise without getting so breathless and could even climb stairs without feeling like I was hauling the earth behind me. It was a time when, after a night's sleep, I'd wake up rested. Nausea was a rarity, and heartburn was a medical diagnosis I helped others with—not something that made me feel like a camp stove. Back then, I hunted down scientific articles like a bloodhound and pored over women's health topics with the kind of avid attention others might have for popular magazines.

Where is that Meshi? I miss her. Will we ever meet again?

Is she in there somewhere?

And yet, at the same time, I'm getting excited to approach the day I get to meet my little baby. I'm like a child standing on tippy-top-toes in front of a gumball machine, ready to taste and see the assortment of marvelous colors before me. Who is this little person kicking, moving, and playing inside of me? What's she like? Will her name, meaning *bright light* and *life*, fit her personality?

During this season of anticipation and change, I wonder at the process of transformation not just in myself, but in the little things around me. Does a purple peony realize her day-to-day growth from a seed? Does she ever find the process of becoming and blossoming is bothersome? How does it feel, on that glorious day, when she unfolds her soft petals and opens her yellow core wide, sharing her beauty with the world around?

Though my own space to bloom will be more secluded, I hope the next 10 weeks will help me prepare for it—growing in me the ability to be mesmerized by all that my baby is, from her first breath.

⇒⇒⇒ LET'S TALK ABOUT IT ⇐⇐⇐

Being and Becoming

> *What the caterpillar calls the end of the world,*
> *the master calls a butterfly.*
> —RICHARD BACH

Dear friend, you may remember earlier we used the analogy of a chrysalis to describe pregnancy and your preparation for your baby's arrival. This is a unique time centered around transformation, preparing you for something—someone—new. Although looking forward to what's ahead and new can be super exciting, it can also be bittersweet.

Letting go

Anytime you accept newness, you also let go of something in your present. So, if in this process of becoming a mommy you feel some sadness and grieving, let yourself be okay with that. You don't have to be happy with all the changes pregnancy and motherhood bring. You may be letting go of relationships, habits, your priorities, where you work, your job title, or even where you live. In a way, grieving is the process of giving honor to how these things served you to this point, for better or worse. They may have given us purpose or helped us pass time, cope with life, learn, or even have fun. So, pause and think about how you're doing and what you're feeling.

There will also be times as a mother when you grieve and miss elements of your prepregnancy life. Please don't feel guilty about this. The idea that in motherhood all things are perpetually blissful and wondrous is a myth![5,6] Although motherhood has *so* many precious, funny, and lovely moments, these are mixed in with poop, sleepless nights, crying, and more poop. Who in their right mind would enjoy all of that? Remember, you can be a wonderful mother even if you don't love poop, and even if you miss parts of your prior life or self. Not being thrilled with all aspects of motherhood doesn't mean you're a bad mother or that there's something wrong with you.[5] It also doesn't mean you don't love your child. It just means parenting is hard.

As you consider these changes in your life, go ahead, acknowledge sadness for what is past or passing. Grab a box of tissues, find a safe space, and give yourself permission to cry. Tears can lighten the soul.

Looking ahead

And when you are ready, I'd also invite you to take a few moments to be curious about what amazing discoveries lie before you as well. Soon, you'll see new expressions of yourself, discover new parts of yourself, experience new ways of life, and do new things you never thought you'd do. Allow yourself the freedom of laughter or tears. While processing these changes, don't hesitate to reach out—sharing the joy and anticipation with a friend and confidante, or seeking advice or comfort from your support people or therapist. We are stronger together.

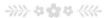

If, during this soul-searching, you find that your medications for mental health conditions are less effective, be sure to let your mental health or maternity care provider know. Are you feeling more sad, uninterested in what you normally enjoy, worried, or irritable? Are you experiencing more pronounced bipolar mood swings? Sometimes medication doses need to be increased in the last few months of pregnancy because of your increasing blood volume.

Digging Deeper

Transformation in a chrysalis is no small feat. What looks like a chill vacation from the outside is truly brimming with change. Did you know that before a butterfly can test out its new wings, it must first fight, struggle, and wriggle out to freedom? Thinking now about your own metamorphosis, pause for a moment. Take three or more deep breaths. *Really*. Then, try the following fill-in-the-blank reflection activity, either by yourself or with a loved one, using it as a springboard for thought and conversation. Enjoy!

- » I am most excited about _____
- » I am nervous about _____
- » I am looking forward to _____
- » I am scared about _____
- » I am sad about _____
- » I am letting go of _____
- » I am holding on to _____
- » I am hopeful that _____

WEEK 31

Baby

- Is about 16 ½ inches long.
- Weighs about 3 ¼ pounds.
- Now is able to control body temperature.
- Is getting chubbier—more roundness to cuddle!

Mama

- You may have weakened pelvic floor muscles from hormonal changes and a growing belly. Urinary stress incontinence (leaking urine when you laugh, sneeze, or cough) is common.
  - Check with your maternity care provider to see if Kegels could help you (A-3c).
- Perhaps you are noticing the instinct to get your surroundings ready for the big arrival.

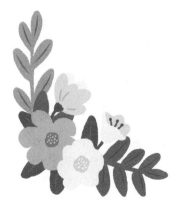

The Lucky Ones

Sometimes, I call my grandmother, who now lives in Oregon, eager to catch up and to tell her I miss her. I love to update her on our life in exchange for tabloid gossip, lottery jackpot totals, inspiring Sunday sermons, controversial questions, and daily house-project mishaps. Feeling her void today, I picked up the phone, dialed, and scooched my pregnant self against a pillow in preparation for a long, meaningful, and entertaining conversation. After all, this is the woman who called my husband "sexy" when he tried on a fitted biking shirt someone gifted him one Christmas.

I waited for the familiar prerecorded, "Leave a message after the beeeep," and then began leaving my customarily long message intended to give her the time needed to pick up. To my delight, *Anya* (mother), as everyone calls her now, wasn't out chopping down a tree, hauling a load of bricks, or returning a borrowed cart from the nearby grocery store—yes, all of which have happened before.

"Hello—hello?" Her warm voice was hurried, laced with the worry she might have missed me.

"*Kezi csokolom* (I kiss your hand)," I answer with a smile, using the respectful greeting all good Hungarian children use with their elders.

I soon gave a rundown of the most recent events in life and pregnancy, which prompted my grandmother to share of her younger years and the start of her own family. Sure, I've heard this story a million times, but like any juicy retelling, I can never get tired of it.

About seventy years ago, as a lively seventeen-year-old with waist-long, thick braids, she fled Hungary with her mother and brother to escape the terrors brought by the Soviet Army during World War II. They first immigrated to the neighboring country of Austria, saying goodbye to all they knew and loved, including her dear father, a military commander who had vowed to protect his homeland at all costs.

A hard and dangerous journey, it also held surprising and humorous moments. Like when they were in the forests just within the borders of Hungary, and Anya used snow to wash her hair. She giggles at the memory of how tangled it became and how, seeing her struggle with the resulting knots, some Hungarian soldiers camping nearby stopped to help her untangle her tresses.

But wait, weren't they supposed to be busy with other matters?

Re-fluffing the pillow behind me, I listened as she reminisced about meeting my grandfather, Lajos, a few years later while in Germany. He was a suave, yet fiery, mustachioed Hungarian gentleman, twenty years her senior. Together they, with other expatriates, often twirled and danced until dawn, during a season in which he worked at the immigration office, and she endeavored to piece together a home out of practically nothing. For lack of space in their tiny studio, they hung all sorts of things—from shoes to wet laundry—and shared a small, twin-size bed, which did not prove to be problematic, because they were busy making love throughout the night, anyway.

"I was much younger than you were when I got pregnant," she continued. "Nineteen—"

Wow, and I barely feel ready now!

"—and I was a refugee. It was a time when people needed to be resourceful, and so we made diapers out of bedsheets and gleaned potatoes from hospitable farmers. Many women chose to deliver their babies at home because hospital infection control was so terrible. So, the midwives sterilized instruments in boiling water and helped pregnant women labor while fathers paced the floor outside."

I told her we, too, were hoping to have a midwife at the hospital delivery, but Dan would be sticking right by my side through it. In fact, let's hope our childbirth class has taught him a thing or two on how to actively support me during labor. *There's no way this fellow's getting off that easy.*

"Why should he be there?" she asked, completely confused. "When I had my babies, we thought it was a woman's business."

Unfathomable.

As we laughed over our differences in childbearing preferences, I wondered if we would have felt the same way had we slipped into each other's timeline.

Promising to call her soon, I said my goodbyes and hung up the phone. It's amazing how fondly Anya remembered her refugee days. She and my grandfather were in love, they had a healthy baby girl, and they counted themselves the lucky ones. They were alive, didn't have to worry about air raids, and that's all that mattered. And it's partly because of her courage, perseverance, and positive outlook that I am granted the luxury to prepare for my little baby under such different circumstances.

Making a Splash

As a high schooler looking for free entertainment in the Pacific North-west, I loved driving through puddles on the side of the road. A girl's got to do what a girl's got to do when everything's wet—all the time. I'd steer our old mammoth station wagon to my nominated puddle and giggle when the car slows as the wheels wade through the liquid resistance.

One particular puddle I'll never forget. On my way home from downtown Eugene, I had turned onto a main street up a steep, ever-green-lined hill. I passed the landmark corner store, not suspecting the beauty I'd glimpse just beyond it.

Then, there it was, glistening before me. The most perfect puddle I'd ever seen. It was long. It was deep. And it was waiting there, just for me. My eyes grew wide with excitement, and I stepped on the gas. I sped up, gaze locked on my target, and steered my big beast of a vehicle over toward the edge of the street.

"Woohooooo!" I squealed, marveling at the massive tidal wave crashing onto the sidewalk. *That was incredible! World, did you see that?*

Sure enough, someone did. From a front-row seat, no less. As I drove past and up the hill, I looked back in my rearview mirror to etch the size of that puddle in my mind's eye for all eternity. But what I saw instead was a soaked bystander who had been caught in the torrent of my shim-mering creation. Scowling in her tan trench coat, she dripped water from every inch of fabric.

Oops! Too embarrassed to turn back and apologize, I vowed to look more carefully the next time and sheepishly continued up the hill, but-terflies in my stomach and a lump in my throat.

—✿—

I didn't know at the time that years later, I, too, would find myself wet. Though not from water, nor from a puddle. Nope, far worse. Sure, I knew that in pregnancy, pelvic floor muscles can weaken, but did I expect it? No. Had I been doing my pelvic floor exercises to prevent it? It has definitely *not* been a priority. Which leads to this memorable moment in our sex life: an innocent cough (a symptom of a minor cold) and a stream as effortless as my precious, man-made tidal wave years prior.

"I always thought—" Dan confessed "—our child would pee on our bed before you would."

Super embarrassing.

I suppose, though, what goes around comes around. We could only laugh at what has proven to be yet another weird moment in pregnancy. Puddles in my bed in Northern California? Well, this certainly isn't the Northwest, but it is pregnancy.

⋙ LET'S TALK ABOUT IT ⋘

Your Pelvic Floor

Ah yes, our dear pelvic floor. It's so important for daily functioning, and yet amazingly, most of us don't even understand what and where it is. Let's shed some light on this mystery, shall we?

Essentially, let's think of your pelvic floor as a basket of layered muscles, fascias, and ligaments spanning your pubic bones and tail-bone.[1,2] Through continuous (yet typically unnoticed) coordinated muscle contractions and relaxation, the pelvic floor supports the organs in your pelvis and abdomen so they can function properly, allowing you to soar through life.[2] The pelvic floor also plays a vital role in childbirth and your sex life.[2] Yep, it's got an impressive resume.

While a well-functioning pelvic floor provides us great benefits, a dysfunctional one (due to weakness, tightness, or injury) can cause a broad range of problems such as those highlighted here.[2,3] Although we'd all rather focus on other things, one in three of us ladies will develop pelvic floor dysfunction sometime in our life—whether in pregnancy, postpartum, or even in menopause.[4,5]

PELVIC FLOOR DYSFUNCTION

Symptoms include urinary incontinence, fecal incontinence or constipation, pelvic pain (either during sex, or not), pelvic organ prolapse, and pelvic girdle pain.

If you are noticing any symptoms of pelvic floor dysfunction, the good news is there are countless nonsurgical options to help—including deep breathing (a vital element), pelvic floor therapy (likely involving manipulation of internal muscles or biofeedback), and even pessaries.[2,6-8] Surgery is, of course, a last-resort option, while catching it early and using preventative maintenance is an excellent way to go.

Lifelong pelvic floor health

So how can we care for this beautiful part of our bodies? Well, having a healthy pelvic floor involves these key ingredients: regular physical activity, keeping your weight healthy for your height, using correct sitting and standing postures, avoiding repetitive heavy lifting, drinking plenty of water throughout the day, practicing deep breathing, and avoiding constipation.[2,8,9] If you're noticing problems, get timely help (with neglect, it will only get worse), and if you've been given pelvic floor exercises, be sure to follow through with those.

Some mamas or mamas-to-be even proactively decide to go to a pelvic floor physical therapist in pregnancy and postpartum. In pregnancy, these therapists can address your various concerns, such as preventing or treating urinary incontinence, treating symphysis pubis pain—and get this—they can even help you learn how to push properly for labor![7,9,*] Postpartum, you may especially want to consider an evaluation if you had a vaginal delivery with vacuum or forceps or had a large baby, since pelvic floor dysfunction is more common in these cases.[2,8,10]

---

* Kathy Kates, FNP-BC, personal communication, June 19, 2021

Bottom line? You have a fancy tapestry of muscles in and around your pelvic floor. Take care of them, and if you notice any issues, seek out a careful assessment by a skilled healthcare professional. It will spare you unnecessary suffering and help you enjoy your life and baby more freely. You go, mama!

Digging Deeper

Are you ready to better understand your incredible pelvis with all its wonders? Find the pelvic floor in month seven's illustration of mama and her baby, and then flip over to A-3 & 4 for:

» More illustrations of the pelvis and pelvic floor (A-3c);

» Information on pelvic floor concerns, such as stress and urge incontinence, and pelvic pain (A-3c); and

» Instructions for perineal massage, an effective way to protect your perineum from labor trauma and chronic perineal pain after delivery (A-4f).

WEEK 32

Baby

- Is about 17 inches long.
- Weighs about 3 ¾ pounds.
- May hiccup, surprising mama with pulsatile movements in her belly.
- Drinks about two cups of amniotic fluid a day, preparing the gut and urinary system for newborn life.

Mama

- Physical intimacy often occurs less frequently, since it becomes more challenging.
  - Try different positions and get creative with ways to be intimate.

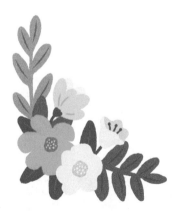

Life Jacket for Two?

Like many pregnant mamas, I've been trying to imagine what to dress my new bundle in for the ride home. You know, *the* perfect outfit that will caress her tiny belly and touch her soft arms and legs for the very first time. For that glorious day, it's got to be unique as a sunrise, special as a good friend, cute as a bunny, and comfortable as a good pair of slippers—not to mention, foolproof for a new mother. *Am I being unreasonable?*

It just so happens, my mother found *the* little, blue, button-down sweater romper in which she dressed me for my trip home from the hospital. She rummaged through old storage boxes, found the treasured item, and removed the musty smell by washing it several times before drying it in the sunshine. And now, over the phone, I'm told it's as good as new, ready to be shipped over and passed on for my own baby's ride home.

It's ready for *my* baby's ride home? *What?* I never even asked my mom for outfit ideas, let alone put in a request for my old one. I don't need any help picking out something special or want any pressure to dress her in anything specific, thank you very much.

Gripping the phone by my ear, I was silent for a moment, but not long enough to hide my annoyance. "I don't need a blue snowsuit for California weather." *On top of that, it's blue! Everyone must have thought I was a boy when they first laid eyes on me.*

"Oh, okay sweetie," she responded quietly. "It was just an idea."

Well, now I've done it. I hurt my mom. I didn't mean to, but I didn't wait long enough to calm down.

"Can you send me a picture of it so I can see what it looks like?" I mustered, trying to offset my earlier snappiness.

"Of course," she said, grace infusing the words.

I thanked her, we hung up, and I let my pregnant belly sink me into our old living room couch. *Good one, Meshi.* What's wrong with me? Why am I so frustrated—over a blue romper, no less? It seems so extreme.

I put up my feet, rested my hands on my convenient belly of a table, and wrinkled my brow in thought. Perhaps the romper represents something greater. On the one hand, boy am I grateful to have a mother this supportive and involved. What a gift she is to me! And yet, on the other hand, sometimes I don't feel like I have enough room to breathe. I don't always want to show off my growing belly or update her on my baby's every movement. It's as if I've lost all sense of privacy and space. My mother has been looking forward to this for so long, and all that energy and love is like a great cascade of water crashing down over me. I fear I might drown or be washed away in Class IV rapids.

Anyone have a lifeboat or life jacket to spare?

If I Could Bear It

As I consider the upcoming birth of my baby, I can't help but wonder if there is a better alternative to a vaginal or surgical delivery. *There have got to be other options, right?*

My inquiring mind propelled me on a little research expedition to explore the ways of the animal kingdom. Sure, it might not be applicable for me, but sometimes my curiosity can't help itself.

Much to my surprise, I found some animals have undeniably improved upon the human experience when it comes to pregnancy and birth. Take the seahorse, for example. Did you know among seahorses, the males are the ones who get pregnant and give birth? Granted, it's a bit of a cop-out since the female dumps the eggs into a small tail pouch of his, but still. It's nice to see males sharing in the load of reproduction beyond just squirting forth a little sperm. And for the record, I wouldn't mind having a cute pouch of my own where my little seahorses could sit and simply spill out when they were ready. To think, thousands of minuscule babies would float around me in the sea like sprinkled stardust.

If you can't pawn off labor to your partner, there's another great option to consider. Turns out, it was long believed that black bears give birth while hibernating. That's right, the female rests for months before labor and then delivers while in ultra-deep sleep mode. She doesn't even bat an eyelash.

While this is now under debate, what I wouldn't give to find my cubs nestled against my fur after a snooze! No need for surgical incisions, to feel the pain of contractions, or to be aware that the precious vagina has stretched far more than I could ever care to consider. Instead, I'd just be surrounded by soft adorableness after a simple, beautiful, and effortless birth. *Sign me up, please!*

Why isn't this the way nature intended?

⟫⟫ LET'S TALK ABOUT IT ⟪⟪

Vaginal Births, Cesarean Births, and VBACs

Well, friend, by now you must be thinking more about evacuating this little one. Although we can't know whether your baby will decide to make his or her grand entrance exactly on the estimated due date, the goal is to stay pregnant until at least 37–38 weeks, so your baby is more mature (considered *early term*), and even better, until 39 weeks (considered *full term*). Certain medical or obstetric complications may warrant delivering your baby sooner, but that's the exception rather than the norm.

So relax, sit back, and let's help you prepare for what's to come, specifically by covering the pros and cons of a vaginal delivery and Cesarean birth. After all, the method of delivery has both short- and long-term implications for you, your baby, and future pregnancies. At first blush, some may think a Cesarean birth is by far the preferable option. It seems easier, and if it's a planned one, you get to "save the date." However, as you'll see, there are some important considerations that make this choice not quite so simple.

Vaginal delivery pros and cons

Did you know that for most women and babies, a vaginal delivery is the safer option? For one, this route avoids major abdominal surgery. Moreover, when your little one travels through your vaginal canal, he is exposed to a beautiful assortment of bacteria (*vaginal flora*) that enhances fetal gut health and may decrease his risk of breathing problems, asthma, and even allergies.[1-3]

True, vaginal deliveries do have several drawbacks that are more likely than with Cesarean births. These include an increased chance of pain or tearing in the vaginal area, pelvic floor weakness (sometimes with urinary or fecal leakage), as well as certain injuries to your baby's bones or nerves.[4] The good news is most of these, if they do occur at all, are usually minor and temporary.

Cesarean birth pros and cons

Despite the awesome benefits of a vaginal delivery, the national Cesarean birth average is currently quite high—at about one in three women.[5] Yes, Cesarean births are sometimes necessary (like with placenta previa), and they can be lifesaving. For those of us in this position, let's be grateful we live in a time when we have this option. Often, though, many women undergo Cesarean births unnecessarily (more on this soon).

While women with Cesarean births are less likely to deal with the cons listed earlier for a vaginal delivery, they likely will have more difficult postpartum recoveries and longer hospital stays. A Cesarean birth exposes a woman to a higher chance of infection, hemorrhage, blood clots, injury to nearby organs, and emergency hysterectomies.[4,5] With this method, babies also miss out on all the fantastic benefits from the vaginal flora mentioned earlier.

Cesarean births can also cause future issues, like pelvic pain and *adhesions* (when two normally separate tissues stick together).[4,5] They can even affect future pregnancies by increasing the chance of *uterine rupture* (the scar area breaking) and additional scar tissue formation along the incision site with each Cesarean birth.[4,5] The latter can make it harder for future placentas to attach properly (called *placenta previa* or *accreta*), which can negatively affect your baby's growth and development.[4,5]

> *⁓⟫⟩ ✿ ✿ ✿ ⟨⟨⁓*
>
> Time to start preparing for that special day! Check out A-4a for more on how to prepare and what to expect, A-4h for notes on packing your hospital bag, and A-4g for help creating a birth plan (wish list).

Why are Cesarean births so common, then?

Despite these concerns, Cesarean births continue to occur more frequently than necessary because women are not given adequate time to labor, are told they need the surgery because they have a "big baby," or they are just not given enough prenatal information about the option of trying for a *vaginal birth after C-section* (*VBAC*).[6,7] Appalling as it is, studies have shown that even institutional racism and biases have led to Black pregnant mamas getting more Cesarean births than white mamas.[8]

So, if you're hoping for a vaginal birth, it's important for you to know that your chance of Cesarean birth is heavily influenced by your birthing location and maternity care providers. Be proactive! Find out what your anticipated birthing location's rates are by asking your maternity care provider or by looking it up online (using research organizations like the Leapfrog Group). The goal is to only get a Cesarean birth if it's truly needed.

VBACs

For those of you who've had a Cesarean birth before, you may be surprised to hear that a vaginal delivery may still be an option for you. Talk to your maternity care provider if you're interested in trying for a vaginal delivery. It's worth the conversation. Although research supports VBACs, you may still have a hard time finding a birthing location that offers it, since it can take time for maternity care practices to catch up. Don't give up! Unless you're in an emergency, you've got time to look at your options.

With VBACs, the hospital or birth center's main concern is the ability to do an emergency Cesarean birth in the rare chance of uterine rupture. As long as it's been 18 to 24 months since your last birth and you've had a *low transverse* (side-to-side) or *low vertical* (up-and-down) type of incision, your risk will be less than 1%.[9,10] VBAC would not be a safe option for you if you've had a prior uterine rupture or if you've had other types of uterine incisions (since these rupture easier).[9] The great news is, the more successful VBACs you've had, the rarer uterine rupture is.

So, the bottom line? If you are a first-time mama and can avoid an unnecessary Cesarean birth—go for it! Make sure your maternity care provider feels the same way and works in a practice that has low Cesarean birth rates (the gold standard is 23.9% for low-risk women).[11,12] Doing so will make it easier on yourself, your baby, and any future pregnancies. If you've had a prior Cesarean birth, you may have the option of trying for a vaginal delivery. As always, speak up and ask questions to help you make those important, informed decisions.[10] And remember, you've got this!

Digging Deeper

The appendix includes resources for you if you are interested in decreasing your chance of Cesarean birth (A-4c) or enhancing your Cesarean birth experience (A-4d). For tips on setting yourself up for a wonderful vaginal delivery experience, check out A-4a. Below, you'll also find a list of various questions on the topic that you can ask your maternity care provider. These have been adapted from the Childbirth Connection website.[13]

» What is the reason you recommend I get a Cesarean birth? How will it benefit my baby and me?

» What are the risks to my baby and myself if I have a Cesarean birth? How likely are they?

» What are the possible benefits of a vaginal birth?

» If I continue with my plan for a vaginal birth, what problems might occur and how likely are they? Could I still run into these problems with a Cesarean birth?

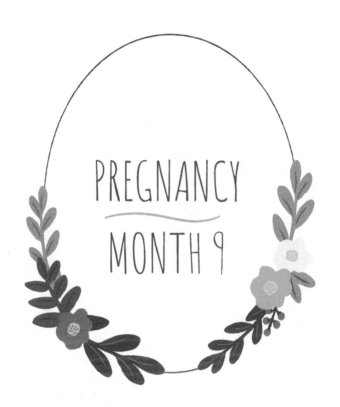

PREGNANCY

MONTH 9

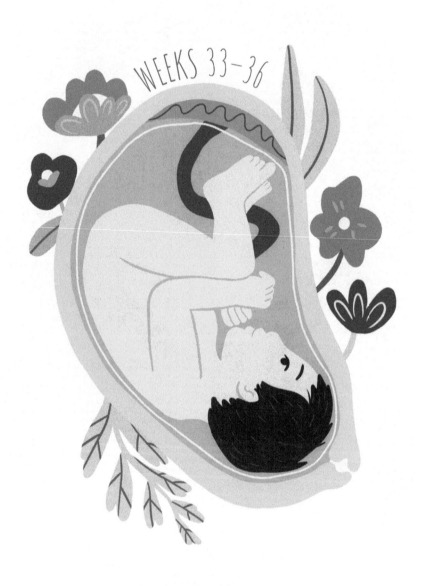

WEEK 33

Baby
- Is about 17 ¼ inches long.
- Weighs about 4 ¼ pounds.
- Can digest milk and absorb nutrients.

Mama
- Exhaustion is super common.
- Work likely interests you less.
- You may have more heartburn due to—you guessed it—your growing belly.
  - Talk to your provider if an over-the-counter antacid, like Tums, isn't doing the trick anymore.

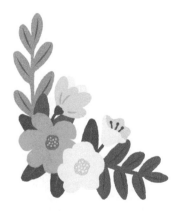

Friends Are Like Hot Soup

Friends are like bras: close to your heart
and there for support.
—ANONYMOUS

There is nothing like a hearty meal, the warmth of friendship, and the compassionate sharing of wisdom to warm one up on a cold night. Amid the chill of a December breeze, I stepped out our front door and began the short walk to my friend's place a few houses down, accompanied by the twinkle of Christmas lights strung along our picket fence.

A few friends, who also work in the medical field and live in the area, had planned an intimate gathering in honor of my growing baby girl. The evening promised to be a time of good company, a homemade dinner, and a chance to glean insights from a midwife and two family physicians, each experienced in delivering babies. Count me in!

As I neared the house, I could already see Gwen, the midwife, through her window, her short, blond ringlets bouncing as she washed mugs and warmed tea for our special evening. Standing in the cheery glow of her porch lights, I didn't have to wait long before Veronica (a family physician and my other neighbor) opened the door wide with a smile. She ushered me in with her typical bubbly excitement and a big, welcoming hug. Inside, I took in the sight of the homey decorations and the joyful faces as Elise, the other family physician, set the table.

Being among good friends is a balm for the soul.

After the soup was done simmering, the bread was warmed, and our hunger was thoroughly piqued, we gathered at the dinner table to enjoy a perfect winter feast. Spoonful by spoonful, I let the hearty, tortellini soup and the hot, buttered sourdough warm me from the inside out. Pushing away the thought of seconds, since my appetite was far greater than the space in my stomach, I contented myself with the plan to get the recipe. With each bite, it's as if I had swallowed winter around me—and I was sure I'd be ready for more soon.

Finished with dinner, while apple tarts baked in the oven, we made our way to the living room and sank into plush couch cushions around the colorful, ornament-filled Christmas tree. I scanned my friends' faces, eager to receive their wisdom. *Okay, ladies, tell me: How the hell am I supposed to survive birth and motherhood?* And that evening, that they did. My friends spoiled me with all sorts of useful gifts of wisdom—advice I basked in, trying to tuck every word and thought into my memory before it flew away.

Veronica began by sharing what she herself received from a close friend when she was with child: "There is a profound juxtaposition of work and rest in labor and in motherhood. Labor is not actually all work—it's full of rest too."

Well that comes as a surprise.

"During contractions," she continued, "a woman pushes herself to her max, and in between she gets to experience complete relief and rest. Live in the moment, and don't fight labor. Instead, let your body experience these different sensations. It will help you prepare for what lies ahead."

But fighting unpleasant sensations sounds so much easier.

"Also, remember this same process when you're a new mama. Motherhood will bring intense moments your way. Let your body rest whenever you get a chance."

Motherhood, intense? Uh-oh!

"Thanks, Vero," I mustered. "I'll try to remember that."

After a few seconds of silence, Gwen spoke up. To my surprise, she simply said, "You'll do great in labor, Meshi."

What on earth makes her say that?

"Actually," I confessed, "I'm worried I'll freak out and start panicking."

"Don't worry," she said with a gentle smile, "fear is normal and healthy. Labor can humble us all. Who wouldn't be scared? There may be times when you'll want to panic, and when that happens, just work to regain control. Let your support people help you. The most important thing now is to set yourself up for success: rest up now and be well-fed in early labor."

I thanked her for validating my fears instead of brushing them off, and made a mental note: *I am not alone, and there are things I can do to prepare.*

Elise spoke then, while colorful Christmas lights shone through the window and the smell of fresh pine intermingled with the sweet aroma of the baking dessert.

"Labor and birth can be a spiritual journey if you want them to be," she remarked. "It can be a time where you learn about God and extract deeper meaning for your life. This is a good time to identify your personal spiritual goals for labor and share these with those who will be with you during it."

Really, labor as a spiritual experience? I suppose it could be.

While warming my hands on my mug of tea, I thanked her, determined to reflect more on this idea. But before I could ponder the profound concept, I had one last surprise—an additional thought from Veronica, an ever-generous friend.

"The irony of labor," she said, "is that it's both everything and nothing."

Oh, this sounds deep.

"When it arrives, labor is profound and all-encompassing, permeating every crevice of your body and mind. And yet, even with its monstrous reality, when you meet your baby, its significance shrinks away into the abyss. What once was will pass and will be no longer. So, when you're laboring, remember—it will not last forever. It *will* pass. In the end, you will find yourself not just with something good, like hot soup waiting for you, but with something far grander—your child."

In the silence, I thanked them, awed and grateful for the honor of having such wise and caring friends. "I don't even know what to say," I added, choking up a bit. "I hope I can remember everything you shared when I'm in the thick of it."

When I reached home that evening, I clutched each bit of advice to my heart as I wrote them down—catching each word of wisdom before it could escape into the frosty, light-adorned night.

Cirque du Soleil

As a rare treat to see a live performance, Dan and I stepped into Cirque du Soleil's enormous, bright, and warm yellow tent and began squeezing our way down our packed row to get to our seats. I must have clubbed the entire line of seated guests with my belly, but since I only stepped on a few toes, it counts as a successful entrance in my book. The lights dimmed to dark, and the music soared through the tent as the spotlight traced the stage.

Out swarmed green, blue, and orange chiseled bodies swathed in tight clothing and adorned with masks—even grown men in full-body leotards. *Now there's a sight to remember.* Dressed as animals and insects, the acrobats crawled, rolled, climbed, and danced before us to thunderous and rhythmic music. I didn't even know where to look next. These figures slithered, curved, and crawled around anything and everything Dr. Seuss could ever rhyme away—a ball, a wall. A cat, a hat. It's as if they were defying the laws of gravity right before my very eyes. As a mere, ordinary human, there's no way I could ever do that without tipping over or breaking my nose.

Man, by contrast, my day job is far too boring.

The troupe surely hosted a night to remember, to say the least—one almost as memorable as the night before. If I could shrink the enthralling Cirque du Soleil experience down into a one-square-foot aquatic tank, I'd end up with whatever my baby was doing then. She kicked, somersaulted, and moved so much inside of me that I really could, in no way, think about sleeping.

I became her stage.

I was a captive audience in my own body. She was giving me the ride of my life, my womb her red trampoline, causing mighty earthquakes from inside out. But she must have misunderstood; I would have been perfectly satisfied attending only one Cirque du Soleil performance.

All I wanted was a good night's sleep, not a circus act.

⋙ LET'S TALK ABOUT IT ⋘

Connecting with Baby

Feeling your little one's movements inside can be quite an experience, right? Before too long, you'll have much more fun and tangible ways to connect. In fact, connecting and bonding will look different every month as your baby develops—and will get way more exciting as time goes on.

After delivery, it won't take long for you to realize that you gave birth to a precious, yet helpless and needy dumpling. It will be normal for your baby to want to be held *all* the time. Go with it. It's impossible to spoil a baby under the age of six months. All she's ever known is being inside of you. Your presence (or another loving person's) comforts and teaches a key life lesson: "I'm safe. I can trust my parents and my caregivers."

Your baby will be an adept communicator—she will use everything she's got (sounds and behaviors) to stay close and make sure you have no chance of forgetting her. *Ever.* Even if you're deathly exhausted. In no time at all, you will notice that one of her favorite communication styles is crying. She'll cry when she's hungry, sick, scared, hot, cold, tired, over-stimulated (*yes, that's a thing*), has a poopy diaper, or just wants to be held.[1] And get this: she will also cry because, well, she's a baby.[2,3] That means she will even cry when there is nothing wrong at all.

A season for tears

Baby behavior studies have found that these little ragamuffins cry a lot in the first four to five months of life (called the ***period of purple crying***).[2-4] A baby will probably cry more during this time than in any other part of his or her life. Crying starts around two weeks after birth, peaks in the second month, and can come out of the blue (no matter how great of a parent you are or how perfect you thought your baby would be).[2,4]

Remember, it's a season and won't last forever. On average, these crying sprees last 30–40 minutes (sometimes up to a few hours) and happen more in the late afternoons or evenings.[2-4] Your crying machine will probably resist soothing, and her face will look like she's in pain.[2,4] No, this doesn't automatically mean she has colic. This means you've given birth to a baby, not a fish. And again, it doesn't mean you've failed as a mommy.

So how do you know what's going on? Well, it's lots of trial and error—no, not what any of us perfectionist parents want to hear. Soon, though, you'll better understand your baby's *cues*—the body movements and noises your baby uses to communicate.

Common cues

To give you a head start, check out this list of common cues to watch for. *If hungry*, she'll put her hands to her mouth, suck on anything around, and root.[1] *If playful*, she'll relax her face, open her eyes, look at you (or something she wants to play with), and perhaps even kick her little legs (**engagement cues**).[1] *If ready for a break* from playing or the environment, she'll close her eyes, turn away, look tense, and maybe even cry, arch, or twist her body away from you (**disengagement cues**).[1] *If her tummy hurts*, she may pull up her legs to her chest. *If she's sick*, she'll get fussy and often also show other signs of illness like fever, runny nose, or diarrhea. What's amazing is that over time, you'll know your baby so well that interpreting her cues will become second nature!

Bottom line? With the birth of your baby, you'll become a baby detective. Although hearing your baby cry can feel frustrating and overwhelming, try paying attention to the cues above. If there is a time when your baby is crying constantly, it's a good idea to check in with your pediatrician or medical provider to make sure there's not anything else going on.[2] Remember, in the first few months, 95% of the time, this unpredictable type of purple period crying is not because your baby is abnormal, nor are the gods out to get you.[2] It's just a part of normal baby development.[2]

Digging Deeper

Becoming a baby whisperer takes time, practice, and patience. Don't you worry, though, you'll get there before you know it. To help you, in "Soothing Baby and Regaining Your Cool" (postpartum week 2), we'll explore ways to soothe your baby and how to cope when you're at your wit's end. In the meantime, check out A-5c for fun ideas on how to bond with your little sweetie. You'll find answers to questions like:

» Can I bond with my baby while formula feeding?

» What is skin-to-skin, and is it something for only mama to enjoy with baby?

» I'm interested in infant massage—can you tell me more about it?

WEEK 34

Baby

- Is about 17 ¾ inches.
- Weighs about 4 ¾ pounds.
- Develops *alveoli* (air sacs) in the lungs, making breathing possible.
- Develops the sucking reflex.

Mama

- Your amniotic fluid has peaked. It's about four cups.
- Blood volume has reached its maximum, having increased by 40–50% during pregnancy, or more in the case of multiples.

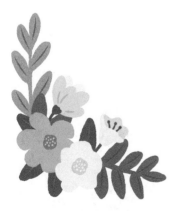

A Belly Button to Make You Jealous

Up until today, I must admit, I underestimated the power of an unflashy, humble old belly button. But now I know—pregnancy does weird things to people, and this I shall never forget.

When my last patient of the morning left, I scarfed down my lunch and went out to begin my usual lunchtime walk. The tree-lined sidewalk meandered through a nearby business park filled with gray, oversized, box-like buildings, and past patches of token lawns. I can't say it's the prettiest loop I've ever been on, but it does the trick—I can get out and waddle with true, pregnant-mama sass.

Before I could even get past the first row of parked cars, I spotted, out of the corner of my eye, a woman staring at me from her car window. Yes, staring. As in, her head swiveled to follow me as I went. *That's weird. Did the back of my dress fall off?* As casually as I could, I reached back and confirmed it was still attached, and continued on.

I couldn't have been more than twenty feet past her when I heard her truck door open. She began to yell after me.

What in the world?!

"Hey—*Hey!* I like your little package—your baby bump—and your belly button is so cute!"

Not sure what else to do, I turned around, saw her waving from the sidewalk by the open truck door, and hollered, "Thank you!" before continuing my path toward the business loop.

What just happened? Did a lady really just get out of her vehicle and yell after me because of my belly button? I stared ahead at the bushes around the bend, completely stunned by how people say and do the weirdest things around pregnant women. *I just don't get it.* To make it stranger, this was actually the third belly button comment I'd received—just today. Truthfully, I think I might be getting a little self-conscious.

How can so many people forget to use discretion and common sense when it comes to commenting about pregnant bodies? It's as if they reverted to their adolescence—no, wait—their preschool days, when no one had any clue about social graces. Would it be too much to first consider how a comment could make a pregnant woman feel?

And what am I supposed to do about my belly button anyway? It's impossible to hide.

I have a little cherry topping my round cake, just waiting to be frosted with comments. The only thing that could save me now is maybe securing it down with a piece of fondant.

Life after the Stork

I'm not exactly sure how the stork ever got mixed up in family planning. It's quite peculiar if you ask me. Was it perched on its rooftop one afternoon, and then somehow became inspired to make a career change? Was it perhaps admiring its reflection in a pool of water, when it took note of its strong, long beak and realized these natural qualities could do the world some good? Or was it that the stork just always loved tiny, soft little humans?

I'm not sure if we'll ever know, but wow, it must have been a handy alleged occupation when it came time for my grandparents to explain the birds and the bees to their children. I wish I could have seen how it all went down.

Did they keep a straight face and look their children in the eye when they uttered their big bad lie? *For the sake of the kids, of course.* "Children, it's simple. [Insert clearing of the throat.] For us Hungarians, the stork brings the babies."

I can picture the mesmerized look on their little faces, as each child marveled at how we were fortunate enough to form such an unexpected alliance with fowl. I wonder if the children asked any of the questions I'm dying to ask: Did these newborns like zipping through the fresh air, naked and suspended by a little sling? How did the stork know where to deliver which baby? Where in the world did the stork find the baby for delivery, in the first place?

As a nurse practitioner, I'm also curious if this scenario meant deliveries were only made once an order was placed. *Now, that's what I'd call good customer service.* Such a business model must have been quite handy for women who couldn't decide on a birth control method. Despite their indecisions, they would never have to worry about ending up with a surprise baby on their front porch. Yet today, about half of all U.S.

pregnancies are unplanned—a figure I'm sure would be far lower if the stork had served the States, too, after he presumably retired from his career in Hungary.

Perhaps I could convince the stork to unretire. Just for a while, at least. It would bring me some peace of mind since I, too, am still deciding on what birth control to use after my baby is born. This reality is sort of embarrassing to admit. As one who prescribes—and often inserts—birth control for countless women, I feel I should be further along in this process.

I know that if I'd sit me down, a pregnant lady, in the office, I'd explain that spacing pregnancies matters and if I get pregnant too soon, my next pregnancy would be at higher risk for developing complications. Getting pregnant too quickly would also mean I'd have less time to enjoy and get to know my new child. As I learned to do, I'd ask myself, *Meshi, what are you looking for in a method, and what have you tried in the past?** Then I'd show myself the smorgasbord of hormonal and nonhormonal, more effective and less effective, convenient and less convenient methods out there. *There's something for everyone,* I'd tell myself, *and if you don't like it, no worries, we can try something else.*

Easy, right?

Sure. It seems the only sensible thing to do next is—track down that stork. Maybe retirement isn't panning out, and it desperately misses us Hungarians. But, if that falls through, then I really will need to stop postponing a decision. I owe it not just to my little one but also to Dan and myself.

⇝ LET'S TALK ABOUT IT ⇜

The Naked Truth about Birth Spacing and Birth Control

When you've been pregnant for as long as you have, birth control may be the last thing on your mind. You may have even forgotten sex can lead

---

* Christine Dehlendorf, MD, personal communication, February 15, 2019 to pregnancy. Sure, you've got other pressing things on your mind—like fumbling through car seat installation, wrapping up work, figuring out pet-sitting for your dog while you're having your baby, and countless other details.

Adequate spacing

However, picking an effective birth control method—and adequately spacing your pregnancies—is a huge gift to your little blossom and your family. You've been growing this brand-new human for a long while, and when he arrives, he'll want to cuddle close and have some special time with his family. While you will stay the apple of his eye forever, your attention is especially important until he's old enough to dart away from you (which is at roughly one and a half to two years old).

Waiting at least 18 months before you get pregnant not only helps you have this special time to focus on your child and family but will also minimize your risk for complications like preterm birth, low birth weight,

> Find your birth control match to help safely space your pregnancies.

and other serious obstetrical complications in your next pregnancy.[1-3] Now if you are older (35+) and feel like waiting 18 months is too long since time is of the essence, then it's reasonable to try to get pregnant when your baby is 1 year old (but certainly not less than 6 months!).[1-5] Another consideration is that if you end up having a Cesarean birth and are desperate to try for a VBAC next time, you'll want to have at least 18 months between deliveries to give your uterus time to heal properly and minimize your risk of uterine rupture. Consider sharing these facts with your partner, too, so you both can take birth control seriously.

Reproductive coercion

If, however, you are struggling with an unhealthy relationship involving reproductive coercion—where your partner interferes with your birth control use or pregnancy wishes—be assured: you have the right to make reproductive decisions for yourself.[6,7] Please talk with your maternity care provider or check out the resources in this book that are designed to help you have control over your reproductive health, and the freedom you deserve. One way to accomplish this may be using an "invisible" birth control method from the list in A-5b. (If you haven't already, you may be interested in reading more about relationships that hurt in B-5f.)

Choosing a reliable method that works for you

Okay, so birth spacing is important—but how do we accomplish this? Truthfully, it won't happen by accident. Get this: You can become fertile again before you even have a period! What's more, some non-breastfeeding women can ovulate within six weeks of giving birth.[8] Statistically, if you let fate have a year of your life and you have sex regularly, it will opt to get you pregnant 85% of the time.[9] So, technically, women can become pregnant all the way until they hit menopause, which is usually in their early 50s—in other words, light-years away.

When it comes to planned pregnancies and pregnancy spacing, the optimal solution is to choose and use a reliable method that works for you. You may be surprised to hear that picking a birth control *method* doesn't necessarily mean picking a pill. Thankfully, we now have so many more options, which can be both more reliable and more convenient— key factors that are especially important for you ladies with certain health or mental health problems for whom an unplanned pregnancy could be riskier.[9,10]

Regardless of your risk level in an unplanned pregnancy, go ahead and take a moment to prioritize your pregnancy spacing and health. Explore your options and find what fits your needs. You won't regret it!

Digging Deeper

If you're still undecided or want to weigh some pros and cons for each birth control option, check out A-5b for an illustrated chart and more tips on finding the right method that works for you. The section covers answers to questions like:

» What are the most effective birth control methods?

» Do I have options if I don't like taking hormones?

» Is it possible to find a method that I can keep to myself?

» Are there mental health considerations when picking a method?

» How do I know when the Lactational Amenorrhea Method (LAM) is no longer effective?

WEEK 35

Baby

- Is about 18 ¼ inches long.
- Weighs about 5 ¼ pounds.
- Creates *surfactant* (a special lung chemical) to keep the lungs open while breathing as a newborn.

Mama

- Typically, blood pressure will return to prepregnancy levels in this trimester.
- You may be surprised to find yourself more ready to go through labor or have a Cesarean birth.

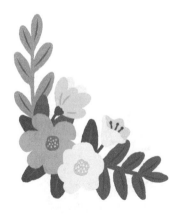

God, I Have a Better Idea

Dear God,

I have some great news! After reflecting about my upcoming labor for days and weeks, I've finally figured out an intriguing alternative for birthing. Please hear me out. I think you'll love it as much as I do. No, it doesn't require transforming me into a black bear or Dan into a seahorse. Rather, it would simply mean tweaking the current labor scenario—oh, just a tad. Labor can remain a miracle but could become something fully lovely and not at all tarnished by a pregnant woman's usual fears or pain. Now, doesn't that sound wonderful?

Consider this—

She with child casually reclines in a location of her choosing, whether it be against a loved one's chest, a soft pillow, or a fresh field of flowers—a body flourishing. Uncovering her belly, she begins joyfully watching for the peculiar yet expected changes to emerge on her figure.

In anticipation, she looks a little closer and sees, indeed, her dawn has come—time to become and blossom. Her baby is almost here. Little velvety leaves and soft, colorful petals peep out, then grow, as the delicate green vines emerge and intertwine on top of her belly like the morning dew. Her body relaxes, her belly button smiles, and the sweet aroma of jasmine bursts forth as her foliage changes to all the colors of spring. Her petals gently unfold on her flowering body and unveil her warm little darling.

Oh, what a love!

—See, it's so peaceful, joyful, and best of all, God, it's pain free. Could you please arrange for this to be the revamped method for birthing? I'm sure all it would take is a mere little breath on your part. Oh, and no big rush—I've got about four to five weeks.

I sure am grateful for your consideration.

With love,

Emese

"Massage" Time

When a woman hears the term *perineal massage*, she's got to wonder: Where on earth is the perineum? (Is it next to the auditorium?) Plus, how do you massage it? And why even bother?

As for the first question, it's that small region between the vagina and anus. And for the last, it turns out, if you care for this friend for the month or so before you deliver your first child, she'll repay you kindly by decreasing your chance of tearing and experiencing perineal pain after delivery.[1] All a woman's got to do is run her fingers along the rim of her vaginal opening for five to ten minutes a day, a few times a week, and over time, apply some pressure to stretch it a bit. Seems like an incredible bargain if you ask me.

I recently embarked on my own expedition to show my perineum the love it deserved—only to find out that it's a bit trickier than I expected. I grossly underestimated the coordination I needed to reach this area around the obstructive bulge of my belly. Moreover, which finger should I use to apply pressure?

In that blessed day of reckoning, I decided it was time to call in the reinforcements. *It's the least Dan can do since I'm about to deliver his child.*

Ever since, he's been graciously helping me out with this so-called perineal massage. "Massage," really? As if! "Quasi-torture," more like it. It has nothing to do with the relaxing image that comes to mind when I hear the word *massage*. Most of the time, I just catch myself cringing and holding my breath. Forcing myself to inhale slowly and deeply, I mutter a few choice words and blow away my discomfort.

I've been so focused on my own experience during the event that it never occurred to me to consider Dan's. Apparently, it has been hard for him, too.

Painful, in fact.

No, not because it is so hard for him to see me in discomfort, which would have been nice to hear. But rather, he's pressing down so hard that his own fingers are starting to cramp.

For a quick guide to perineal massage, check out A-4f.

"Are we almost done?" he asked with a ragged breath. "This is hurting my finger."

What? Give me a break. Listen pal, you're busy stretching my precious perineum and you're complaining about your finger?

The thought sounded so ridiculous that I couldn't help it—I burst into uncontrollable laughter.

⫸⫸ LET'S TALK ABOUT IT ⫷⫷

Demystifying Baby Feeding

As this journey of growth unfolds and your body continues to bloom, you may have found that it's not just your belly that has stretched during this process. Two lives tucked inside one body is a unique time, packed full of all sorts of funny, emotional, and strange experiences—experiences that extend all the way into mommyhood as you become an expert on your ever-changing newborn. Learning about your baby—including her feeding preferences and cues—is a process filled with trial, error, and a dash of instinct. Every baby is unique, so have patience with yourself in this part of your journey.

You may remember that in "Feeding Your Milk Monster" (week 28), we explored the pros and cons of feeding your baby breastmilk and formula, and the considerations that may impact your decision. Today, let's chat about the experience of feeding your baby—regardless of which method you choose.

Once your baby's born, you'll quickly see that your life will revolve around feeding, burping, and diaper changes. Since initially she will be a night owl, this cycle will happen around the clock and without any real rhythm. The more help you can get during these early months, the better! Ask people to make you scrumptious meals, shop for food, take your dog on a walk, and hold or burp your baby so you can have time to yourself, with your partner, or with your other child(ren).

Whether you are breast- or formula-feeding, you'll be figuring out the logistics, such as the meaning behind your baby's various cues, how

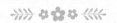

Breastfeeding can parch mamas—be sure to always have a water bottle or large glass of water by your side!

to hold your baby during feedings, and even how to prepare or store milk safely.

Breastfeeding considerations

If you're breastfeeding, your baby will first be consuming your glorious "liquid gold" colostrum and then your mature milk when it comes three to five days later. Sometimes, your milk may take even a little longer if you've had a Cesarean birth, a longer labor, or if you have certain medical conditions like diabetes.[2] You'll be figuring out how to keep your breasts happy, express milk with a pump, and latch your baby properly to your breast (so it's not painful and she can get milk out efficiently).

Formula-feeding considerations

If you're formula feeding, you may need to experiment with different bottle nipples and formulas to find one your baby likes and tolerates. If

WHAT'S A MILK BANK?

Milk banks collect and distribute human milk to infants in need. Awesome, right? So, if for some reason your baby needs supplemental milk, you may not need to jump straight to formula. Donated human milk may be an option. Be sure to ask your labor and delivery nurse, lactation consultant, or maternity care provider for more info.

And for you mamas who end up producing more milk than you know what to do with, donate it! It's easy, free, and can be so satisfying. Your contributions would help other mamas and sustain life beyond your own baby.

Whether receiving or donating, ensure your milk bank adheres to strict safety and pasteurization standards by finding one affiliated with the nonprofit Human Milk Banking Association of North America.[3] The ones meeting these safety standards are endorsed by the American Academy of Pediatrics.[4]

you plan to avoid breastfeeding completely, then after delivery be sure to avoid any nipple stimulation like the plague. That means wearing a bra even at night, not expressing milk, and showering with your back to the water. And if you've always wanted to feel like a cabbage patch, here's your chance: place clean, cold cabbage leaves in your bra—some women swear by it. If you go this route, you'll need to switch them out when they warm up.

No matter which method you choose, feeding time may end up being your favorite activity together with your baby because it can be so special, quiet, entertaining, and intimate. If it is a little overwhelming at first, don't worry. Learning new things can be exhausting and stressful, so hang in there and keep at it. This is a great time to gather information about your postpartum resources, such as lactation consultants and breastfeeding groups. Lactation consultants can help all mommies, even those who are bottle- or formula-feeding.

Digging Deeper

If this topic of feeding your mini milk monster intrigues you and you'd like to prepare more, check out A-5d for more great information. There you'll find answers to questions, including:

» How do I know my baby's hungry?

» What is cluster feeding, and does it mean my baby's starving?

» Should I lay my baby down while bottle-feeding?

» I'm tired—can I breastfeed my baby while I'm lying down?

» Is burping my baby a huge waste of time?

WEEK 36

Baby

- Is about 18 ½ inches long.
- Weighs about 5 ¾ pounds.
- Has more fully developed kidneys, allowing urine to be better concentrated.
- Starts to replace *lanugo* (fine, downy hair) with *vellus hair* (like peach fuzz).
- Moves into a head-down position for birth—fingers crossed!

Mama

- Your uterus has expanded upward to reach your rib cage. Once your baby "drops" lower into your pelvis, you'll breathe easier but may begin a sexy waddle.
- Soon you may be basking in the glories of maternity leave.
  - Turn in your leave paperwork when it's time.

To Tahoe?

I've had a lot of worries in my life,
most of which never happened.
—MARK TWAIN

For months now, I've been debating whether to spend my last month of pregnancy up at Lake Tahoe with Dan while he completes a required fellowship rotation in sports medicine. Usually, it's recommended that pregnant mamas stay close to home their last month of pregnancy in case they go into early labor. As such, it has been a great source of tension between Dan and me and has provided an excellent opportunity to slam our bedroom door whenever I see fit.

"What? You expect me to travel up to the mountains, and stay three and a half hours from home, right up to my due date?"

Slam.

"Just tell them your wife is pregnant and you can only go for two weeks. What do you mean, you can't?"

Slam.

"What if I go into labor in the middle of a snowstorm? Don't you care about me and my needs?"

Slam.

As time has shown, this door had been solidly crafted and perfectly hung to withstand my new coping method. In fact, it has served me well all the way to today—when I can't put off the decision any longer.

I'm a simple soul. I don't think I'm asking for too much—just a little control. Predictable weather patterns and familiar maternity care providers would be a great start. I just want to nest, not fly the coop.

If I were a bird, I'd be settled down amid the bright golden leaves of a pomegranate tree. If I tired of that, I imagine I'd fluff up my motherly self until I looked like a great plume of feathers and then people-watch for hours and days. I certainly wouldn't be flying away on some great migration.

After all, what if my baby decides to come early? What if I can't get to the hospital, so I deliver in a jeep during a blizzard? *What if. What if. What if?* My worries kept coming, tempered only by the fact that I don't want to spend the last few weeks apart from Dan.

So, I teeter-tottered back and forth between my options until one day I had my answer. I got an email from my friend Anna—not only a true gem but also a tough, Alaskan woman who, during many a summer, put in long hours with a commercial fishing crew. Since college, we'd kept in touch, and now, as a relatively new mother, she wrote:

I think you should go stay with your husband in Tahoe . . . assuming you can manage the elevation change, and I would expect that after a few days you'll adjust just fine. I visited a friend who has a six-month-old and she was saying it feels like her husband and her are just roommates looking after a baby now.

So, I can't say from personal experience, but I think it would be good to treasure your last few weeks alone together. As far as wintry places—they are beautiful in the sunshine! Bundle your hot pregnant body up and go for walks in the snow, do big-belly yoga moves, cook your husband some tasty dinners, sing songs for your baby, and rest—put your feet up.

I'm pretty sure I should have been putting my feet up more. It doesn't necessarily feel like exercise, but your heart is pumping blood for two humans—it's pretty hard work. It kind of sounds like a wonderful chance to rest and refocus (you could think of it like a spiritual retreat?) before your little one comes out into the daylight.

You are going to be such a wonderful mother.

I'm off to attend to the endless list of things to do when the baby is finally sleeping.

Love you,

Anna

Wow, exactly what I needed. With a cleansing exhale and a smile, I turned to the bedroom door and giggled. I won't be needing its help any longer. Yes, it really could be a fun and beautiful time at Lake Tahoe—a time full of love, play, and sleep. Goodness, to think my fears almost kept me from pursuing this incredible opportunity! And if in the rare chance pregnancy complications arise, I guess I'll just have to trust God and go with it.

A Life Lesson

We're snuggling in a lovely cabin in the hibernating town of Truckee, California, near Lake Tahoe. And I feel just fine. Yep, I feel just fine! At most, I'm a little winded when going up stairs, but then again, what pregnant woman isn't used to that by now?

To think this trip was such a source of anxiety, concern, and marital friction over the past eight months. What a lesson! Yes, stop freaking out. I suppose most of us have our own "Tahoe" worries, either while pregnant or not. Yet how much more freeing are those days when we choose to live by our values and not our fears!

Right before we left on our trip, I had my 36-week appointment with the midwife. (Yes, the dogs are still there, and no, I'm not about to ask that one stretched across the couch to make way for mama. I'll just stand by the door, thank you very much.) Happily, my little one is now oriented head-downward, and her heartbeat and growth are both still on target. Phew!

Unfortunately, though, it seems my blood pressure is creeping higher as I get further along in pregnancy. The readings are in the upper end of the normal range, and I don't have any protein in my urine or symptoms that indicate I could be developing preeclampsia. But Dan and I will need to monitor it daily here in Tahoe—just to be safe.

Although it's tempting to start worrying about the *What ifs* again, this time, I'm determined to carry with me the lesson I just learned. I need to just relax and enjoy my life. *Breathe.* Oh, and did I mention— relax? It does the body and the blood pressure some good, and besides, I'm not in control of my life anyway.

≫≫ LET'S TALK ABOUT IT ≪≪

Getting Real about Labor and Your Expectations

*I think, at a child's birth, if a mother could ask
a fairy godmother to endow it with the most useful gift, that gift
would be curiosity.*
—ELEANOR ROOSEVELT

Have you started wondering what the big day holds—the day when your little one's born? It's normal for women to be excited yet also nervous or fearful about certain aspects of labor. This is especially common if it's your first baby, you've had a difficult prior delivery, or you've heard of or watched nerve-racking labor stories or videos. So, let's have a little heart-to-heart.

When going into labor, it's vital to keep sight of your ultimate labor goal: to have a healthy baby and mommy. The rest of the details on your birth plan (wish list) are icing on the cake. Remembering this can be pivotal for perspective in the moment.

Although we don't quite know what this birthday journey will look like, we do know that sooner or later, somehow, your baby will exit. What a glorious thought! Whether you feel highly prepared or underprepared, and whether this will be your first delivery or your fourth, the birth process will almost certainly surprise and challenge you, labor will teach you about yourself, and you will be forever changed by the experience.

Be like water

To get ready for this unique journey, it may be helpful to hold in your mind the image of water—an element that is soft but strong and that flows around or over any obstacle. So too, in labor, let yourself trickle (rest) when it feels good and let yourself surge with the rapids when power is necessary. Water knows how to yield but also to cover, completely saturate, and move great things. In labor, in motherhood, and in life, the practice of letting go and being pliable like water gives you a huge advantage. Try to visualize this daily.

Just as a drop of rain falling on a mountain doesn't worry about its course to the sea, so, too, take one moment at a time in labor. Don't think ahead about how you'll possibly make it through the end. Be in the moment. Give yourself grace if you get tired, discouraged, scared, teary, angry, upset, or whatever. Remember, your support people and labor staff are there to help you refocus and keep going. Usually, when you feel like you can't go on any longer, your job is almost done! You'll be meeting your baby soon.

Give yourself, and your baby, grace

When labor asks unexpected things from you, there's no need to fret. Do what you need to do, accepting what you need to accept, to accomplish what you went there to do. There is no shame in labor, nor cause for judgment. Instead, be proud of what you have achieved. You have already grown a whole person, remember?

Sure, if you have any specific, personal goals in labor, give it a fair shot. Maybe you want to get to four centimeters dilation without medication, or to relax more during contractions. Go ahead, share these goals with your labor support people, and discover what strength you have inside of you.

When you do meet your little one, forget the movie images of the picture-perfect newborn. Yes, labor takes a toll on your baby, not just you! Your darling may look a little disheveled, may be somewhat blue, or have Bart Simpson's head shape. Have grace for your bambino and know he or she will look much cuter in a few days.

If, after birth, you feel strange, are shivering, or are "out of it"—don't worry! Hopefully your support people or labor staff will remind you this is fully understandable. You, my dear pregnant mama, will have just given birth. Now that's what we can all call an accomplishment!

The exciting day is approaching when you'll get to meet your baby! If you end up having your little one prior to your estimated due date (which may happen), skip forward to postpartum week 1. You may also enjoy reading the last few "Let's Talk About It" sections.

Digging Deeper

Giving birth will forever be a memorable day. You'll bring to labor a full array of unique strengths, in addition to those of your support person(s). In fact, go ahead and take a moment to list your strengths. Also, if you are ready to hear more about labor logistics, take a peek at the contents in A-2 and A-4. There, you'll find answers to the following questions, and so much more:

» In what ways can picking the right support person improve my labor experience? (A-4a)

» What does a contraction feel like? (A-4a)

» Is labor going to be nonstop pain? (A-4a)

» Can you give me some ideas for getting more comfortable during labor? (A-4a & b)

» When should I call the hospital? (A-2)

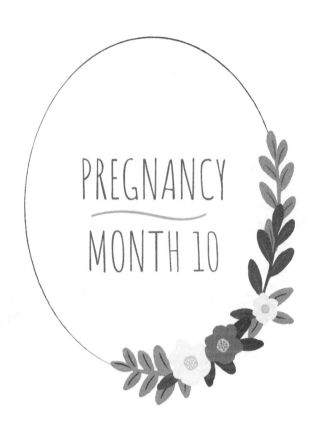

PREGNANCY

MONTH 10

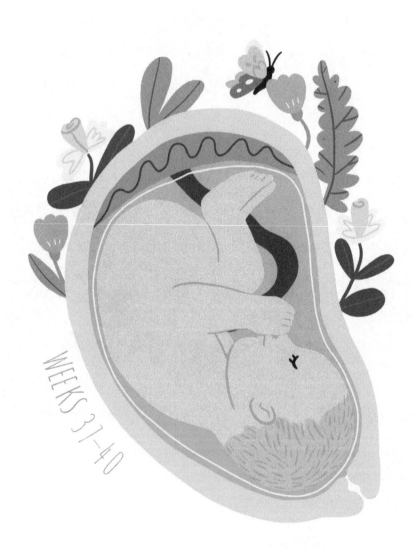

WEEKS 37–40

WEEK 37

Baby

- Is about 19 inches long.
- Weighs about 6 ¼ pounds.
- Is early term!
- Fetal lungs are mature and ready to breathe.
- Moves lower into your pelvis.

Mama

- The increased blood volume may cause ankle and hand swelling, as well as carpal tunnel syndrome.
  - Put your feet up (literally), wear only comfy jewelry, and try a wrist splint if needed.
- You may notice mixed feelings about upcoming labor. So common!
  - Talk to your provider about your specific fears and concerns. She or he can help you prepare for a good labor experience.

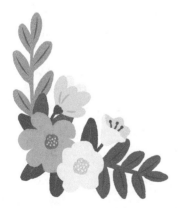

Twist and Shout

The town of Truckee, California, is nestled in the mountains at about 6,000 feet in elevation, 13 miles to the northwest of Lake Tahoe. It's a place where people still say *hello* with a smile and *thank you* when you least expect—a place where desperate hitchhikers are, indeed, rescued along the roadside and where your Safeway checkout clerk, sporting a '70s mustache, sings "Twist and Shout" while bagging your milk and bananas. This year, it is also a place where there is so little snow that the pinecones around our cabin far outnumber the tourists.

I drive around town, hopping out here and there to capture something on camera, such as the Ace Hardware that has grown into a sporting goods store, and the advertisements for a sturdy bear box—something every homeowner apparently needs.

Driving past the historic district, I head down 89 South to explore the wooded outskirts. Past rushing rivers and towering pines I go, as the patches of snow on distant peaks seem to beg for Mother Nature to bring on a steady flurry. In the background, my radio blasts honky-tonk music, telling me a story about the good old days and someone's golden dream.

Will I look back at this part of my life and think of it as the good old days?

I'm not sure, though I have found that living amidst the wilderness is doing something magical—working wonders on my mental preparation for delivery. At every turn, I am inspired by rugged, daring people who are communing with nature. They swim in the outdoor pool and blast down black diamond ski runs. Vibrancy courses through their veins.

Do I have that kind of inner strength and resolve? That raw realness I'm seeing around me? I just had to find out. So, I purchased a monthly pass to the local gym, which includes access to a reasonably well-heated outdoor pool—a perfect litmus test. Since then, like many locals, I've been swimming laps while the air crackles at 25 degrees. Carefully tip-toeing across the cold and wet deck in my two-piece, I watch the vapor of my breath uncurl as I toss my towel onto the bench and climb into the pool. With each stroke, I've been proving to myself that I, too, have a little bit of that innate human strength tucked within me—a bit of resolve I can tap into during labor.

My strength is mounting, and I want to declare, to I don't know who, "Come on, bring it on! I'm ready." I feel like putting on a pelt coat (is that what people wear in January?), tracking a deer, and building myself a hut somewhere in the middle of nowhere.

I'm ready to travel down the path of all the mothers who have gone before me. The path unmarked, unknown, and whose course only becomes clear once traversed. Now, I must trust that we—my body and my babe—are programmed to do this in unison and that my pain will have a purpose, for it will lead to something great: my daughter.

I can hardly wait to meet her.

A Fairy-Tale Adventure

Today, it's as if I'm living in a gingerbread house. I shuffle over to the chalet window in Dan's sweats like I do every morning, and, pulling open the plaid curtains, I press my nose against the frosty window like a little child. Has it snowed yet?

This morning, I found to my delight that—yes!—it has. Icicles hang from the edge of the A-frame roof while soft, rolling mounds and wisps of white span my view. It's as if a storm of cotton candy has blown through and blanketed the town. The sight of the long-awaited confection, frosting the world, kindles within my soul a certainty that almost anything is possible—even childbirth.

After breakfast, I put on my cross-country skis and head out for a little contemplative exploration, Meshi style. Dampened silence surrounds me, and all I can hear is the swish of my skis against the crinkling snow. Amid the grand, towering pines and glittering expanse, I feel so small—like a woodland elf. This may as well be a fairy tale.

Hmm, a fairy tale . . . Now, if this were such a story, what would the subject be? Oh, I know, the adventures of pregnancy and my wanderings hither and yon, not knowing where my firstborn will emerge.

Yes, that's it. And how has the story unfolded, leading here?

Let us begin in Cupertino, where the protagonist (yours truly) has recently moved. Though she continues to dream about the rolling vineyards of the verdant Santa Rosa, her old stomping grounds, and of her friends and her yellow house. So, this pregnant wanderer grabs a satchel and fashions herself a rainbow so she could commute back to the area in color and style. After a step onto the multicolored arch, away she'd go!

"Splendid, if I do say so myself," she beams. Adjusting the bag slung over her shoulder, she glides across the rainbow. "I wonder what surprises I'll find when I step with this faith into labor?" Below, she glimpses the expanse of the glistening Bay, reflecting the colors of her arched path. While admiring the sight, she retrieves a cluster of magical grapes from her bag and plops the whole bunch in her mouth—so her cheeks were full as a chipmunk's. As she chewed and chewed these bubblegum-like delights, her belly began to grow larger and larger, and her body felt lighter and lighter.

"I seem to be turning into a hot air balloon!" she exclaimed with a lighthearted laugh and curious eyes wide open. Carried on the breeze, she now soars south toward Petaluma, passing the countryside, the chicken farms, the poultry factory, and the upturned faces of people on the hills.

Will this be the place? she wonders, as she waves. *No*, she decided, *it's just not quite right.* The wind picked up, and she let it carry her higher and higher, like a feather, northeast toward Lake Tahoe where snowflake flurries swirled in the air.

Cradled by the chilly breeze, she came to rest in a . . . snowman-drawn sleigh? Yes, surprising but welcome—a ride replete with heated seats, mittens, a plaid quilt, and complimentary earmuffs. How nice! The sled set off with the jingle of bells and slid on toward Lake Tahoe, gliding across the mountain passes.

Dan should be around here somewhere, she thought. How convenient!

As I pulled myself from the daydream, I could hear again the swish of my cross-country skis below me, under the weight of my big, warm belly.

My outdoor trek had been sparkly and peaceful—just what I needed. I traced my tracks all the way back to our gingerbread cottage, to rest a bit more in my imagined adventures as this fairy tale's pregnant wanderer.

But still I wonder: Where *will* I have my baby?

⇻⇻⇻ LET'S TALK ABOUT IT ⇺⇺⇺

Protective Mama Bear

As your big day draws closer, your wonder about life on the other side is surely mounting. Today, let's help you prepare in a new way by exploring your role as protective mama bear. Of course, you've already started making important decisions and lifestyle choices to keep your baby safe—changes that will morph and unfold in exciting ways over time.

Overall, mamas are naturally expert protectors of their precious young. Go, mamas! Although their feats can be jaw-dropping and awe-inspiring—such as when a mother summons super-strength and lifts a car off her trapped child—more often, protection comes in the form of unflashy, yet intentional, daily actions and choices. These might include keeping a baby close in a wrap or carrier, placing him on his back to sleep, buying a car seat, keeping the crib free from blankets and toys, eating organic, getting vaccinated, asking people to wash their hands prior to holding your baby, or even moving to a safer neighborhood. While parenting, these and many more decisions are made each day to keep our little ones safe.

However, as you navigate these choices, it won't take long for you to discover that while some are relatively straightforward, others are much trickier to tackle. Finding that healthy degree of protection is a fine balance and may be harder if you are a first-time mama, are anxiety-prone, have experienced certain types of traumas or loss, or routinely focus on the unsettling news about our struggling world.

Finding balance is a process. When faced with topics like circumcision, childhood vaccines, day cares, child care providers, camps, sleepovers, and social media, you may frequently find yourself thinking:

What's the right decision? and *Am I overreacting?* Often there's no easy answer to the right path forward. While this is frustrating, be encouraged—we can do this together! When faced with tough calls, talk to your partner and the trusted people in your life. If you need more information to make an educated decision, make time to seek answers from credible sources.

For instance, if debating recommended childhood vaccines, ask your healthcare provider about the potential benefits, risks, side effects, effectiveness, and ingredients, as well as their schedules and the options to modify them. If you choose not to vaccinate, find out the potential health risks and day-to-day implications, such as its impact on school, travel, medical care, or your community (like the elderly or those with weakened immune systems). Some parents are surprised to hear that if a young, unvaccinated child gets sick with a high fever, your healthcare provider may recommend seeking out medical care earlier and initiating more expansive (sometimes invasive) testing, given your child's susceptibility to certain serious illnesses.

Once you decide about a certain issue, plan on frequently assessing the impact that choice has on you and your baby, partner, relationships— your life! Be willing to learn from your experiences and be ready to tweak your boundaries and your protective grip as needed in the years to come.

Maternal gate-keeping

Now, mama bear, please know it is easy to end up being unnecessarily hyper-protective of your cub. In the phenomenon called *maternal gate-keeping*, a mama's actions and behaviors metaphorically open or close the gateway to involvement in her baby's life.[1-3] Sometimes, mamas close the gate on (or discourage) their partner's involvement, either consciously or subconsciously protecting the baby from the partner.[1-3] While this may be for good reason (if, for instance, the partner is unable or unwilling to safely parent), often a mama's "gate-closing" simply stems from the cultural, personal, or religious beliefs that mamas know best and she is the expert parent.[3,4]

So, what does this gate-closing look like? Well, it includes micromanaging, criticizing, redoing tasks, and even setting inflexible standards or trumping decision-making.[3,5] These acts can cause tremendous pain for the partner, make him or her less confident in parenting, strain your relationship, and ultimately cause your partner to be less involved in the future.[5,6]

To avoid these problems, be proactive when your baby arrives. Pay attention to whether you invite or discourage your partner's participation in your baby's care. Ask for your partner's opinion about baby-care matters, give compliments for a job well done, and although it may be hard, give

RELATIONSHIP TIP

Free yourself from the heavy burden of parenting alone! As a mama, you do not need to assume sole responsibility for protecting your little wonder. Work together. This builds your relationship and generates more creative solutions. Tap into awesome parenting classes, couples therapy, and support resources to help you get on the same page.

your partner a chance to get to know the baby and figure out what parenting is all about.[3,5] In other words, extend the gift of time for baby care. Of course, it won't always be done *your* way, and that's okay. Breathe, practice patience, and count to 100 (or 1,000!) if needed. You're providing a beautiful chance to bond with your partner while growing closer through this shared adventure—and you're giving yourself the opportunity to learn a trick or two by standing back.[6]

Digging Deeper

Ready to take the next step to protect your dumpling? Remember your resources. A wonderful parenting ally will be your baby's healthcare provider, such as a pediatrician, family practice physician, nurse practitioner, or physician's assistant. Generally, if your baby has serious health problems or is born preterm, working with a pediatrician is a good way to go. To prepare for success:

» Ask your maternity care provider about how to find a healthcare provider for your baby.

» Check out potential candidates' websites to help you better understand their level of experience and philosophy of patient care.

WEEK 38

Baby
- Is about 19 ½ inches long.
- Weighs about 6 ¾ pounds.
- Has fingernails that reach the fingertips.
- Continues to plump up.

Mama
- Braxton Hicks toning contractions occur more frequently around this time.
  - Call your maternity care provider if you are experiencing symptoms listed in A-2.
- You will likely become more tired and uncomfortable as the days pass. You may feel more "ready" than ever to deliver.

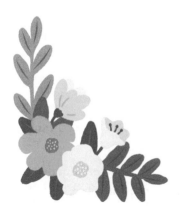

Fish Woman

After working up the courage to climb out of my toasty bed, I headed into the bathroom to shower before breakfast. Soon, the warm water ran down my back and rounded front. What a lovely way to start the day. I can hardly wait to eat breakfast and journal by the fireplace while peering out at the white-tipped trees.

As steam billowed around me, I began to hum and lather myself. My, how different my body is now than 38 weeks ago! With some effort, I slid my soapy hands down my arms and then legs.

To think, a woman's body can grow a real baby. That's absolutely incredible!

I was basking in this thought when I noticed it.

Wait just a minute—

Something feels weird. Running my fingers along my side, I discovered what could only be—skin tags. What on earth? I pinched my skin and tried to get a good look at these unwelcome newcomers but only became cross-eyed in the process. Me, with skin tags? How long have those been there? Surging hormones were changing my skin without even asking. How rude.

The minute Dan walked through the front door after work at the ski patrol station, I shared my horrifying discovery. "Dan, look, I have skin tags—on my skin!"

I'm not sure where else skin tags could have been, but the idea was so unbelievably impossible that clarifying seemed a wise choice. I lifted my shirt and showed him the evidence as my eyes began to well up.

"Hmm," Dan responded, carefully thinking over his next words. "Little scales."

Reaching out, he brushed away my tears.

"My very own fish woman," he added softly. "I love fish. You know that. Now I have one that doesn't even require a fish tank," he said with a smile. "My own walking, 190-pound fish woman."

He could have at *least* called me a mermaid.

Nonetheless, the picture was amusing and stirred up one of those wonderfully cleansing laughs, the kind that shakes my entire belly.

So what if I am a fish woman? What can I do about it?

Life will never be the same again anyway, and neither will my body. It's changing and—after delivery—it will be changed. But maybe looking like a sea creature serves some greater purpose. Maybe it will forever remind me that I'm now also a mother and have a child to love.

When Is It My Turn?

*Just as a woman's heart knows how and when to pump,
her lungs to inhale and her hand to pull back from fire,
so she knows when and how to give birth.*
—Virginia DiOrio

According to perfect strangers in my Tahoe spin class, I am now *all belly*. I think I would have to agree, especially when I'm trying to shimmy past the other spin bikes to climb onto my own. "Shimmying" is not really something a pregnant mama like me can do anymore. I frequently underestimate my girth and find myself in a conundrum—much like when one tries to park an SUV in a compact parking spot. It's embarrassing.

On the other hand, when family or friends see my newest profile pictures, they refer to me as "a ticking time bomb," and say I'm "due to pop at any moment." I can't say I like either of those analogies. The first one makes me feel dangerous, and the other, well, let's just say the word *pimple* comes to mind. Why couldn't they call me a whippersnapper instead? I'd feel like a sassy, round firecracker, ready to fill the silence with some action.

I feel so close to delivery, yet still, I wonder: When is it my turn? It seems like everyone has delivered but me. My good friend and pregnancy-confidante, Bethany, has been on the other side of labor for months now. Around me, so many other women are going about life with their babies in their arms. Am I the only woman left on this entire planet who has yet to deliver? I want my baby out, but then do I really have the energy to labor right now?

Last night I had some contractions every 20 minutes for two hours, but then we all fell asleep—my contractions concluded. That won't do. It's so hard not knowing when all this is going to begin. It's as if I'm about to run a marathon but have absolutely no idea what day the race is and when the starting pistol will fire off—tonight or in two weeks?

⋙ LET'S TALK ABOUT IT ⋘

Waiting on Baby

There's a Hungarian proverb that goes something like this: "Patience creates roses." It's something akin to the saying, "Things take time." It takes ten months to make your baby, and it may feel like the last few weeks are another ten. Labor may feel like yet another ten. Time is elusive, at times sticky, at other times slippery.

You may be one of those women who has had intermittent contractions for weeks or has waddled around a centimeter dilated for a while now. Your body is tangibly showing you it's gearing up, and you feel like it could happen any minute. Or perhaps you have not felt anything more than occasional Braxton Hicks toning contractions and you wonder if your body is acting normally. In fact, both are normal, and neither will predict when you will go into labor or how long labor will be.

In the meantime, the waiting game can feel difficult, annoying, and irritating. This is especially common if you're past your due date or are feeling super uncomfortable. You wonder how you should plan your day. Should you go out to lunch with a friend? Can you run an errand in a nearby town? Do you have time to start a small house project?

To pass the time

While waiting, keep busy, but only a little. Staring at the clock will only make you feel like you've stepped into a time warp. Take the pressure off and think of this season as your "due month" instead of focusing on your "due date."* Plan small, refreshing activities that you can cancel easily if needed. If your water breaks while you're out grocery shopping, no big deal. You'll have a good story to tell your child one day.

Here are a few other notes and guidelines to help you stay well and be prepared: If flu season is upon you or another virus is surging, it's wise to avoid sick people and crowds, since it's tough to labor while you're sick, and it's easy to pass illnesses on to your newborn. Weather permitting, plan outdoor rendezvous instead of indoor activities. Also, stay close to home so you can easily get to your birthing place of choice (though if desperate, remember a hospital won't turn away a laboring woman). If you love to exercise, feel free to do so, just take it easier than normal so you have energy reserved for later. Last, remember to leave space for plenty of resting and naps. This is not the time to catch up with all your long-lost high school friends, remodel your kitchen, or adopt a puppy. You've got something great to accomplish, so stay focused—good practice for what's to come.

Where's the finish line?

For those of you yearning for the birth day, you'll be happy to hear that it's sometime in the next four weeks. Based on national and international recommendations, you'll get to stay pregnant up to two weeks past your estimated due date (42 weeks).[1-3] After this, you are *postterm*, and the placenta may not support your baby as well, increasing the chance of complications for you and your baby.[2,4]

So, if you are beyond your estimated due date, your maternity care provider should discuss your options on how to proceed. Don't be alarmed, however, if this conversation comes up as early as 39 weeks! As usual, get your familiar, inquisitive-mama prowess going and collect the information you need to make an informed decision.

As part of that conversation, it's important to remember that, barring medical or pregnancy complications, there are numerous benefits to you and your baby when you let your body go into labor on its own.[5-7] Yes, your body has all sorts of tricks up her sleeve. By basking in your body's

---

* Kim Sterner, RN, CNM, NP, personal communication, January 14, 2022

WHAT IS MEMBRANE SWEEPING?

This simple process can encourage your body to go into labor on its own. Membrane sweeping, done by your maternity care provider, involves the insertion of one or two gloved fingers into the cervical canal (*internal os*), then rotating the finger(s) in a circular motion along the bottom of your uterus.[10]

This technique separates the amniotic sac from the lower part of the uterus, which releases fatty prostaglandin F2α and phospholipase A2 proteins. These beauties may get contractions going within the next few days.[3]

Note: this method can be used once your baby is full term (39 weeks) and your cervix has dilated some; it can even be repeated, if necessary, though the optimal timing and intervals are still a mystery.[10]

The cons? It may feel uncomfortable, could cause cramping and bleeding afterward, or could possibly increase the chance of your bag of water breaking prior to labor onset.[13] But hey, for those desperate mamas ready to meet their little ones, this can be a relatively easy way to initiate labor!

beautifully orchestrated ensemble of associated hormones (like oxytocin, endorphins, catecholamines), mamas are set up to have the "easiest transition possible—physiologically, hormonally, psychologically, and emotionally—from pregnancy and birth to new motherhood."[6]

Labor induction

Induction is a process by which medications or mechanical methods are used to begin your labor (often between 41 and 42 weeks in the United States).[3,7,8] Sometimes this means jumping right into the induction method, like getting a human-made version of the oxytocin hormone (like Pitocin) by IV, while other times the cervix needs preparation, or softening, first.[3,8,9] This cervical softening can be done using medications like misoprostol (CYTOTEC) or dinoprostone (CERVIDIL), or mechanical methods like membrane sweeping, *amniotomy* (breaking your bag of water) or balloon catheters.[3,8-10]

Inductions can be offered at different times and for different reasons. For example, women can get induced because they have medical problems or pregnancy complications, they don't go into labor on their own, or they are full term and want to give birth already! In other words, they can be **medically indicated** (opted for because of medical or pregnancy problems) or **elective inductions** (opted for because of reasons other than medical or pregnancy problems). The three U.S. professional midwifery groups caution against elective inductions since they disrupt a mama's normal physiologic process of labor.[5,11] It's also helpful to know that the very common Pitocin-induced labors tend to be long. They also require

WORDS OF AFFIRMATION

Did you know your mind can serve as a powerhouse of strength during labor? Our thoughts change the way we feel and behave. So, mama, check out these inspiring truths. Pick a few favorites and write them down on an index card to have handy for labor. During each contraction, repeat the statement in your head, like a mantra.

- I am strong. I am calm.
- Release and relax.
- Open, surrender.
- I'm doing it.
- My body was made for this.
- I am not alone. Women are birthing with me right now, all around the world.
- This contraction will be over in a minute. I can handle anything for one minute.
- Contractions help me meet my baby.
- I can't go around it; I will go through it.
- God is my strength.

continuous electronic fetal heart rate monitoring and administration of IV fluids, both of which limit a mama's flexibility for various labor positions.[7]

Now, getting an induction on the books can be exciting for some women but discouraging for others. If you're in the latter group, don't worry, often all your baby needs to hear is that you mean business, and she decides it's time to cooperate! Scheduling inductions helps hospitals plan for what's to come, ensuring women don't get overlooked or neglected. It doesn't necessarily mean your body is not going to go into labor on its own.

As always, it's vital to have an in-depth talk with your maternity care provider about your wishes, the reason for and timing of the induction, and the associated risks and benefits. Remember, for some women, induction may increase their risk for Cesarean birth.[7] If you decide to hold off on an induction for a while longer, most maternity care providers will recommend additional monitoring of your baby after 41 weeks. Three common methods include (1) *nonstress tests* (NSTs), which check how your baby's heart rate changes when she moves around, (2) *biophysical profiles* (BPPs), which combine an NST with an ultrasound, and (3) *modified BPPs*, which combine an NST with a measurement of the amniotic fluid volume; each method simply involves placing an external device or ultrasound probe on your cute belly.[2,12]

So, as the Hungarian proverb says, let your patience grow your little rose. Treasure this special moment as much as you can. Soon, you will no longer be pregnant, and as hard as it may be to imagine now, you will likely come to miss some aspects of it.

Digging Deeper

While you are waiting for the big day, there are a host of things you can do to prepare. Check out A-3j for a list of twenty suggestions to help you pass the time, including stocking up on snacks, wrapping up work, installing your car seat, and finding some cute postpartum lounge clothes. To make the most of this time, seize the day in small, manageable ways. Trust me, you won't regret it!

WEEK 39

Baby

- Is about 19 ¾ inches long.
- Weighs about 7 ¼ pounds.
- Is now full term!
- Now has a fully matured liver.
- Has established breathing patterns of 40 breaths every minute.

Mama

- Sleep may be more of a dream than reality.
  - Use your body pillow, ask a loved one for a massage, and rest when you can.
- With your belly in full bloom, large meals no longer fit.
  - Eat smaller portions and snack throughout the day.
- You're nearly there! The exciting moment of meeting your baby will be this week if you're having a planned Cesarean birth; otherwise, it's around the corner!

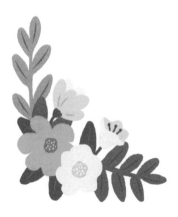

Musing and Anticipation

I can't believe I'm finally 39 weeks pregnant. I could go into labor any time.

To think, I'll finally deflate sometime soon. No more "eating for two," or having people commenting on my size and body. No more heartburn, hidden toes, toilet seat warmers, Saint Bernards, dreams of the Wild West, or nights like "The Princess and the Pea." Goodbye perineal massage, unprovoked crying, and feeling short on space. Soon, I'll be cuddling close to Dan, and sleeping flat on my back whenever I want.

So excited.

Even so, pregnancy has had highlights I will miss. I've had the opportunity to grow a real-life, 3D human inside of me. Through these months, the world has spoiled (and sometimes smothered) me with special treatment all because, well, I'm *with child*. Come to find out, the world agrees—pregnant women deserve this attention. Through the journey, my courage overcame timidity, my humor grew in moments of awkwardness, and I now give myself more permission to cry when it feels right. I've discovered pregnancy offers such an opportunity to grow in flexibility, to release control, to become less selfish, to focus on beauty, and to trust God, if we so choose.

Still, as I think about the path that remains ahead of me, I find it easy to worry over the uncertainties: What will labor and birth be like? What will having a baby do to my marriage and other relationships? Will I ever feel like myself as a mom? Will I get my body back? Will I feel isolated after delivering?

Although it's common for each pregnant mama to have her own set of worries, I remember we *are* tougher than leather and can grow and adapt like the yellow-blossomed succulents along the California coast. With resolve, I steer my thoughts to what I'm looking forward to the most: I'll get to meet my little one in the next few weeks! Soon, I'll get to see what she's like, and she'll finally teach me what it means to be a mother. Goodness, I'll even get to shave my legs, tie my shoes, and find pants that fit. I can hardly wait!

Is It Time?

Three days before my due date, contractions began during the night. Feeling like a bad period cramp, they came and went at first every 30 minutes and then every 5 to 15. After a few hours, I moved to the couch and tried to sleep as best as I could, dozing and periodically updating Dan, who mumbled something like, "Let me know if they are five minutes apart," and continued sleeping.

What a help.

By morning, realizing that these contractions meant business, Dan canceled his last day of work, hurriedly packed up, and smashed all our belongings into the car. We turned off the cabin heater, put the keys into the lockbox, and off we zipped down the salted road while the garage door closed behind us.

We had hoped that my sister, Lili, would be able to travel up from Los Angeles to join me at my labor, which would logistically be tricky even if I began labor in Cupertino. Now, as we rushed down the mountain highway, I dialed the phone. The snowy banks slid past as I waited for her to answer.

"Hey—I've been having contractions all night," I blurted as soon as she picked up. "Over the past few hours, they've been every five to fifteen minutes."

"What? Really? Do you think I should come?" she asked, excitement mirroring my own. "What are the chances your contractions would stop?"

"Well, it's hard to know, but probably things will continue since they've been going all night," I muttered, shifting in the seat as another one came.

"Okay, I'm on my way," she said in a rush. "I'll be there by evening."

"Did someone order a Lili?" my sister asked as I opened our door that night.

It was nine-thirty, after a long drive, and it was as if I had a fairy godmother at my doorstep—a luxury every pregnant woman deserves.

Amid our laughter, I welcomed her inside and then gave her the latest updates. Unfortunately, shortly after our call, my contractions slowed and then screeched to a grinding halt. I had hoped this meant my baby was simply being polite and was trying with all her might to wait until Lili arrived.

However, my little trickster decided to do nothing more than stay safely tucked inside throughout my sister's entire visit. Yes, through all *three days* she stayed with us. During this time, we mostly read, slept, and ate. So anticlimactic! At the end of it, we named this trip a successful "dry run" and waved goodbye as she parted for her return flight.

What happened to all the contractions? How could they just stop like that?

Ever since, Dan has been asking me if I've had any contractions.

"No!" I finally snapped. "Have you?"

I've also received a flurry of texts from well-meaning people asking how things are going, which basically means all day long I'm telling people the same disappointing news: "There is nothing new to report. I'll keep you posted."

I guess in the meantime, I can get some other things situated, like reviewing relaxation techniques and laboring positions with Dan. And of course, more of that blessed perineal massage.

⋙ LET'S TALK ABOUT IT ⋘

Helping Your Older Child Adjust

Dear friend, things are getting down to the wire—how exciting! I bet you have so much on your mind. To help your homelife transition go smoother postpartum, let's take a moment to discuss helping your other child(ren) adjust to your little baby. Soon, a brand-new family member is going to sweep in, take all your attention, and shake everyone's foundations. Who wouldn't be a bit off-kilter after finding this addition to the family is a crying and eating machine who sleeps during the day and wails at night?

Most likely, your spectacular, blooming self has already offered plenty of opportunity to talk with your child about what's to come. If you haven't had much time or it's been a while, take a moment to check in. Your baby inside is changing everyone's life, and although it's exciting, your child may not always be thrilled. You may notice mixed or negative feelings toward this intruder, like resentment or jealousy. Rest assured, this is common, especially if you have younger children who want to play, be close, and have mama or daddy's undivided attention. You'll find older children may have an easier time but are still going to want to socialize, get to sporting and extracurricular activities, and be able to talk or hang out with you. After all, they love you! And so, when these times together are threatened, children can act out, fight, have more tantrums, and if younger, they may even temporarily regress developmentally (use baby talk, become "un-potty-trained," or suck a thumb).

Ask questions

To help support your child, be proactive and check in regularly. With younger children, snuggle up and read a children's book about the "big brother or sister" or "the new baby." Ask questions along the way. Depending on your child's age, your questions could include: How do you feel about a baby coming (or being here)? Why do babies cry? What do you think a baby likes to do? What do babies eat? What is it like being an older sister or brother? For older kids, find a good moment for those heart-to-hearts, whether in the car, on a walk, over dinner, or at bedtime.

Offer reassurance

To help your child feel loved and secure, be sure to say *I love you* often and remind him that this will never change. It feels like a no-brainer, but it's easy to forget in the chaos. It can also help to refer to your baby as "our" baby and ask your child to pick out or organize baby things or to come alongside you as your "helper."

Set aside time

Although life will be busy once your baby's home, make time for your older child(ren) daily. This is so important. It may seem impossible at first, but don't worry, soon you'll become an expert multitasker. You'll be feeding your baby while reading a story to your child and will be balancing multiple kids on the lap you thought only had room for one. Mamas are amazing! If you miss a day, have grace for yourself and try again tomorrow.

Whenever possible, allow yourself to ask for help with the baby so you can sneak away for that special together time with your older child(ren). Your baby won't know the difference, but your older child will. It doesn't have to be long, just make it intentional and free of electronics. Children also love it when they can do special activities with loved ones—like baking, visiting the park or zoo, or going on a scavenger hunt—so see if these can be worked into the schedule. All these intentional moments reassure children and help them along this crazy, beautiful, messy home adventure.

Digging Deeper

Looking for other fun postpartum ideas for your child? You could buy a small gift to give when your baby comes home or create an entertaining postpartum activity box to make your child feel special. Items to gather for such a box might include:

» For younger kids: playdough, crayons, coloring books, pipe cleaners, silly putty, books, stickers, stuffed animals, stamps, and puzzles.

» For older kids: books, journals, cookbooks for kids, STEM or model kits, puzzles, modeling clay, or even a digital camera to help your aspiring journalist capture those special moments.

WEEK 40

Baby

- Generally is between 18 and 21 inches long.[1]
- Generally weighs between 6 and 8 pounds.[1]
- Is preparing for his or her debut—may be any day now!

Mama

- Congrats, your body has reached its maximum weight gain!
- Compared to prepregnancy, your breasts are now larger and about three pounds heavier.
- Your uterus is now 500–1,000 times larger than before you got pregnant.
- Your maternity care provider will recommend delivery by 42 weeks. Some women who don't want to wait that long choose to get induced earlier.

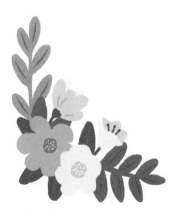

Change of Plans

What began as a familiar morning trip to the bathroom became, in a moment, anything but. My dazed waddle over was interrupted by the strange sensation of a warm fluid trickling down my inner thigh. *What in the world?* I continued walking, but there it was again. Am I peeing on myself or . . . ? Is it happening, finally—the day before my due date? Is this the big day? Thrilled at the thought, I headed back to our bedroom.

"Dan," I said, giving his blanketed shoulder a shove. "I think my water broke."

"Really?" he muttered from underneath a mountain of pillows.

"Yes!" I shared, a spring in my voice. "I felt a strange trickle down my leg."

Silence.

I crawled over to him on the bed like a big bad wolf and peered at his peaceful, slumbering face. His eyes were still closed, and his breath was calm, as if nothing had happened. *Is he really still sleeping?*

A few more determined nudges and an eternity later, he sat up and started acting like a real doctor. He checked to see if there were any signs of my water breaking, and concluded yes, it probably did. Hooray! When will my regular contractions start coming? Oh my goodness, it could be any second!

Soon, though, the wave of excitement settled into a lake of anxiety in my stomach. This is already derailing my labor plans, since my baby is no longer protected by that lovely aqueous bubble. Even if the contractions don't start, we'll need to minimize our risk for infection by ensuring she's born within a couple of days and by limiting the cervical checks that determine my dilation.

But what about my birth plan? I've always imagined I'd labor in our apartment until I was at least five to six centimeters dilated. Accompanied by soft music, I'd sit and sway on my yoga ball, I'd let the warm water of our shower soothe me, and then I'd try all sorts of spectacular labor positions Dan and I had learned. Only after that would we go into the hospital for the final contractions and pushing.

All this would have been fine if Dan could check my dilation. But now, he'd be estimating instead of checking. And if those estimates aren't right, I could arrive at the hospital so early in labor that it might prompt unnecessary medical interventions. My heart sank.

Still, being the stubborn woman that I am, I decided there was no time to waste. After all, my contractions could be only minutes away! After much poking and prodding, I convinced Dan that it's time to get out of bed for good and coaxed him into fixing us a nutritious breakfast. *And voilà!* Half an hour later, we scarfed it all down and headed outside for a long walk along nearby trails, hoping to kick-start the contractions.

Easier said than done.

Throughout the day, I climbed up and down countless flights of stairs and meandered along the trails—for miles. In the evening, we updated our midwife by phone, and she agreed we could wait until morning to give my body a bit more time to go into active labor. However, if I didn't, I'd need to go into the hospital to get augmentation—a dose of artificial hormones to get my contractions going.

That is not part of the plan!

Scared and a little angry, I went to bed. Maybe miraculously, the contractions would start in earnest. Eventually they did, arriving between five and fifteen minutes apart. Great! Except, I was also supposed to get rest—and rest wasn't happening.

Eventually, I'd had it.

"Dan," I asked with a nudge, "could you give me a massage?"

"Now, honey?" his words were thick with the fog of sleep. "Are you sure?"

"Yes, I've been having contractions for hours and I'm so tired. I need to sleep, but I can't unwind."

He paused, sighed, and rolled over to face my back. With a hefty dose of good intention, he drizzled nearly half a bottle of massage oil on my skin. *This is going to be great!* I thought. *He is obviously committing to a very long massage.*

If only.

Haphazardly, he glided his hands along my back like on a slip 'n slide. Swoosh, swoosh. And then—nothing.

"Dan, wake up," I pleaded. "You barely massaged me."

Another quick, meaningless stroke followed by a snore.

"Dan, can you please massage me?"

"Honey, I'm so tired. Just let me know when you really need some help."

"What? I thought I just told you."

"I mean, when you're in labor."

A pang of panic shot down my spine. *Oh no! I've made a terrible mistake. This is my doula—my support—for labor? What does he mean, ask for help when I'm "in labor"?! I'm in labor now.* Here I am, contracting, and he is oblivious to my needs. How is this going to work? I want to deliver without any pain medication, but I won't be able to do it without his full effort. *God help me.*

Thankfully, He did. For the rest of the night, I dozed off between contractions, glistening under the moonlight.

The Climb

> *There is only one way to eat an elephant. One bite at a time.*
> —OLD AFRICAN PROVERB

By morning, I had not begun active labor. My body had failed me. In the hospital parking garage, fear and frustration gave way to tears. Eyes swollen, I hugged my yoga ball and walked toward the entrance, dread mounting as labor loomed like a craggy mountain. But I'm already so exhausted, how could I ever reach the summit? None of this is according to plan!

Little did I know that would be the case with the entire day's journey.

First off, the nurses tried to determine if, indeed, I had broken my bag of water. This proved to be way harder than expected. It took two test strips, a lot of waiting, and eventually, an ultrasound showing decreased fluid around my baby to finally confirm I didn't just pee on myself yesterday morning. *See, told you so.*

Next up was checking my dilation.

Yes! I'm sure those contractions did something.

Nope, long and closed, my midwife shared.

Zero? Damn.

And the next bit of news was even worse.

"Your biggest enemy today," my midwife warned, "is fatigue."

Great. In tears, I stared at my IV, listening to my baby's soft heart-beats amplified through the monitor. What happened to laboring in the comfort of my own home? I sniffed back the tears. While I have no idea how I'm going to get through this, I *do* know crying wouldn't change much.

Still in disbelief over the course of events, I listened to the midwife explain the various steps we could take to have our baby—hopefully, in the next 24 hours *and* without a Cesarean birth. She noted that often, the cervix must be ripe (softened) before it will dilate from artificial hormones. So, we could begin there. Or we could try going straight for the Pitocin, hoping the synthetic hormones prompt contractions and dilation. But if that doesn't work, it would both waste time and increase my risk of infection.

Unsure which path to take, we called our faithful friend, Veronica, seeking advice. She assured us that for women like me, there's no need to soften a cervix before starting the hormone. The water-breaking signaled I'm ready for business.

What a relief! This was the first bit of good news, and there was more to come—she offered to make the two-hour drive and be my doula. Grateful for the offer, I accepted, surprising even myself.

The next thing I knew, I looked like a telephone pole: lines hanging from my left arm, attaching me to a monitor. Water and hormones entered my bloodstream, and a screen validated my pangs in the form of peaks and valleys marching across a screen. Wireless monitoring continued as the four of us—Dan, myself, my baby, and the IV pole—walked laps around the Labor and Delivery unit.

A few hours later, I heard a quiet rap on my labor room door. Veronica arrived with a smile, lugging a grocery bag full of thoughtfulness—chips, pineapple pieces, orange juice, and flowers. Yes, everything *will* work out. Somehow.

With the Pitocin at work and seemingly ever-present contractions, my sense of time faded. My two dedicated doulas alternately massaged my back and fed me snippets of food, washed down by sips of orange juice.

Five hours later, it was time to check my cervix to see how effective, if at all, the hormones had been.

"Meshi, let's evaluate your expectations before they check you," Veronica wisely urged. "How dilated do you think you are?"

"Oh, seven centimeters would be nice."

"Now remember, we just want to see a change, *any* change, to show your cervix is responding to the Pitocin. *Any* change is a good sign."

"Okay," I said, not giving it much thought, knowing I must really be about nine.

The midwife came in to check and, with legs butterflied out, I waited an eternity to hear a number—any number above five.

"Three centimeters."

Wait, what?! After all the pain, the moans, the grunts, the position changes, and I have seven more to go? You've *got* to be kidding me. In the silence of disappointment, my body begged for sleep. Just let me pause life—take a break. I promise I'll come back.

"How about a change of scenery?" Veronica suggested. "Perhaps a shower?"

"Sure, if you can get me there," I muttered. "Just cut my shirt off." No, I didn't wear a button-down, and this old gray tee shirt with ruffles, well, it doesn't seem so cute anymore.

Once there, I sat down, dousing myself over and over, as I stared at the ceramic tiles. Veronica sang in the background, a soft and soothing Celtic-sounding melody, while I watched drops of water stream down my big Mama Earth–like belly. My soul quieted and though it felt like only minutes, it turned out to be about an hour of relief.

Eventually, my nurse checked me and said I was six to seven centimeters but still had "a ways to go yet."

"How long is 'a ways'?"

"Well, typically, people dilate one centimeter an hour."

Wrong answer. Despite the fog, the number clicked. *Three hours?* No way! Not if I have anything to do with it. By then I had already been battling a nearly irresistible urge to push—something that would almost certainly tear my cervix unless I was fully dilated. How could I possibly fight my body for another hour, let alone three?

Thankfully, Dan and Veronica had my back, literally, and with united forces kept this crazy laboring lady from pushing.

"When can I push?" I pleaded, after what felt like forever.

"Don't worry," she answered. "When it's time, we'll know."

How's that supposed to help? Well, I guess it's better than "three hours." Willing the time to pass, I proceeded to vomit (in a bag) and poop (on myself)—which surprisingly, didn't even phase me. Covered in my poop? Don't care. Just let me push.

When my faithful doulas called in my nurse to check me again—I was fully dilated! Women's bodies are full of surprises, let's not forget. And so, no, it wasn't three hours, it was one. All I had was a little anterior lip left on my cervix that could resolve with a few contractions. My body *finally* did something well!

As if in a dream come true, I watched the nurses, like little fairies, transform my room into a place more suitable for a newborn. They turned on the baby warmer, unfolded the sterile field, and laid out the instruments. I'd seen such organized chaos during my nursing rotations and knew: Something big was about to happen. Nurses don't scurry around for no reason.

It's like everything kicked into overdrive. My midwife had not yet returned, all Ob-Gyns were busy elsewhere, and a nurse was going to have to catch the baby.

I laid back for my final cervical exam and waited for the news while Dan and Veronica (who have both attended many deliveries) put their gloves on, just in case.

The anterior lip had resolved, and I was ready. Ready!

Thank you, God.

At that moment, a random Ob-Gyn flew through the door and threw on a blue gown. Donning her sterile gloves, she said, "You can push."

Really?

"I can push?"

"Yes." Relief poured over me as I finally stopped fighting my body. I pushed.

"Now wait a moment so your perineum can stretch."

What? I have to wait again?

"Now you can push."

Another push and another wait. Ten minutes later, our daughter was out! Praise God, praise Dan, praise Veronica, praise everyone who prayed for me.

They placed our little Smurf on my chest, and I slid her small, blueish face closer to my breast. It took but a few tries to convince her my nipple might be more promising than her thumb.

So, you are the one who somersaulted inside of me.

I just held her then, not even really fathoming what had happened. I had a baby and felt barely alive. They gave me some fluids to drink while they made a small vulvar stitch. Ten hours after the start of the Pitocin, I had brought my seven-pound, thirteen-ounce baby into the world.

Several hours later, when it was time to transfer to the postpartum unit, I gratefully accepted the offer of a wheelchair that Dan, thinking way too highly of his wife, was confident I didn't need. "We'll just walk down," he says. *You must be kidding me. Not after all I've been through, thank you very much. You bring that damn wheelchair. Now.*

And so, after making me a tad bit more presentable to the world, off we went, Dan wheeling us down the long, maze-like corridor to our postpartum room.

When we had settled in and we could rest, I fed my precious daughter as best as I knew how and then pressed a magic button for nurses to bring her to the nursery. I never thought I'd have done such a thing, but at that moment, I desperately needed one thing—sleep.

I couldn't believe it—it certainly didn't go as planned, but we reached the summit! With no more contractions to conquer, I closed my eyes and fell asleep with an ice pack between my legs, content to know that there was nothing else I needed to do. My precious daughter had *finally* arrived.

⋙ LET'S TALK ABOUT IT ⋘

Nearing the Birth Day

Well, you're likely realizing you've been in your chrysalis for a very long time. It may even be getting a bit stuffy. Be encouraged! Great news is coming your way—you're about to see what's on the other side. Already, intense emotions and physical sensations are cultivating your mama roar—the spirit and passion behind phrases like: "Let's get this baby out of me, already!" "My back is killing me!" or "I can hardly wait to find out what my baby's like." What great energy to channel into your labor and your baby's delivery!

Perhaps, though, you also find yourself a little (or a lot) apprehensive for what lies ahead. This, too, is quite common. An amazing experience is coming your way, which will change your life forever. It's only natural to have some fear or worry. To remain centered, trust in your body's wonderful design to birth, tap into your spiritual roots to strengthen your soul, allow your birthing support person to advocate for you when the time comes, and have confidence in your chosen maternity care team's skillset. This is also a lovely time to sneak in some special moments with your partner or other children.

Before you know it, you'll be on the other side, having received two poignant treasures—a precious newborn and a victory! From that moment forth, whenever you celebrate your baby's birthday, you will likely also, in your heart, be celebrating what you accomplished. Dear pregnant mama, you've come so far on this journey and are ravishingly strong!

USE YOUR VOICE

To help you have a beautiful labor experience, ask your maternity care provider any lingering questions you may have about labor, inductions, and what to expect after delivery. While in labor, speak up, make your questions and concerns heard, and make your needs known. Go, mama—you can do this!

Digging Deeper

While you wait in anticipation, take a moment to ponder your upcoming day—its uniqueness, its impact, its meaning. Visualize the courage you will find within yourself as you take on what, if your first, is a rite of passage—when you join the ranks of the women who also have experienced this profound physical and metaphysical transformation. To better prepare:

» Brush up on the stages of labor, birthing positions, and comfort measures for labor. (A-4a & b)

» Review when to call your maternity care provider. (A-2)

» Encourage your labor support to fine-tune those awesome support skills. (A-4e)

BABY'S EARLY MONTHS

WEEKS 1–15

MONTH 1

Baby

- Is learning about new surroundings and how to trust.
- Has unpatterned sleep, wake, and feed cycles.
- Can clearly see objects 10–12 inches away.
- Mainly functions using reflexes like sucking and grasping.
- Often breathes irregularly: at times rapidly, at times slowly.
- Has jerky arm movements.
- Prefers feeding on demand.
- Loves skin-to-skin cuddling and being held!

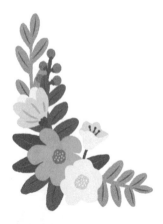

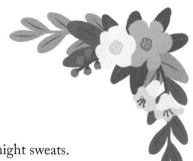

Mama

- You might experience hot flashes or night sweats.
- Breasts produce colostrum until mature breastmilk comes in (3–5 days postpartum).
  - Don't worry! Breastfeeding or pumping will help your milk come in.
- For about three to eight weeks, you will shed *lochia* (outer uterine discharge). Though it will begin bloody, it will eventually turn yellow-white.
- Within two weeks of delivery, you will lose about 10–13 pounds. Goodbye, extra fluids and placenta!
- If not breastfeeding, you may ovulate as early as four weeks after delivery.
  - Don't forget your birth control.
- You might temporarily have greater trouble with urinary incontinence. Remember, kegels and pelvic floor physical therapy can be lifesavers.
- Your immune system will soon return to its prepregnancy state. Mamas with autoimmune conditions may notice flare-ups for several months postpartum.

WEEK 1

Heading Home

They wheeled me down the hospital corridor, I, the proud mother cuddling my new, soft bundle, who smelled so good. Dan and I posed by the exit to capture the traditional hospital photo op, the very last moment before we took our baby past the automated sliding glass doors into the expansive world beyond. As we got in the car, I kept wondering how we actually got permission to take this little person home. Were we *really* qualified?

The drive home had never before seemed so long or treacherous. Cars whizzed past on either side while one even wove in and out of lanes as if trying to stitch together the highway before us. My heart skipped a beat, and my protective mama instinct appeared out of who knows where. *People! Don't you know I have a brand-new baby in here, only two days old? Slow down!* Well, that's what I would have shouted out the window with a scowl had the hospital provided us with a complimentary megaphone. But instead, I restrained myself, prayed God would protect, and marveled at how I could love someone this much already.

Soon after getting home, we decided a simple stroll would be a pleasant way to start off our first day back. After all, we're two grown adults—adding a baby to the equation couldn't change things that much, right? But boy were we wrong! I quickly realized I had no idea how to dress my baby for the California weather. I mean, surely she could freeze out there in the 55-degree air!

Finally, two hats and three blankets later, we emerged with our baby wearing the blue romper my parents dressed me in on the day I left the hospital—yep, the one I never thought I'd use (go figure). Perplexed by how to fit this layered human football into a stroller or baby carrier, I decided to simply carry her—with a kung fu death grip, of course. We walked past the trees casting their shadows on the sidewalk, crossing paths with the neighbor's prowling cat.

Ah, the soothing outdoors does the tired soul so much good. Speaking of tired, it's not just my soul that could use the rest. Each step seems monumental, and we're not even past the first stop sign. And why are my quads killing me? Come to find out, I squatted for about an hour and a half during labor. *I suppose that sounds vaguely familiar.*

No sooner had we reached the apartment after our walk than Dan got antsy. He was ready to introduce our baby to our landlords who live below us on the first floor, and who've become friendly acquaintances, frequently sharing conversations and their homegrown zucchinis in the months since we moved in.

"Dan, you seem so thrilled," I remarked, "it's like you want to show off our baby to anyone in the world."

"Not to anyone—" he said with a shake of his head "—to everyone." His response said it all. How lucky that my husband is this excited about his new baby girl.

"Sure, go ahead," I said, trying very hard to be the relaxed mother I so desperately wanted to become. "But please be very careful going down the stairs."

Next thing I knew, the door was closing behind him. Away he went with my baby, essentially ripping off one of my appendages. She was a mere fifteen feet below me but seemed a million miles away.

All I could do was cry.

A Glimmer in the Dark

That night in our home became one to remember. After the sun had set, and not too long after drawing down our shades, my quiet angel started to cry. Nonstop. Don't ask me how she was blessed with that sort of lung capacity, but she was. And cry without ceasing she did—all night long—each tearful sob and scream reducing me, her new mama, to a mere ragdoll.

I picked her up and kissed her round, wet cheeks.

"*Mi a baj kicsikém?*" (What's wrong, my little one?)

Holding her close, her chin resting on my shoulder, I walked her around the bedroom, rubbing and patting her tiny back. And when that got old, I sat down on my yoga ball, hoping I could gently bounce our woes away. *Nothing.* All she could do was wail and shriek as if she were trying to digest a tire.

Oh my goodness! Is this what normal babies do? Or is something wrong? Is she hungry? Is she in pain? Is she hot? How am I to know?

Dan was recovering from a cold (with earplugs, I'm sure), so I had decided to take one for the team rather than wake him. I paced the dimly lit living room floor with my unhappy love, sometimes up and down, sometimes circling the perimeter. Her intense cries reverberated off the hardwood floors until I thought surely my eardrums would shatter. No amount of dancing, *shhh*ing, walking, rocking, breastfeeding, or singing comforted her—for 10 hours straight.

By then, *I* wanted to cry. I couldn't believe this is what I signed up for. Is this the price of love? I think we made a mistake. A terrible one. If this is what mothering is, I don't think I'm cut out for it.

Finally, at about 5:30 a.m., she fell asleep—probably from sheer exhaustion.

How could I possibly do this for another 18 years? Did Mother Atlas ever feel like this? I flopped onto our bed, pulled up the covers, and drifted off in the blessed silence. For the next few hours, crying monsters (who also needed me) surfaced in my dreams. I woke up drenched, exhausted, and in a fog. *I'm so tired of hearing crying—all the time. I don't want to be needed anymore.*

Boy, was I relieved when later that day, my mom and sister arrived to our rescue for a few weeks. *Thank God!* Maybe I can finally sleep. While I lay in bed, I could hear them bustling about and chatting away in the kitchen while they prepared lunch. They then sat down at the table outside of my bedroom.

"Meshi seems a little weird," Lili whispered to my mom.

Hell, yeah! You think? Not sleeping for days can make a person feel so strange and sometimes scared. Will I ever feel like myself? Am I capable of adequately caring for someone so little and vulnerable? What if I drop her? What if I make a mistake?

"It's normal," my mother assured. "She'll be back to herself very soon."

Really?

Phew, what a relief!

ᐧᐧᐧ LET'S TALK ABOUT IT ᐧᐧᐧ

Coping with Your Beautiful Mess

Congratulations! Regardless of whether you had a vaginal or Cesarean birth, epidural or not, this is truly a huge accomplishment! Your life is now officially turned upside down. You're figuring out your baby's needs, if the poop is a normal color, and maybe even how to help the rest of your family adjust to this newest family member.

In the meantime, your body has already begun the recovery process from this monumental event. For some body systems, this recovery can take six weeks, but for others (like the cardiovascular system, pelvic floor muscles, or your mental health), this can take longer.[1] Although you may feel a bit out of whack during this process, don't despair. It won't always be this hard. Of course, if you are especially concerned about something, reach out to your maternity care provider.

> **DIY PERINEAL ICE PACK!**
>
> Mix ½ cup corn syrup with ¼ cup sugar. Put in a doubled-up, unlubricated condom or baggie. Keep in the freezer and use as needed. Thank you, pelvic floor therapists, for perfecting this recipe over the years!

Since we listed the common physical changes in the prior milestone section, let's look at what's going on with your emotions and mental health. Go ahead, grab some popcorn, an ice pack, water, and your stool softener, and read this section with your partner or support person. Ready?

Okay, so you may have always envisioned yourself blissfully soaring through motherhood with a smile, doting on your baby, singing your way through the day, *La la la la la. Isn't this* all *wonderful?*

But unfortunately, most women who have these expectations are in for a surprise. Up to 75% of mamas worldwide experience something called **baby blues**. It's a normal and temporary situation—different from postpartum depression—in which you experience emotional fluctuations and passing negative feelings. Overall, you may be happy and excited, but then may cry or be irritable, tired, anxious, and scared at random times.[2-6] It usually starts a few days after birth, could last up to about the time your baby's two weeks old, but then disappears.[2-6] Buckle your seatbelt, dear mama, you're in for a short ride—no, it doesn't mean you're losing your mind.[†]

It's understandable that baby blues can develop, since the changes occurring in your body and life right now include massive hormonal fluctuations.[3] However, if your symptoms last longer than two weeks, you're unable to cope easily or function normally, or you are having distressing feelings most of the day (including thoughts that scare you), please contact your maternity, primary care, or mental health provider as soon as possible instead of waiting it out.[5] In these circumstances, prompt assistance is hugely important.

Given all of this, it's no wonder postpartum is the perfect time to ask for help—yes, *really*—even those of us who find it hard to ask for help or have difficulty accepting it. It's okay if it's a struggle; we all do sometimes! It is especially important right now to put yourself out there and ask for help so that you and your child(ren) receive what is needed.

BABY BLUES SYMPTOMS

Crying, weepiness, sadness, mood swings, irritability, impatience, fatigue, insomnia, poor concentration, worry, anxiety, and lack of concentration.

Also, it can be a game changer to sleep, eat (nutritiously, if possible), and get outdoors. Even opening a window can refresh you and connect you to the world you've always known. As for your partner or support people—Dad or other loved ones—order some takeout, hold the baby between feedings, and start practicing how to change a diaper. Who said blowout poops can't help you bond with the little one?

[†] Julie Jorgenson, LMFT, personal communication, July 2, 2021

Digging Deeper

Dear mama, to help foster your mental health and well-being postpartum, check out the resources in B-4. There, you'll find answers to common questions like:

» How may a parent's untreated mental health problems affect his or her baby? (B-4a)

» Can partners also struggle with postpartum mental health problems? (B-4a)

» What is postpartum psychosis and how common is it? (B-4a)

» What practical tool can I use to proactively monitor my mental health? (B-4b)

WEEK 2

I Wish Upon a Star

Star light, star bright,
It's been only two weeks since my little love was tucked inside of me, and out of who knows where, nostalgia hit me. It dropped into view much like a shooting star—swift and unexpected. It must have streaked its glorious tail across my subconscious and—*puff*—landed in my lap. I'm pretty sure I'm covered in stardust now because all I can think about is how much I miss being pregnant.

First star I see tonight;
I don't understand. How could this be? What more could I want than my little one here with me? She's my sweet, precious girl, the purpose behind my pregnancy. I no longer wonder what she'll be like because, well, here she is—in my very arms. Her tiny hands fit in my palms and her entire being nuzzles into my chest.

I wish I may, I wish I might,
And yet, my heart longs for the 10 months past. How I miss the days when I was big and round and could feel her kicks and hiccups from within. I ache for when we lived so close, we barely fit—when I could wear her inside of me. I miss the special attention from the world, even the annoying advice, the unexpected belly touches, and the "eating for two."

Have this wish I wish tonight.
With birth, it seems, I gained a daughter and lost a pregnancy. It's as it should be, and yet—now, I wish upon a star and yearn to have it back.

Finding Myself

I found you! Finally. Yes, *you*, silly. Where have you been all these days? I've missed you. It's so nice to feel your familiar presence again.

Peeking into the mirror, I am awed by this wonderful shift in my sense of self. A shift that came about from one beautiful, key ingredient for life—sleep.

This morning, propped against my fluffy pillows, I felt like a queen residing in her chambers. The sunshine etched my bedpost with gold while I reclined and watched my sister and mother take on all the official duties of the courts. You know, cooking, laundry, diaper changing, baby cuddling, and burping. Sinking into the sweet embrace of sleep, I counted my blessings. Yes, every mama needs help for at least a few weeks after the royal birth.

Another lovely change has been the level of our little lady's nightly tirades. Desperate to find the cause, the King and I issued a royal decree banishing from my diet all dairy products involving cows' milk. It turns out their milk—like nuts, caffeine, and chicken—is a common allergen for babies, and it may take a couple of weeks to clear out completely from breastmilk. In the meantime, we're entertaining all sorts of interesting, tasty, and horrid alternatives like goat, almond, coconut, and soy products. A true adventure for the palate.

Although I can't say it's easy to cut out foods I love, the switch already seems to be helping her. Last night, I got one beautiful, uninterrupted stretch of sleep—for four whole hours. *Four!* What I wouldn't pay for this to happen again. I think I'd even drink goats' milk or eat twice-baked potatoes with vegan cheddar and sour cream.

⟫⟫ LET'S TALK ABOUT IT ⟪⟪

Soothing Baby and Regaining Your Cool

Giving birth changes everything. Likely, by now you've realized how determined your little one is to make his needs known. When things don't go smoothly, no worries! Parenting is not about perfection; it's about perseverance. While there is a lot of trial and error involved in parenting, there are a few tips that can make things easier. So, let's dive into the ones that involve soothing your baby, and what to do when you're at your wits' end.

Soothing baby

To begin with, babies love to be held, especially if you're moving around (like rocking, swaying, or walking).[1] Holding him like a statue won't do the trick, or at least, not for long. Count on staying active for the next few months.

Movement can even help to soothe a crying babe, as does repetition. Try singing, rocking, walking, bouncing, patting his back, or whispering *Shh, shh, shh*.[2] Changing your baby's position, feeding him milk, doing skin-to-skin, or turning on some white noise can also help (try a noise maker or a car ride).[3] It may take a few minutes for him to respond, so don't give up too soon. If one of your soothing techniques doesn't pan out, just try something else until he's calmer. Remember, it is possible to overstimulate your baby by trying too many things at once, so simplify if needed.[2]

Although all of us would *love* for our upset baby to stop crying entirely (and immediately), it's not always in the cards.[3] He's a baby,

---

BIRTH TRAUMA

Sometimes it can be hard to connect with your little one if your labor either didn't go as planned or was traumatic. Birth trauma can occur when there was an actual (or perceived) threat of either serious injury or fatality for you or your baby.[9] If you can relate, I'm so sorry you went through this.

While no words can erase the pain, I'd encourage you to please check out the first section in B-4i, which is designed to help you understand what you went through and to get the appropriate care for healing. It can make a world of difference for your mental health and for your ability to bond with your little one!

after all. Consider it an accomplishment even when it's only a decrease in the intensity. If you're in the throes of a marathon crying episode, let other people help and feed *you* in this exhausting process. Better yet, have them try their luck at wielding their magical baby powers.

Also, remember you may be able to avoid massive baby meltdowns by being proactive and staying attuned to your baby's cues.[3] In the early months, try carrying him throughout the day (save your arms and use a baby carrier) and pay close attention to disengagement cues, especially during social events.[2,4] Once you see him needing a break, remove him from bright lights and loud noises, and keep him from being passed around like a football.[2,4] Your careful attention can save you both a lot of angst.

Regaining your cool

Let's be honest, a crying baby is very stressful, overwhelming, and frustrating.[5] Sometimes *we* just want to cry. When you're at your wits' end, needing a break—listen to your needs and do just that. Put your baby safely in his crib and walk away for a few minutes.[6] This will give you a chance to cool down. Although we don't plan on harming our little loves, as parents, we get pushed to new limits. In desperate moments, we find it is hard to be patient and easier to lose control.

Make a point to practice this habit of a glorious pause, since doing so will not only help you feel better, but it will also help avoid *shaken baby syndrome* (**SBS**). With SBS, head trauma is caused by a baby being shaken, which can result in lifelong neurological damage like blindness, cerebral palsy, and learning disabilities—or even death.[7,8] We need to be extra cautious in our baby-handling in the first year of life, since babies have weak necks, planet-sized heads (relatively speaking), and delicately developing brains. So, join me in being proactive with our little ones and with ourselves so we can tend to their needs, build relationships, and make our nest a place of nurture.

Digging Deeper

Who knows how many times you were interrupted by your little one's crying before you could finish reading this section? Yes, it's a great opportunity for practice! This is a wonderful time to watch for baby cues and try out some fun baby bonding ideas from "Connecting with Baby" (week 33) and A-5c. You've got this!

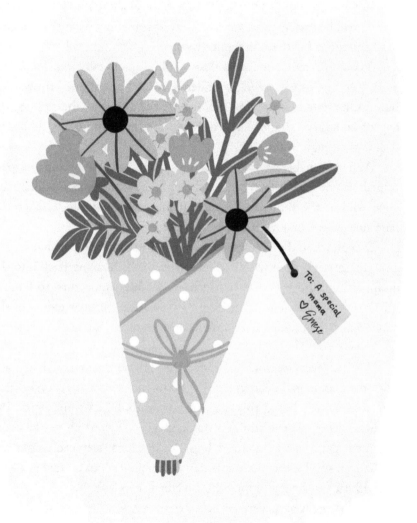

WEEK 3

Cinderella

"Well, Meshi, tonight's a big night. When the clock strikes 10:45, our little one will be *exactly* three weeks old. And you know what that means," Dan announced with excitement. "Everything's going to change."

As our eyes met, hopeful smiles stretched across our faces. *But it can't possibly be that simple, can it?* I wondered, while he continued the nightly, humdrum chore of emptying the dishwasher. I took in the sight of the bag of laundry tied and cinched, ready for the laundromat, and dirty dishes piled high in the sink.

Well, reasonable or not, this is the sort of anticipation our postpartum souls needed. In fact, for a little while now, our imaginations have gone wild at the thought of experiencing something like Cinderella's fairy tale—here, in our very home!

Except, when the time came, we wouldn't see the blue ballgown and a pumpkin stagecoach with curlicue wheels transforming back into the disappointing ordinary. Oh no. Instead, our life would turn to fantasy. That's right. A little *bibbidi-bobbidi-boo* here, and a little wielding of the magic wand there, and what do we have? Hours and hours of more sleep, *without* crying.

We had every reason to believe this enchantment could happen. Multiple people had been promising us for weeks now that everything gets noticeably better at this age. They couldn't all be wrong, right? The implications were delightful. To think, maybe we won't always be overwhelmed. With just a few more hours of precious sleep each night, we might even survive the intense demands of parenthood! Giddy, and with belly aflutter at the joyful thought, I readied myself for bed.

And before we knew it, our little crying machine granted us our first four-*and-a-half*-hour stretch of sleep—just as she turned three weeks old. I guess fairy tales can come true.

Forget the Breast?

I finally understand why a minority of women exclusively breastfeed beyond a few weeks. It's a hard and unrelenting job, which continues into all odd hours of the day and night. It demands everything from a mama—her attention, her body, and her time. Add in other factors—like a baby's latch, tongue tie, or weight, and a mama's own health, work schedule, and milk supply—and it gets complicated fast.

Watching my baby breastfeed, I recall a passing conversation I had with my lovely Ob-Gyn mentor, Dr. Spivak, right before I went out on maternity leave. The scene plays across my mind as my darling and I rock back and forth.

"Have a wonderful time getting to know your little one," my mentor had urged. She then leaned toward me, her dark-brown, tight curls swaying with the movement. "I also just want you to know," she shared, "breastfeeding is very hard. I didn't realize how hard it would be until I started. It may be the hardest thing you do."

Could it really be that difficult? I had wondered.

Now, though, I can say with certainty that—yep, she was right. Despite working with women who breastfeed, I definitely underestimated how hard it really would be. After all, we women have breasts hanging from our chests. Shouldn't it just be instinctual? But no, it requires stamina, patience, and determination to not give up despite the steep learning curve. It truly is a labor of love—but then, so are most aspects of mothering, I suppose.

Grappling with the all-consuming challenge of breastfeeding, I've been asking myself—is it really worth it? I opted for this route because of the pros, but all I can really see right now are the cons. So what are the pros again?

For one, I get to have bigger breasts without the surgery. *Nice.* Two, in California, it gives me a legitimate way to opt out of jury duty. *True, but neither of these are good enough reasons to continue this nonstop milk-fest.* Three, my baby and I reap spectacular immune benefits, and it gives us another way to bond. *Ah yes, that's good—real good.*

Emerging from my internal debate, I reposition my little girl for burping. She rests her chin on my shoulder, and I lean my head against hers, deciding I might as well carry on. No, I don't know how far we'll get, but I do want to try my darndest—day by day, moment by moment. Maybe we'll get to the six-month benchmark, but maybe not.

In the meantime, I will forge ahead. As a person climbs a mountain one step at a time, so I fashion a liquid armor for her, drop by drop. I wonder how far she and I can get.

⸺⟩⟩⟩ LET'S TALK ABOUT IT ⟨⟨⟨⸺

You and Your Baby-Centered World

Phew! What a whirlwind it has been, right? At this point, you're tired and are juggling so much to keep everyone alive. Yep, this is survival mode. This is also a time when new parents tend to become preoccupied with their baby.[1] You live and breathe your little one and may melt when you see her cute dimples. With all this newness, you may even be getting a little (or a lot) worried about all sorts of things related to your baby, even if you've never struggled with anxiety before.

You may wonder: Is she getting enough milk? Oh my gosh, is she breathing? Am I going to drop her? Am I a good mommy?[1-3] If you think about it, this *obsessive-compulsive disorder-like* baby infatuation and fixation is nature's way to keep you baby-captivated.[1] It enrolls you in a crash course on your little one and can help you figure out how to provide for your baby's needs as a new parent. This mindset is super common, especially in new parents, and can also occur if you struggle with OCD at baseline.[2]

Unwanted thoughts and compulsive behaviors

In this season, many parents notice obsessive—sticky—unwanted thoughts about harm coming to their babies.[4,5] If you can relate, *breathe*. Sometimes, parents' distressing, repetitive, intrusive thoughts may include the belief that they will be the source of the harm—even though their desire is the exact opposite. If you can relate, please know there is no need to feel guilty or ashamed. This doesn't mean you are a bad parent or that you will harm your baby. Distress itself in this circumstance is a reassuring sign of your desire to keep your child safe. The other good news is that for many people, obsessive thoughts resolve in the first few weeks postpartum.[5]

Sometimes, to soothe these distressing thoughts, people turn to *compulsive behaviors*: repetitive actions that often take up a considerable amount of our time and limit the normal flow of our day. They may include watching your baby sleep *all* the time, rigorously tracking your baby's feeds, or even trying to get your baby on a strict schedule.

Here's the good news: Overall, most parents get more relaxed and less anxious by three to four months.[1] And, yes, they feel more confident in their parenting abilities, too.[1] It's on your horizon!

In the meantime, don't stress about the fact that you're somewhat more concerned about such baby matters, and remember to invest in self-care, even if for a few moments each day. For those of you mamas with all-consuming anxiety, who struggle with OCD, or who have distressing, intrusive thoughts or compulsions, don't go it alone! This is the perfect time to seek help and reassurance from a trusted mental health specialist (see B-4c). There's so much hope for you, too!

Digging Deeper

Sleep has got to be the one activity we mamas crave the most. It also happens to play a vital role in improving and rebalancing our mental health. Check out the resources below to rejuvenate and rebalance. They cover questions like:

» How can I get any sleep around here? (B-3b)

» Every time I put my sleeping baby down in the crib, he wakes up. Help! (B-3b)

» Is swaddling my baby a good idea? (B-3b)

» Can you remind me of practical ways I can nurture my mental wellness? (B-4f)

WEEK 4

We, Her Marionettes

> *Spies and parents never sleep.*
> —Linda Gerber

Our baby, or "mini maestro," as I like to call her now, has become quite an adept conductor for our nightly, in-home performances. She simply sounds her passionate shrieks, accompanies them with her dramatic lip quivering, and just like that—it's showtime. Her soprano-pitched musical score carries throughout our nest, and calls Dan and me, her marionettes, into action.

Already?

Although never adequately prepared or in costume for our performance, we begin the opening act in desperation. We bounce, waltz, and pace the mini, nine-pound prodigy to her liking, passing her back and forth between us as she demands. This routine we continue for hours—long after she stops crying. Just in case. Her musical accompaniment has long faded, and silence has settled.

There now, see how sweet and innocent she looks while asleep?

This is the standing intermission. Our cuddling conductor rests in aching arms. Heaven forbid we wake her, even if for a sip of water.

As showbiz goes, we now understand the show must go on—always—even if we would prefer a night off. *Could we turn in early, just once? Nope, sorry, tickets are sold out. The act is booked.*

After the intermission, we have the second, and most technically challenging, act—the transition from our arms to her spot in the crib beside our bed. We tiptoe underneath the dimmed lights to the room. Concentrating with each slow step, we try our best to avoid those randomly creaking floorboards that could startle the mini-maestro and sign us up for another performance.

Squeak.

Oh no!

Pause.

I hold my breath, and with an eye on her still-peaceful face, I lean over and lay her down gently in her crib. *Success.* Okay, now it's time to kick it into high gear as we try to mount our bed with sophistication.

Are you crazy? Stop breathing. She could hear you!

Oh no, she's stirring. Freeze, wherever you are! Yes, too bad if it means dangling off the mattress. With all your might, just hold it. We can't risk you tumbling to the ground. It would make far too much noise.

Phew! She's asleep again.

Our much-anticipated grand finale consists of a graceful final pivot into the horizontal position. It takes poise. It takes strength. And yes, it certainly takes guts. Dan and I then lie in that familiar corner of the bed, successfully smashed together like two sweaty, overworked dancers too scared to get comfortable. We made it. Proudly, we snuggle together in the dark, dead silence.

No encores tonight, please. You might wake the baby.

That Contraption

Sometimes, I wish I could sneak away for a few moments just to have a little time for myself. I'm not quite sure what I would want to do first. Shower? Shave my legs? Sleep? Eat? All these options sound so luxurious! How on earth would I ever decide?

I suppose before I drop everything to figure it out, a reality check would be helpful: Getting some time to myself is logistically tricky, since my sweet milk monster is hanging from me every two hours to feed. Breastfeeding is my life, and who knows when that will ever change? My sole identity has been whittled down into being a milk station, and I can't get away for longer than a sigh. Sure, giving my baby nourishment, whether breastmilk or formula, is a sacred task, but it takes so long. And it happens so often. I constantly have the Breast Friend breastfeeding pillow strapped around my waist, as if hoping this life preserver–like invention will keep me from drowning in the seas of motherhood.

If only there were a way out. Let me think, here. Wait a minute, I've got it! If I could just store up some breastmilk, so Dan or a babysitter could feed her, I might get somewhere! What a glorious day that would be. The thought sounds so exciting I could frolic through a field of flowers.

Okay then, today's the day. *Carpe diem.* Or I guess, in my case, it's *carpe papillae*—seize the nipples. To tell you the truth, I'm nervous about putting an innocent and ultrasensitive body part into the hands of an inanimate object. What if it malfunctions and clamps down on my breasts with invisible teeth, never letting go?

Still, it may be the door to freedom . . .

In the end, desperation won out over fear. It was time. I picked up *that* machine—the double electric pump—and reluctantly placed my precious nipples where I thought they belonged. Wary, I just sat there. Nipples, are you still okay? *So far, so good.* I then turned on the pump and slowly ramped up the suction. Not bad, not too painful, but I must say—it felt weird and utterly humiliating. All I could do was watch my nipples jostle back and forth to the sound of the machine suction. In fact, I felt quite industrial, somewhat like a cross between a human and a cow. A cow-human? A *cuman*?

So, this is what it's going to take, huh?

Well, I'm doing it! Although I couldn't understand how all this effort could lead to such little milk coming out, hope filled my soul as puddles appeared in the bottles. Maybe this would, indeed, grant me a single, undisturbed chunk of time to myself.

⇢⟫⟫ LET'S TALK ABOUT IT ⟪⟪⟸

Postpartum Depression

So, dear mama, the daily grind continues. It's your sacrificial hard work (hopefully, with help) that's paying off and helping your baby grow bigger every day. Nice job! Now, let's reflect on how you're doing and what you might be going through. After all, your emotional well-being not only affects you but also your baby and family: when you are well, you can thrive, connect, and meet your baby's constantly evolving developmental needs.

In "Coping with Your Beautiful Mess" (postpartum week 1), we talked about baby blues, and today we're delving into the topic of postpartum depression (PPD). It's the most common complication of childbirth, so consider grabbing your partner or loved one for this part—you'll both learn something, guaranteed!

You may be surprised to hear that PPD can happen to any parent and may occur anytime in your baby's first year of life.[1-5] In fact, did you know that this first year is when parents are at the highest risk for developing depression?[6] At least one in seven moms and one in eleven dads have PPD, and it often peaks at around three months after birth, or even a few months later for dads.[7-12] It's seen worldwide, spanning cultures, races, ethnicities, and socioeconomic classes—meaning there is no single type of person who gets PPD.[1,3,12]

You're more likely to get PPD, however, if you're stressed, single, or younger[6,13]; have spotty support[3]; had a difficult and/or traumatic birth or a low-birth-weight or preterm baby[3]; or if your baby is in the NICU.[3,10,11] These make for incredibly stressful and taxing times. PPD is also much more common among those with a history of abuse or violence during pregnancy, as well as those with a personal or family history of depression or anxiety.[3,13-15] Unfortunately, this covers a lot of us! Though it is unknown what exactly causes PPD, neurotransmitters, sensitivity to hormonal shifts, and the immune system's inflammatory response may be contributors.[3]

PPD Symptoms

So, how do you know if you have PPD? Well, tip-offs include sadness, apathy, and not enjoying the things you once loved. You may also experience anger, guilt, tiredness, pain, difficulty concentrating, changes in your appetite, sleep problems (trouble either sleeping or staying awake), or even suicidal thoughts.[3,14,16,17] Yep, it's a long and varied list. Remarkably, the main way PPD manifests in some mamas is through anxiety, irritability, or mental confusion—not the stereotypical "depression."[17] Or it may be feeling overwhelmed, alone, and just "not your normal self."[17]

PPD in dads

Dads, depression may present differently for you. It often develops gradually, around three to six months after delivery, and the biggest risk factors are if mama is struggling with depression, you yourself have a history of severe depression, or you experienced depression or anxiety during the pregnancy.[5,8,9] Tip-offs include overworking to escape, getting more irritable, experiencing rage or anger, being exhausted, or feeling hopeless; additionally, some either pick up or increase a habit of coping through drugs or alcohol.[9,18,19] Again, the main symptoms may not be the "sadness" typically associated with depression.

> ->>> ✿ ✿ ✿ <<<-
> PPD looks different
> for everyone.

There's hope!

If you can identify with these symptoms, there is hope for you! The good news is that, though serious, this condition is treatable with professional help, lifestyle changes, and practical support at home. Reach out to your healthcare provider (whether a maternity care, primary care, or mental health professional) right away to get started on your road to recovery. Of course, if you ever feel so hopeless and down that your life is on the line, call 911 or 988 or go to the nearest emergency room.

Also, please know that ignoring your suffering, trying to tough it out or will it away, or just working to think positively does *not* fix anything—it only delays you feeling better. These delays could even result in chronic depression. Though untreated depression is like a "thief that steals motherhood" (or parenthood), making you miss out on special bonding times with your baby, this doesn't have to be your story.[14] So, go ahead, dear friend, tap into your bravery, and get help. Your little one and your family need *you*!

Digging Deeper

Hopefully, reading this section has helped you better understand how common PPD is for parents and that it's nothing to be ashamed of. It's so important to be proactive and nurture your mental health, as well as to check in with yourself regularly, especially in your baby's first year of life. If you're in a relationship, don't forget about each other—communicate your needs and watch for those PPD tip-offs. Also, B-4 contains answers to common questions like:

» I think I might have PPD—I'm overwhelmed and not sure where to go from here. Help! (B-4c)

» If I ignore my PPD, how might it affect my little one? (B-4a)

» How is PPD treated? (B-4d)

» Can I be on psychotropic medication while breastfeeding? (B-4e)

» I have bipolar—what's important for me to pay attention to postpartum? (B-4a)

MONTH 2

Baby

- Starts connecting with people through smiles, noises, and gazes.
- Is more trusting and expects responses to cues.
- May calm self by sucking thumb.
- Keeps eyes open for longer, and sees farther (8–10 feet).
- Begins to relax the arms, legs, and fists.
- Likes being held and looking at patterns (especially those in black and white).

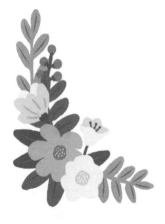

Mama

- Lochia discharge may continue, though it changes from lighter pink to yellow-white.
- Most pregnancy-related physical changes will return to prepregnancy levels.
- You may need certain medications readjusted if dosages were changed in pregnancy.
- The process of hair growth will restart. In the first few months, though, you'll first notice hair thinning or even large chunks falling out. No, you're not going bald!
  - Cut down on shampooing, use a wide-tooth comb, and part your hair creatively. Time for cute headbands, scarves, and hats.

WEEK 5

Who's That Girl?

Damn, girl! I can't believe it. Who's that gorgeous thing staring back in the mirror?

Okay, I admit, my reaction may have been a tad bit over the top, but what can I say? With weeks of motherhood comes perspective.

Wondering if Mrs. Glam was real or only a figment of my imagination, I slid open the bathroom window and ushered in the morning sun. I leaned in closer to the mirror, my gaze met by reflected blue eyes and a heart-shaped face.

"Perfectly stunning, if I do say so myself," I whispered under my breath. Nope, I wasn't wearing a little black dress, hadn't caked on makeup, or hadn't even put on the most ordinary of jewelry. It was just me, au naturel, finally wearing a clean tee shirt, sweats, and a smile. Add to that two barrettes, freshly tweezed eyebrows, and the disappearance of the *Rocky Horror Picture Show* circles under my eyes and—voilà!—practically ready for the runway. If this is not a true mommy miracle, I'm not sure what is.

My secret? Three two-hour chunks of sleep and a dash of exercise! Could it be that I'm finally transitioning into a new season of motherhood?

Cherish It

> *Parenting: The days are long but the years are short.*
> —Anonymous

Every day, Dan and I take an informal poll about whether we think we will survive this whole parenthood gig. For the first time in days, the jury voted a unanimous, "Yes!" which was inspired by our baby stretching her nighttime feeding out to every three hours. Aside from my engorged bombshell breasts, my body couldn't complain.

In fact, I felt so rejuvenated that former passions of mine appeared out of nowhere and came back to entice me. I began to dream of once again working to empower women about their health and of spending more time writing. I couldn't believe it. Going back to work in a few months was an exciting prospect. Who knew these interests were all still smoldering inside?

At the same time, this excitement worried me. I don't want professional aspirations to distract me from this special season with my sweet one. No matter how exhausted I normally am, everyone gives me this single piece of advice: treasure this time because it goes by quickly.

But what exactly is it that I'm supposed to treasure? The sleepless nights? The intense crying fits experienced by both my darling girl and myself? The two-minute showers? The breastmilk-stained clothes? The sexless nights? The endless loads of laundry? Or perhaps it's the sense of being isolated to the fringe of society?

After ruminating on this mystery, I think I have finally figured out what there is to treasure. It's the tiny fingers and toes, the soft hair on her head tucked under my chin, the delicious smell of my newborn, and the gentle noises while feeding. It's the sleepers patterned with pink elephant drawings, the animal mobile dangling above her crib, and the tender lullabies.

It's a time of innocence. The time when my little one can be cradled in one arm, when she doesn't crawl away, say no, or prefer her friends over me. It's about watching her discover the world around her—like when she realizes those pudgy fingers nearby actually belong to her.

It may be that we mamas are to also cherish our own self-discovery. Who would have thought I could get so attached to a little human whom I have seen for only thirty-some days? How unexpected to hang on her coos, to be amused by her uncoordinated, flailing arms, and to be mesmerized by her escapes from her swaddle.

In so many ways, we mamas are traveling in slow motion on a swift train. So long, hard, and challenging are the days that we forget we are really zipping through life. It's far too easy to forget this is our one journey with this one child whom we received from heaven above. If I'm not mindful, it will all be over. And I will have missed my chance to cherish any part of it.

LET'S TALK ABOUT IT

Nutrition for Mamas

Fueling ourselves with nutrient-dense foods is one of the most amazing gifts we can give ourselves, especially during the early weeks of our motherhood adventure. It gives our bodies the tools to carry on and function well. Some of you mamas may agree, envisioning how your family has been feeding you traditional postpartum foods to help you heal, restore balance, and minimize your risk of future illness.[1] Perhaps you have been on the receiving end of cultural practices such as consuming "hot foods" like milk and chicken, salty foods, and special herbs or specific dishes.[1] If so, isn't it incredible how helpful it can be to have supportive family or friends who feed you, even if you aren't keen on *all* their traditional practices?

Most of us mamas, however, have noticed how much easier it is to focus on feeding our baby than ourselves. We're so distracted that we forget about our own needs and are grateful to get a few pathetic, nutrient-light snacks to eat once or twice a day. Let's see if we can improve on that. Maybe feeding your little one can be a trigger for you to drink water and grab a nutrient-dense snack or meal for yourself. After all, your baby eats about every two hours, and this is a great goal for you, too.

When you can, eat a rainbow of foods rich in fruits and veggies, whole grains, and proteins. Your body will thank you by giving you more energy while improving your mood and health.[2] Who knows, you may even have energy to walk down the block and back! If you're breastfeeding one baby, you'll need about the same number of extra calories postpartum as in pregnancy (330–400 calories above your prepregnancy needs) to help you get back to your prepregnancy weight.[2]

Remember, though, the key is to not get discouraged when you have a bad day. Keep trying to eat well. You deserve it, and nutritious eating can make you a powerful beast of a mama!

LOOKING FOR FOODS AND SUBSTANCES
TO BOOST YOUR MILK SUPPLY

Well, it's not quite so simple. These *galactagogues* (substances that increase milk production) are still veiled in mystery; there haven't been enough well-designed research studies to determine which actually work and are best.[3] For now, consider starting with the foods some mamas have found helpful (shown in the list below) and asking your lactation consultant or maternity care provider for their recommendations, too.

- Grains: oats, quinoa, barley, millet
- Veggies: beets, carrots, sweet potatoes, dark leafy greens
- Fruits: apricots, dates, figs
- Legumes: lentils, beans, chickpeas
- Nuts and Seeds: flaxseed, almonds, cashews
- Healthy Oils: coconut, olive, sesame, flax
- Other: alfalfa, fennel, fenugreek, caraway, dill, and brewer's or nutritional yeast

Digging Deeper

Today, try some lactation cookies or flip back to B-1e for some scrumptious, healthy snack options and recipes (including directions for a fresh, green smoothie and Peanut Butter Pow! Balls). For more information about nutrition postpartum, including during breastfeeding, hop over to B-1d to get answers to common questions like:

» I don't have much support around me. How can I make sure I don't starve in the next few weeks?

» In terms of nutrition, what do I need to think about while breastfeeding? Is coffee okay? What about alcohol?

» My baby is fussy all the time—could what I'm eating have anything to do with it?

WEEK 6

Sleep Train

Who would have thought that so much of my well-being could hinge on my baby's sleep habits? Those nights when she strings together her sleep cycles like an iridescent pearl necklace, I'm overcome with gratitude and relief; the nights when they're piecemeal, I feel like curling into a ball and letting gravity roll me away to wherever its whims may lead.

So, imagine how thrilled I was when I caught wind of the next sleep milestone: around six weeks of age, babies' brains are developed enough that night sleep patterns appear—allowing them to catch a single, four-to-six-hour chunk of sleep. Yes, it's true!

For the last few weeks, I've wondered how I would react when this monumental day finally blessed our home. Would I even remember how to sleep for so many hours? Well, last night a concrete answer replaced my curiosity. Our "little firecracker," as Dan calls her, slept until five in the morning. Yes, you heard me—five! You'd think I would have had a heart attack or thrown a party, but no—with my head buried in my pillow, I never even noticed what was happening. I slept right through the entire miracle!

Yearning to experience this again the following night, Dan and I climbed into bed with our baby in his arms. Now, all we needed was for her to fall asleep. Sometimes I wish I could just kindly ask for her cooperation, explaining sleep is necessary for her brain development, and we mean business. However, realizing we need a more age-appropriate approach, we decided it was time to board the sleep train—destination Dreamland. Sure, it's perpetually running behind schedule, but despite how late it may be, it eventually reaches the train depot.

All aboard! As passengers and conductor, we each took our positions. As usual, I stretched out, turned over, and nuzzled deep in a sea of flannel blankets while Dan rested against our headboard, cuddling our sweet bundle. And just like that, we were off.

Sh, sh, sh, sh, sh, sh, he whispered.

With rhythm, he began to rock and calm her while I let myself be carried along.

Sh, sh, sh, sh, sh, sh, sh, sh, sh, sh . . .

The bed gently rumbled beneath us as we chugged along, mama and daughter lulled to sleep.

Sh, sh, sh, sh, sh, sh . . .

Fortunately for us, our devoted conductor fought mightily his heavy eyes and stalwartly escorted us, his beloved passengers, on. We must have zipped past spectacular night sights: city lights, multitudes of leaping sheep carefully counted, or perhaps even that famous cow known for jumping over our moon. Although I would never know, I was so grateful for the ride.

Sh, sh . . .

Sh . . .

Grand Opening

I didn't think it would go like this. We had been looking forward to this "grand opening" day, and here it was, finally before us. As far as I could tell, I felt ready to go. I had stopped bleeding, and my stitches even healed. And when it came to sex, what more was there to consider?

Apparently, for mamas like me, there can be a lot more to consider than I'd thought. Dan and I were blissfully on our way to enjoying the moment when I had to call the whole thing off.

Close the doors! A wave of unexpected emotions had overcome me. Sex, I suddenly felt, would change everything.

I had looked away from him as my eyes teared up. I'm not ready. Physical intimacy would sully a part of my body that had now become a sacred zone—the part of me that created new life and then shared it with the world. My uterus just housed my baby. And my rugated canal? Well, it was her rose-colored passageway into our world.

I'm not sure where all these cascading thoughts came from, but one thing was for sure—I wasn't ready for something so special to be replaced with ordinary activity. *Sorry, we're out of commission for who knows how long.* I need time to process.

"That's okay," Dan had assured me, quietly. "We can wait until you're ready." Though considerate, he was also clearly disappointed.

"I'm sorry. I have no idea how long it will take," I had responded, hoping I wouldn't feel like this forever. But, since these emotions and thoughts were news to me, too, I had no idea when they might fly away. They just landed on my heart like a hummingbird, and, like nectar from a flower, drew new meaning out of my pregnancy and birth.

I suppose my views about my body and purpose had also changed since birth. In my mind, my breasts had become bags of milk from which my baby constantly gulps. For the time being, I couldn't imagine them serving any other purpose. They were taken.

As my precious firecracker lay sleeping, I leaned back against our trusty green couch to recuperate from the emotions stirred up by the events of the day. I closed my eyes and placed my hands on my belly, as I had gotten used to doing so often in pregnancy. However, instead of finding the familiar firm roundness, my hands found something far more yielding and squishy. With rolls. *Oh yeah*. My belly, too, had changed. It's like the rest of me now—a mass of softness, a tender mess, ready to comfort, embrace, and cushion my sweet one.

Will I always feel like this?

⇒⟩⟩⟩ LET'S TALK ABOUT IT ⟨⟨⟨⇐

Diving Back In: Sex after Childbirth

Sex? I know, some of you mamas are rolling your eyes and thinking, *Yeah right*. But since you likely haven't vowed celibacy and others of you are raring to go, let's have a heart-to-heart. Grab some popcorn (and your partner if you'd like) and join me for another uncensored conversation about sex. This time, however, we'll focus on postpartum as a continuation of "Getting It On, or Not, While Pregnant" (week 27).

First off, there is a wide range of normal when it comes to postpartum intimacy and sex. This is an important time to remember sexual desire and satisfaction hinge on how you are doing overall. Your emotions, body, spirit, mental health, body image, relationship with your partner, baby, delivery, cultural beliefs, and even breastfeeding play a huge role.[1-7] A few weeks ago, your baby infiltrated every nook and cranny of your life, and now, you may even be in physical pain after delivery or experiencing health problems. And you're exhausted. Very exhausted. So, although your partner may be ready to have sex yesterday, some of you mamas might not be ready yet—and no, that doesn't mean you don't love your partner.

Taking the plunge

It's often recommended you wait *at least* four to six weeks after an uncomplicated delivery to give your body a chance to heal. Of course, you can start later. In fact, many women wait until two to three months after delivery, and some hold off even longer, sometimes to uphold culturally prescribed periods of abstinence.[1-3,8-11]

Most mamas find their sex lives are closer to their baseline by their baby's first birthday, regardless of whether they had a vaginal or Cesarean birth delivery.[3,8,9] Also know that in the coming years, you'll probably notice a (natural) variation in the quality of your sex life.[12,13]

CONSIDERING HAVING SEX AGAIN

When thinking about resuming sex, remember these three simple rules:
- Have sex only when you are emotionally and physically ready since sex is not just a physical act. It also impacts our souls and selves.
- Pregnancy spacing is important, so make sure you use a reliable birth control method to avoid any "oopsies." For more on this, see "The Naked Truth about Birth Spacing and Birth Control" (week 34), and A-5b.
- Don't forget to use condoms if you're at risk for STIs. Be proactive, for your sake as well as for your baby's.

So, if you're not yet ready for sex, that's okay! Be sure to be patient with yourself and with one another and enjoy being intimate in ways that don't overwhelm you. If it's hugging, holding hands, or just a little smooch, go for it—these release endorphins too! Soon, you, too, will be ready to get your sexy roar going.

If you're ready to get it on now and, better yet, have also received the green light from your maternity care provider—go for it! Remember, going slow is not a bad idea. You may notice new physical sensations and experiences, as well as unexpected emotions. Share your thoughts and feelings with each other on a regular basis and see if you can have fun while it lasts (since your baby will likely cry before you know it).

Common postpartum experiences

If you notice sexual problems postpartum, know you are not alone—they are actually very common. Specifically, these can include aspects of female sexual dysfunction (such as a loss of sexual desire), perineal pain, pain during sex, vaginal dryness, or urinary or anal incontinence.[1-4,6,13,14] These are more likely to occur after a complicated vaginal delivery, or if you have postpartum depression, take certain antidepressants, breastfeed, or have struggled with sexual problems prepregnancy.[1-7,8,10]

Some of these problems resolve themselves naturally in time, while others require some sort of intervention or treatment. If you're worried about any of these issues or never have enjoyed sex—talk to your maternity care provider. There is help for when you are ready! In the meantime, honor your body with grace and patience, and invest in one another even if in seemingly small ways.

Yep, having a baby can even affect your sex life!

Digging Deeper

So, you just heard sex postpartum may feel a little different, especially in the weeks to months after having a baby. To help you along this journey, skip on over to B-5e for handy tips and answers to questions like:

» Since having a baby, my libido is low and it's harder to orgasm—is this common and when will it ever get better?

» Help! It's painful to have vaginal sex.

» What are good lubricants to use, and are there some I should avoid?

» It's so embarrassing, but it's hard to control gas. What can I do?

WEEK 7

Growing Apart

Some days, like today, seem to drag on forever. The past several days have been long, in fact, since they started with my baby and me each contracting a cold. Being sick, she has needed extra attention, comfort, and feedings, and I haven't found a moment to rest.

Today, I must have double-checked the clock a thousand times to make sure it was still ticking—counting down every minute in the 12 hours Dan would be away, eagerly awaiting his standard, six-thirty arrival. Each evening, my ears strain to hear the familiar sounds of the car alarm, the squeaky gate, the footsteps up the stairs, and—finally—the opening door. Like Pavlov's dogs, I start drooling for help the moment the car alarm sounds.

This time, however, despite my desperate longing, Dan arrived half an hour late. I couldn't believe it. How dare he? Didn't he know what I'd been through? He walked through the front door and greeted us with a vibrant hello as he tossed his keys onto the counter.

"Where the hell have you been?" I snapped at my poor, unassuming victim.

Realizing he had walked into a dragon's lair, he hurried to the sink and washed his hands: step one in preparing for his fatherly duties.

"Guess what?" he hollered from the other room, while engaged in step two: changing into his sweats. "The medical residents really liked the sports medicine lecture I gave them today."

"Oh, that's great." I replied in a tone that could hang a man if words were made of rope. He emerged, as ready as he could possibly be, and just like that, I handed my baby off and stormed away to eat, take some medicine, and have a shower if I was lucky.

🌹

It was only after I had taken care of these needs that it hit me. My husband just had a long workday, rushed home, and tried to connect with me over the daily happenings. And my response? I breathed out fire and singed his heart. A pit grew in my stomach. How could I be like that, so unsupportive and hurtful?

I apologized and asked for forgiveness, which he generously extended, as always. He gave me a warm hug, and for the future, we decided to wait with evening sharing time until we both had had a few moments to ourselves.

I think I understand now how people fall out of love, grow apart, and have affairs when they have kids. How empty nesters wake up one morning and don't even know why they married or where to even begin to make up for lost time. It's not like anyone plans it; it just happens slowly. People stop being intentional with their partners. They get distracted. They get tired, sometimes even lazy. They start living for their children and pour out affection until nothing is left.

I don't want that to be us.

In our preparental years together, we basked in good times of laughter and flirting, enjoying our road biking and travel adventures. But even then, as for all people, hard seasons speckled our lives. So, surely we can overcome these challenges, too.

Now, if I could just tame mama dragon's tongue, it would be one great step toward growing together instead of apart. *God help me.*

Thank God for Chocolate

Some days, a frazzled mama needs a hefty dose of encouragement—especially on those days when life unravels around her. Our baby is still sick, which means everything is permeated by imperfection, struggle, and tears. For starters, I just noticed I'm wearing her vomit on my sleeve, her snot is smeared across my shoulder like an effervescent snail trail, and I smell. *There's definitely a problem if I can smell myself.*

To make matters worse: Our house is a complete mess. Another pesky pantry moth appeared in our kitchen, promising countless more still unseen, and the blood of raw hamburger meat leaked out all over our perishables in the fridge. After grocery shopping, I couldn't remember where I parked the car, and at the gym, I showed up in a tee shirt stained with milk rings encircling my nipples. (What's a mama to do? Avoid eye contact and lift weights among tan, buff guys, with rings around my rosies. That's what.)

But then it all changed. My encouragement arrived. Sure, it's as small as a ladybug, but it's also as strong as an earthquake. Ah yes, that hard square of chocolate. There really is nothing like 73% dark chocolate with crunchy almonds. Its rich, delicious taste can transcend it all—messes, moths, and milk stains.

Nope, it's nothing a little chocolate can't fix.

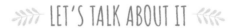

LET'S TALK ABOUT IT

Heading Back to Work or School

When life is already a challenge, going back to work or school can feel all the more difficult. Sure, it may seem like a vacation compared to the endless tasks of mothering, but there's a lot to coordinate to get out the door fully dressed and ready to meet the world. Your feelings about the transition may also be more mixed than you expected. Whether it's just a slight hesitancy, a gentle sadness, excitement, relief, or all-out crying for a week or so before—it's common. Your little one is part of you forever. And now you'll have to keep tabs on his needs partly through the eyes of your caregiver.

Navigating mixed feelings

Working or going to school can bring up all sorts of feelings. Some mommies feel proud that they can hold a job and provide for their families or go to school and invest in their families' future. At the same time, work and school can also bring up feelings of guilt that you're not with your baby 24/7. If this is you and you don't actually need to work as much as you do, consider altering your schedule to fit what is right for you and your family. If you're unable to cut back on your hours, hang in there! This could be for a season, with other options up ahead.

Getting out the door

When it comes time to head back to work or school, plan on waking up earlier to get out the door on time—it will take much longer than before. Say goodbye to those leisurely mornings where you could spend 30 minutes curling your hair to your favorite music. Your mornings will be busier, especially if your baby pulled an all-nighter, is not feeling well, or decided to surprise you in some sort of special way. Just do your best and count it an accomplishment that you made it through your workday—even if your leggings were inside out or your mascara was smudged. If you're breastfeeding, try feeding your baby right before you leave for work.

Staying aware

To help you keep a pulse on how your activities are affecting your family, plan on checking in with your partner, family, self, and baby regularly. Is this working? How is your baby doing? And your older children? If not well, get creative. Perhaps you can work from home, have shorter days, go to school part-time, take PTO days occasionally, come home during lunch, send pictures or texts to your older kids, or see if your partner can change his or her schedule. These are formative years for your baby, and since a healthy family is key to a healthy baby, it's important to take everyone's needs seriously.

Caregiver jealousy

Last, you may be surprised to find yourself sometimes hurt and jealous by how attached your baby gets to the caregiver. It doesn't mean your baby doesn't love you and that you're not special to him. Just remember—it's both okay and important for your baby to get attached to your caregiver. He needs to have that bond built so that while you're gone during the day, he feels safe and loved. So, don't be surprised if your baby takes even a couple of hours to transition back to you after work. Be patient and give yourself a pat on the back for finding such an incredible caregiver. Good job, mommy! Also, expect to glean some awesome tips from your caregivers—veterans have all sorts of tricks up their sleeves.

Digging Deeper

To help you prepare for that big debut, it's a good idea to have a dry run a week or so before to give your caregiver a chance to get to know your baby, get oriented, and practice preparing a bottle and feeding your munchkin when you're out of sight. In A-5, you'll find a whole host of practical tips for returning to work, alongside answers to questions like:

» What should I look for in a caregiver? (A-5e)

» Where can I find a trustworthy caregiver? (A-5e)

» Help! Can you give me a list of important topics I should cover with my caregiver? (A-5e)

» In what ways can I make my return to work or school easier? (A-5f)

WEEK 8

Napping

*There really are places in the heart you don't
even know exist until you love a child.*
—ANNE LAMOTT

As my baby and I lie down to nap in our family bedroom, I realize naps are indeed God's way of telling mommies, "I love you." It's a splendid invention, if you ask me, a treat dolloped with sweetness. It's so exquisite, in fact, that napping with my daughter has turned out to be one of my new favorite activities. It's not only refreshing but also fills a part of me, a void I didn't even know existed. It comforts her, sure, but strangely, also me.

My dumpling lies down on my chest, then turns and lifts, turns and lifts, and turns and lifts her head until finding the perfect inch on my chest. While birdsong flutters through our open window, I begin to gently pat her back with one hand, cupping her little round bottom with the other.

Pat. Pat. Pat.

She's so tiny and adorable.

Her squirming relaxes, breathing slows, and her arms go limp above her head in deep contentment. The wind chimes ring to the gentle breeze outside while we lay there quietly in deep, unspoken understanding. Closing my eyes, I hope this moment will never pass.

Roller-Coaster Ride

A few days ago, we received a congratulations card in the mail, upon which our friend wrote, "Enjoy all the firsts." The thought was so profound and timely. It got me thinking: What sorts of firsts have we had so far in our first two months of parenting? Well, our little one had her first breath, cry, poop, night of sleep, breastmilk, bottle, car ride, and hike.

And how could I forget the first time she cooed softly or reached out toward my face during her diaper change?

Of course, as every mama knows, some firsts we could do without: like blowout poops, food allergies, and colds. Yesterday, we also had another such first—our baby seeing tears streaming down her mother's face. I've been so utterly exhausted, and I just don't know how to manage motherhood. Dan has been working more 12-hour days, which means I don't ever get a break, and my stamina seems to have taken a vacation.

At times like these, motherhood is like being on a very long roller-coaster ride, which twirls, climbs, rocks, and dips. I get emotional highs when my little one smiles and sudden lows when she won't stop crying and I long for sleep. At times, the ride enthralls me and I can hardly wait for what's around the bend. But other times, it seems way too bumpy, jarring, and scary. *Can motherhood give a mama whiplash? Will it always feel this intense?*

I'm not sure who decided to call parenting a "full-time" endeavor, but I beg to differ. There seems to be a teensy-weensy, tiny little misunderstanding. "Full time" implies a normal nine-to-five workday with an hour lunch and a couple scheduled breaks. Parenting, though, is something far more demanding and all-encompassing. Surely at some point, this schedule will become easier to handle . . . right?

⋙ LET'S TALK ABOUT IT ⋘

Becoming Active Postpartum

I'm so glad you're here! I realize your life feels very full right now. And since you've become a professional baby rocker and bouncer over the past few months, any extra movement is likely the last thing on your mind. Yes, that's okay! Remember, becoming more active and restarting physical activity postpartum looks different for everyone.

Some mamas are raring to go a few days after a smooth vaginal delivery, while others prefer to wait a little longer. If you're feeling well, are healthy, and had a smooth vaginal delivery, go ahead and exercise, but take it easy to see how it feels.[1] Don't start with a 10-kilometer run—your baby may have a fun all-nighter in store for you. Rather, tap into your motherly wisdom and preserve your energy.

If you've not been physically active to this point, you're not alone! Decreased activity often occurs because of cultural reasons, time constraints, exhaustion, or having had a complicated labor or a Cesarean birth.[2] It is also common for those struggling with mental health problems or for mamas who gave birth to the world's next marathon crier. Whatever the reason, this is the season to have grace for yourself—not a time to whip your body back into shape!

If you had pregnancy or delivery complications, be sure to check with your maternity care provider before restarting exercise. Otherwise, if you're not sure where to start, try leisurely walks. These can be a lovely way to ease into activity, boost your mood, and avoid isolation.

While keeping a healthy, wise pace, set your sights on the general physical activity recommendations discussed at more length in B-2a. Essentially, aim for at least 30 minutes of physical activity most days of the week, and strength training at least two days a week, to keep your heart, weight, and mind healthy.[3-5] Brisk walking, dancing, swimming, yoga, biking, and hiking are only some of the many fun ideas. Yes, it's okay to sometimes go at a snail's pace while people-watching, kitty-cat-spotting, or hunting for treasures, but remember your body also needs more. These higher intensity activities develop the beautiful, strong body that will carry you through the years of your child's development and beyond.

Digging Deeper

Ready to increase your daily physical activity? After all, it has countless benefits, and you can feel so good afterward! If so, take a peek at B-2c, where you'll find practical info and answers to questions like the following. You go, mama!

» If I had a Cesarean birth, what do I need to pay attention to when physically active?

» I'm so busy, how on earth am I to fit in exercise?

» Is it okay to work out hard if I breastfeed?

» What is diastasis recti, and how is it treated?

MONTH 3

Baby

- Is more alert.
- Is better at communicating (develops distinct cries to signal tiredness, hunger, etc.).
- Starts laughing.
- Can hold head steady when upright.
- Grabs items and sucks on or plays with hands.
- Begins rolling (from back to side).
- Likes toy rings and rattles, and sitting in a semi-upright position while playing.

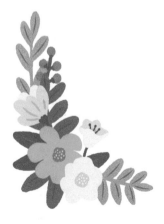

Mama

- You may start feeling a little less exhausted.
- If not breastfeeding, you will likely have normal menstrual cycles by the end of the third month. Otherwise, they don't normally return before six months postpartum, sometimes even longer.
- By week twelve, you no longer have increased pregnancy and postpartum risk for blood clots.

WEEK 9

Panic

I would have never guessed how a small change of circumstance on an otherwise typical morning could abruptly transform me from a calm, reasonable mama into an anxious, ferocious mama tiger. Not wanting to wake my little one from her nap, I had stepped out onto our porch and closed the door behind me to return my boss's call. After we had exchanged pleasantries and discussed my maternity leave dates, I hung up and went to turn the doorknob, only to discover—it was locked!

All sense fled. I was about to bash in anything—kick in a door, knock out a wall—*anything* to get in. With my power surging and my palms sweating, my blood pulsed in a rapid beat. I wanted to scream for help.

My baby was inside, and I was not there to protect her!

No, the house was not on fire. No, she was not in any acute danger. And no, she likely didn't even know I was gone. I peered through the bedroom window, and sure enough, she was sound asleep in her little vibrating chair.

But the full implications of the situation gripped my heart like a vise: We didn't have a spare key, our landlords were on a trip, and Dan was working a long day in surgery. And there was a big, thick locked door separating my baby and me. What if she needed me? What if I wasn't there when she woke up?

I've never had great survival skills, had only completed one measly course of Search and Rescue (which was years ago), and for that matter, I have a terrible sense of direction. And how could I possibly go seeking help while in my bathrobe and some frumpy outfit (which I vowed never to wear outside the house) with barely brushed teeth?

By the grace of God, I had an idea. When all else fails, ask Dan. When my call finally went through, I was grateful to find he knew exactly which window I could climb through if I jimmied it just right. I followed his directions step-by-step, and before I knew it, a tiny sliver of space widened between the window edge and the wall. It worked! My pulse slowed and relief poured over me. My baby was safe.

"Don't worry, mommy is here." Well, this is what I would have said in Hungarian if she had even known I was gone in the first place. As it was, she was still sleeping peacefully, and who wakes a napping baby for no reason? Plopping down on our oh-so-familiar couch, I breathed a sigh of relief and praised God (as I imagine any mama tiger would) for a disaster averted.

Not a Paper Doll

Excuse me, oh body of mine, but do you happen to know where I can buy a pair of skin suspenders? I've noticed a surplus around my center, and I thought they might help. To be perfectly honest, I simply don't like what I see today. Yes, yes, I know—you don't get much sleep, you're sustaining a baby, and you are just happy to be alive.

But still, I'm not satisfied with you. Your legs and arms are so undefined and round. Rolls are constantly attempting escapes from underneath this nursing bra. And your belly? Don't get me started. I just want to shave off two inches and donate it to the starving children my grandmother always told us about when trying to convince us to eat our dinner.

I know I should be more gracious toward you, but it's so hard today. I should have never let the mirror catch my gaze. What was I thinking? I know you're not meant to resemble the magazine models staring you down at grocery store checkout lines, challenging you to a comparison. They tempt you to analyze every inch of yourself and ask you to dissect your body under a microscope. And here I am accepting their invitation. But no! That's a job for a surgeon or, better yet, a medical examiner performing an autopsy.

I just won't buy into the lie.

Bodies are tools, not objects. You, dear self, are not meant to be scrutinized but gently admired—like a reflection on a rippling lake. Those models are imaginary. Two-dimensional. Just paper—airbrushed, edited, and photoshopped. You, on the other hand, are real. You breathe and give life. Your imperfections make you unique and special.

I want to give you grace—to let my criticism float away like a kite, a loose balloon, or Chinese lantern. I know we are all created wonderfully and are to be adored and cherished by loved ones. Yes, even—and especially—by ourselves.

⇛ LET'S TALK ABOUT IT ⇚

Honoring and Accepting Your Body after Birth

You've gone through so much, dear friend, and both you and I know it hasn't exactly been simple. I'm sure you have all sorts of stories to share. The good news is your baby is getting bigger by the day and even becoming more fun and entertaining, right? Although sometimes it can feel like you're stuck in a time warp, these difficult days will soon get easier—often by month three and certainly by six. Hang in there!

A few weeks ago, in "Nutrition for Mamas" (postpartum week 5), we covered some nutrition self-care tips that hopefully you've had a chance to try. If not yet, that's okay! Why not pick one doable self-care tip today? What a lovely way to gift yourself with kindness and energy!

In the meantime, you may have noticed mixed feelings about yourself and your body.[1] It doesn't take much to find ourselves impatient with our bodies, especially if the pressure is on from others.[2] But if we thoughtfully consider these expectations, it's easier to see that this pressure is neither fair nor reasonable.

Your body is beautiful and is doing its very best to serve you! Remember to extend kindness and patience to yourself in this time.

You're not a boomerang, so it's no surprise that you don't just swing back to your prepregnancy self immediately. Your skin around your belly may stay looser for a while, and you may still have some extra weight on. Calling it "baby fat" seems quite cute and appropriate, don't you think?

This is a perfect time to wear some of your maternity clothes. Although marketed for pregnancy, these outfits serve well postpartum, too. Oh, and you may just want to toss that full-length mirror. It doesn't help us be patient with and gracious to ourselves.

While you're waiting for your body to slowly recover, remember that it is a tool for living and loving. Yes, it's time to rethink what beautiful is: you have strong arms to hold, breasts to give your baby milk or a comfy place to rest, a mind to engage, and a heart to pump the very force of life and love through your veins. Consider your stretch marks as nature's tattoo, reminding you how adaptable and flexible you once were in the year of your little one's birth. And yes, these tattoos will eventually become lighter and shimmery, making you shine naturally—almost glimmer!

Digging Deeper

In addition to reimagining what beautiful truly is, identify three parts of your body you are grateful for. If nothing comes to mind, perhaps it could help to take a quick jaunt through "Cultivating a Healthy Relationship with Your Body" (B-4g).

For you mamas who are really struggling with how you feel about your body, please reread "Loving Your Body" (week 12) or talk with your mental health or healthcare provider. Immense freedom comes from loving and accepting yourself—and it benefits not only you but also your family and baby!

WEEK 10

Silence Haiku

Infant sound asleep—
paused life, golden peace. Too still?
Babe inhales. Relief!

Heading Home

Ever since her birth, I've been waiting to introduce my daughter to both her grandfather and my childhood home in Oregon. Finally, the day arrived! I packed us up and headed for airport security, but unlike my earlier trip to the Pacific Northwest, I had no pregnancy declaration and, in fact, no major announcement of any kind. No, this scenario was obvious—I'm a mama with her baby in tow. I have nothing to prove, except to show myself that I can, indeed, travel with a newborn. It somehow feels like a rite of passage.

When we landed, I clumsily boarded the Portland shuttle that would drive us south to Eugene and then on to the home I grew up in. On the way, we passed the familiar 45th parallel sign and drove through the evergreen-lined streets. Until finally, we reached our destination—the yellow, ranch-style home settled on its familiar street corner.

As we were welcomed in and exchanged hugs, it felt as if I had stepped into a time capsule—surrounded by forgotten familiarity. What a pleasant surprise! I slipped off my shoes like we always did and added them to the row along the entry wall where they belonged. Seeing my smaller shoes next to my dad's reminded me of all our brisk evening walks when I'd take three steps to his every stride just to keep up.

A smile stretching across my face, I inhaled and let my surroundings infuse me with a little bit of what was, while making me more fully *me*. There by the fence is where we ran to catch the yellow school bus while still chewing our last bites of breakfast. This is the stiff recliner, with its duct-taped back, in which my father taught me my eight times tables and where he twirled me around when I needed a break. Over there is the bright watercolor my grandfather painted for me of sailboats along Lake Balaton.

I suppose homes are not only where memories are made but also where memories come alive once you're all grown up. Memories breathe again in the sounds. The smells. The familiar cracks on the sidewalk and creaking of the walls. And the pictures. Shades of gray or color, crisp or faded—these framed and unframed memories make my childhood home seem like a living family tree. How I'd love to swing from limb to limb, to be able to soar in and out of these pictures, experiencing for a little longer the fleetingness of yesterday.

But most of all, how I ache to hug my soft, round grandmother again, who lived down the street and died just two weeks after our baby's birth. I wish she could hold us both. I wish we could laugh together mightily just one more time and savor her crepe-like pancakes while watching *I Love Lucy* in black and white.

⇛ LET'S TALK ABOUT IT ⇚

Loneliness and Changing Relationships

Today, dear friend, let's chat about loneliness—something that, despite not being mentioned often, occurs frequently in our world today. This feeling of isolation is widespread, especially among those aged 16–24 and mamas or parents.[1-8] Did you know nearly half of Americans report feeling left out or alone sometimes or always?[1] And get this—one in four people rarely or never feels "there are people who really understand them."[1] My goodness, this is a lot of us!

Defining loneliness

Think of loneliness as "an unwelcome subjective feeling of lack or loss of companionship."[2] It can include feeling like you do not belong to a social network (*social loneliness*), or like you have no intimate relationships (*emotional loneliness*); these feelings can be temporary, situational—during transitions like having a child or getting a new job—or long-standing.[2,3,6] Long-term loneliness can profoundly impact your well-being and that of your child and can lead to physical and mental health problems, such as coronary artery disease, substance abuse, sleep problems, depression, anxiety, cognitive decline, and stress.[2-4,6,7,9] In fact, the adverse health impacts caused by loneliness have been likened to smoking 15 cigarettes a day![2]

> Though parenting involves stressors that tend to push parents toward loneliness, remember, you've got this! Focus on teamwork, communicate your specific needs to one another, and don't forget to praise one another for any accomplishments—no matter how small they might seem. This encouragement has a tremendous positive impact, especially in co-parenting!

Loneliness, you may have noticed, is unrelated to the number of friends or people around you, or even your social media acquaintances.[4] You could be smack dab in a room full of people, have your baby on you 24/7, or even be constantly on social media, and still feel alone. Why? Because "there is [still] a mismatch between the quality and quantity of social relationships that [you] have and want."[2]

Loneliness and parenting

As a mother, you may find loneliness can creep in for all sorts of reasons. For one, you now operate under various constraints—like limited time, child care, and energy, the logistics of nap and feeding schedules, and even the physical separation from others while your little one's feeding or having a crying fest. Having children with chronic health problems or disabilities, or being single, an immigrant, or an ethnic minority parent can also contribute.[4] With all these at play, it can feel as though the world keeps going while you are left behind.

Mamas also tend toward loneliness because the act of mothering affects your other relationships. For instance, if you have a partner, you're likely missing the good old days when you could be spontaneous, have sex multiple times a day, go on dates, and talk for hours. You're both exhausted, just struggling to keep up the daily necessities of life. Unfortunately, this leads to frustration, disappointment, hastier communication, and feeling misunderstood.

As a mama, you may also be feeling lonely because you're missing other friends, family, or coworkers. Since your little one arrived, conversations or hangouts may be less frequent, shorter, more fragmented, and less fulfilling. Maybe these hangouts have been entirely absent. Or perhaps when you do connect, you feel hesitant to share your struggles and raw motherhood experiences, worrying about being judged or misunderstood.[8] Sadly, there is a widespread notion—a myth—that motherhood *should* be wonderful and instinctual. The only way we will ever set the record straight for ourselves and our mama friends is with a little honesty. Find people you trust, and share. By doing so, you're creating a safe space for others to be real—a space for the connection that is a wonderful antidote for loneliness.

So, my friend, whether your loneliness is a fleeting feeling or a persistent one, there is hope! Yes, the early months of motherhood are intense, but know—you have more freedom coming your way. As your baby gets older, he or she will develop more predictable nap and sleep schedules, giving you beautiful flexibility. You'll be able to join mom groups, organize playdates, or go on walks with others. Who knows, you may even find more connection among coworkers, too, if you're heading back to work soon.

Digging Deeper

Looking for some ways to get connected? Check out these suggestions and mark two to start with:

» Get out of the house most days of the week.

» Reach out to a friend or family member.

» Communicate with your partner. What are your needs? What do you need your partner to know for you to feel more understood?[8]

» Go on a date, even if only for one hour.

» Spend time at your local playground to meet other parents.

» Check out local parent resources, such as hangouts, and breastfeeding or parenting groups (held in-person or virtually).

» Invest in your spirituality or get involved in a faith community.

» Volunteer.[6]

» Hire a babysitter so you can spend time with those you miss.

» Check in with yourself after using social media to see how it affects you. If it's not helping, cut back on your use.[1]

» Reach out to your healthcare provider if you're depressed or have social anxiety.

» See if your partner can take paternity leave.

» Move up your return-to-work date.

WEEK 11

Beyond Cardboard and Vinyl

This motherhood journey hasn't exactly fit the picture my mother painted about the wonders of parenthood, I decided while sitting at our kitchen table this morning as my baby napped. Goodness, how many times she covered the subject in depth long before we were ever thinking about having a baby! By the sound of it, it was a type of utopia, and thus, she could hardly wait for us to make her a grandma.

So much so, in fact, that one year, still not ready to dive into parenthood, Dan and I had decided we needed a solid (if temporary) solution to quench her eager, grandmotherly desires. You can imagine the thrill we felt when we spotted our answer to prayer at the toy shop. Without thinking twice, we grabbed it, marched to the cashier, and instantly made our glorious purchase.

I remember that Christmas Eve so vividly. We carefully wrapped our cardboard gift and presented it to my mom with the sincerest excitement.

"This is something you've waited for so very long . . . Well, here it is. Finally."

Bewildered, she began to unpeel the mystery, wondering how something so flat could hold so much promise. And then there they were, his little blue eyes staring back at "instant-grandma," silently begging to be loved. He was cute and shiny. And oh, so durable—something that a new mom like me definitely would appreciate in a real newborn.

Sure, it wasn't quite what she'd pictured, but if the 2D grandson ever got old, we had numerous other reasonable options. Store aisles are jammed full of vinyl or fabric babies—in 3D! They have hair, can smile, cry, crawl, and even hold your hand. And poop. What a gift!

Now that we have moved beyond the cardboard and the vinyl, though, and our own darling stirs in her crib, I can see what these replicas are lacking, aside from breath itself. They are static—missing the joy brought by change and growth.

There is a delight that comes from watching my baby develop, seeing that moment when she realized she owned two hands with countless fingers and so she couldn't stop intertwining them. Nowadays, she loves grabbing anything in sight (like my clothes, hair, and earrings) and, when not death-gripping pieces of me, her new favorite pastime is blowing the most perfect raspberries—causing little bubble goatees to form on her chin.

Yes, that is what these toy babies are missing—the wondrous *becoming* of a little person.

A Smidge of Envy

How I wish my breasts were longer. No, not larger, but *longer*. Like a garden hose, a twine rope, or Rapunzel's hair in its prime. As I sit here and breastfeed (again), I find myself envying women of a certain age—the age at which breasts can dangle like extra appendages, sometimes even extending to the waist or elbows. Simply marvelous!

If only I were so endowed. Just think about it—how it could revolutionize breastfeeding! It would be so much more convenient. During the day, I could take a shower, fix a meal, do the laundry, hop on a stationary bike, or write, all while my baby fed peacefully, suckled, and slumbered in bliss. When my mini milk monster was ready for another feed, I could simply toss a breast over my shoulder, or stretch it to wherever she was, and allow her to latch on to her heart's content while I went about my own life. And at night, my sleep could be uninterrupted and normal again, since for her to enjoy a midnight snack, neither of us would need to budge.

But then again, I suppose that would rather negate the point. I'm her mommy, and she's my baby. She depends on me for survival. I'm intended to be the one person she can count on, whose life does stop, if only for a short while, for her. I'm the person whose purpose is to nurture, love, and cuddle her, ensuring her every unspoken need is met—even if at a cost.

❧❧ LET'S TALK ABOUT IT ❧❧

Postpartum Weight Loss

When your every breath revolves around keeping your baby alive, it's important to take occasional, mini vacations for your own health. For today, let's talk about one key element that can impact both your mental and physical health: postpartum weight loss. Specifically, let's look at what's normal, why a healthy weight is important, and how to get back to your prepregnancy weight. What do you think—are you with me?

Benefits of healthy weight

Remember, it may take a while for you to get back to that lighter, prepregnancy self, especially if you're a bit older. It's worth it, though, since a lower weight can help you be more active, feel better about yourself, pamper your knees, and give you the chance to more comfortably wear the clothes you missed in pregnancy.

To top it off, postpartum weight loss also helps you avoid an unhealthy weight long term, which means a healthier next pregnancy (for you brave souls) as well as decreased risk for diabetes, high blood pressure, and heart problems later on. This is especially important for you if you had gestational diabetes or preeclampsia, because these already increase your chance of developing type 2 diabetes or cardiovascular disease, respectively.[1,2]

How long does it take?

Okay, so what kind of timeline are we talking about for getting back to prepregnancy weight? Well, it all depends on (1) how much you gained during pregnancy, (2) your lifestyle, and (3) your health. The good news is that most mamas lose 10–13 pounds naturally by two weeks postpartum, simply by giving birth.[3] For the remainder of the weight, though, give yourself about six months.

During this time, expect a slow weight loss of about two to four pounds a month. Quick dieting and super rigid eating plans are neither fun nor sustainable, and they may also reduce your milk supply. Instead, think about creating a healthy and lasting lifestyle that gives you freedom to enjoy tastes, traditions, and activities. This will not only benefit you but also show your child what healthy living is all about.

So, what's the trick?

Though breastfeeding mamas may find it helps with weight loss, the two main factors for both losing weight and keeping it off are—drumroll, please!—healthy and mindful eating, and regular exercise.[3,4] Yes, it's that simple . . . and that hard. These vital companions to a healthy lifestyle and weight will also give you the fitness and strength you need to protect your baby once he is mobile and living on the edge.

> ->>> ✿ ❀ ✿ <<<-
> What's the secret to healthy and lasting weight loss? Nutritious foods, healthy eating habits, and staying active.

Please note, if you are one of the many plus-size mamas who has always struggled with a heavier weight, consider following up with your primary care provider. He or she will be able to help you explore whether you might have an underlying medical condition or eating disorder, and discuss weight loss support available to you, including medically supervised weight loss programs or even bariatric surgery.

Well, that's the scoop on weight loss. The key ingredients are mindful eating and regular physical activity—plus a healthy dose of patience for yourself in the process. When you embark on this journey, focus on one step at a time. What can you do today that will make a difference tomorrow?

Digging Deeper

Ready to take the next step? Given what your life is like now, what's reasonable? Is it eating an extra vegetable or fruit? Cutting out the soda or chips? Is it trying to cook a simple meal once a week instead of buying fast food or takeout? Or is getting out for a daily walk an option? Go ahead, pick one simple, enjoyable gift you can offer yourself as an investment in your health.

WEEK 12

Fulfilled?

"Are you fulfilled as a mother?" my sister asked over the phone.

"What do you mean exactly?" I replied, grabbing a bite to eat and buying myself time to think.

"Well, I wouldn't know, but I hear motherhood is supposed to satisfy like nothing else. Does it really create this surreal realm of existence . . . ?"

I placed my plate on the table, contemplating.

"In many ways, I think that's true. But being a mama is hard."

Our conversation turned to other topics, and I found myself mulling over the question throughout the day. Reflecting on the subject, I checked Webster's dictionary for the definition of *fulfilled*.

When I found the spot, it read, "made full."

So, in other words, am I "filled to the full" as a mother?

If it's a question of whether my life feels full, why yes, it *is* full. It is full of love, deep communion with a precious baby girl, sweet smiles, playing, surprises, milestones, diapers, comfort, challenges, crying, worry, poop-stained clothes, dirty dishes, messy rooms, and work. I think that qualifies as full.

Does that mean, though, that I don't miss certain things or that motherhood fills every yearning inside of me? No.

Is that bad to admit? I feel a little guilty for even having the thought.

I miss more reflection time with God, my undivided time with Dan, and our biking together. I miss freedom, work as a nurse practitioner, schooling, non-baby-related conversations, and the opportunity to get dressed up without looking like I just escaped from a tornado. And yes, I do wish I had more space and energy to continue my other interests and remember who I was.

But would I ever wish away this time? Never. That would mean I wouldn't have my baby, and I can't bear that thought, not even for a moment. I'd much rather be filled to the full with my motherly endeavors than anything else, even if it means fighting daily for my survival. I love her so.

Dirty, but Loved

Families are like fudge—mostly sweet with a few nuts.
—ANONYMOUS

No, she's not a firefly or a glow worm, but despite this, I'm starting to think my baby could actually glow in the dark. All I would need to do is place her under those neon, TV-germ-commercial lights, and we'd see millions of new microorganisms covering her soft, innocent skin.

All of this is due, I am sure, to our first large family gathering. I was not expecting the waves of people hovering over my baby, and I just don't know how to handle it. How am I supposed to protect her from getting sick or overly exhausted when everything is chaotic and out of my control? How can I become the relaxed new mom I'd like to be while the things around me make my blood pressure skyrocket?

Today, family members big and small, old and young, swarmed around to meet our new little bundle and decide for themselves who she looked like. Eyes pored over every inch of her little self, as if hunting for evidence that she belonged.

"She has a snippet of Lizzy in her. Look at her hair color."

"She looks likes Meshi's mom and grandmother."

"No, I don't think she has Dan's chin, do you?"

Once she was fully dissected and pieced back together like a family mosaic, they moved on to testing her grip, pinching her cheek, and counting her toes. Only then did they plant warm kisses as official stamps of approval.

Get away, all of you! I just wanted to scream. *Look, but don't touch!*

But I didn't.

There was no casual way of conveying this. Helpless, I conversed with those gathered nearby and followed my baby through the room with a hawklike gaze, wondering: Do I have what it takes to be a mother—to be tough as fruit leather, soft as custard, and flexible as pie crust dough?

I suppose it's a luxurious problem, trying to navigate the smothering attention of an eager and loving family. It's something my sister would call a problem of the blessed. We have a loving community that welcomes our baby so freely and generously.

And my response? Stress. How will I be able to strike a balance between protecting my baby and giving her the freedom to be deeply loved?

When it *eventually* came time to tuck our darling back into her car seat for the drive home, I just *had* to snuggle her close and tell her how I missed her—she who was much loved and covered in layers and layers and layers of perfume, kisses, fingerprints, and germs. Though she never left my sight, I missed her.

I have so much to learn.

⇶⇶ LET'S TALK ABOUT IT ⇜⇜

Mama Guilt

> *If we can't stand up to the never good enough and who do you think you are? Then we can't move forward.*
> —BRENÉ BROWN

As mamas, we want the very best for our babies and children, right? So, we give, and give, and give of ourselves as best as we can to make this happen. Much of our existence orbits around embodying that perfect mama (whoever she may be) who is concocted from our imagination and expectations, from those around us, and society at large.

Sooner or later, though, we run into a teeny, tiny, eensy-weensy problem: our own human limitations. Life forces us to face an onslaught of needs, newness, and difficulties at all odd hours of the day—even as our strength, stamina, and patience wane. Before long, our mothering efforts just seem to fall short.

Dear mama, we all experience these moments of inadequacy. It's not just you! We all get grumpy, lose our temper, make bad decisions, miss our baby's feeding cues, sleep through a pumping session, forget to change a poopy diaper, burn a meal, have a messy house, or smoke again—just to name a few. Welcome to the club!

Defining mama guilt

It's no wonder, then, that we're so familiar with guilt—that distressing feeling of failure and regret we get whenever we believe our actions or thoughts were bad or wrong. You may feel guilty when you actually did something wrong (like fight with your partner or lie), or when you *thought* you did (like taking time out for yourself or setting a boundary). In other words, sometimes guilt is appropriate, able to launch us on a path to positive life changes, while other times it's an unnecessary burden stemming from unrealistic expectations or underlying depression.[1,2]

Guilt versus shame

While guilt is a byproduct of behavior—when we do, or *think* we do, wrong—shame attacks the core of who we are.[2-4] "Shame is," according to researcher Brené Brown, "the intensely painful feeling or experience of believing that we are flawed and therefore unworthy of love and belonging."[4] This deep-seated fear silences and separates us from others so we won't be "found out," and it can lead to depression.[3,4] Unfortunately, when we self-isolate and bury our story, our shame only "metastasizes," making the situation worse.[4] Though shame is different from guilt, we may experience shame by itself or together with guilt. Some of us, for example, may feel an inch tall when we decide not to breastfeed or when we struggle with mothering.

Perfectionism

It may not be a surprise, then, that perfectionism often grows out of shame.[4] We may not realize it in the moment, but perfectionism is rooted in trying to earn approval and acceptance.[4] Yet perfection is an unattainable goal whose pursuit is exhausting and self-destructive.[4] Sure, it's good to do our best and strive for "healthy achievement and growth," but perfectionism is something entirely different.[4] "Perfectionism is the belief that if we live perfect, look perfect, and act perfect, we can minimize or avoid the pain of blame, judgment, and shame. It's a thief."[4] Fortunately, when we embrace who we are and share our story with trusted individuals, shame loses its power.[4] Yes, mama, we have hope!

Aim for "good enough," not perfection

You may be delighted to hear that your baby doesn't need you to be perfect. This is a huge relief, since there is no such thing as a perfect parent anyway. Rather, research has shown that what your baby needs is for you to be a *good enough* parent—which is not only attainable but also preferable.[5] Why, you may ask? Well, when you're imperfect, your baby slowly learns to function in an imperfect world, and that creates opportunities for resiliency to form. Make no mistake, we are not talking about neglect or abuse but rather parents stiving to do right (to love and care to the utmost) yet falling short of this goal.

> ## WHAT DOES A GOOD ENOUGH PARENT LOOK LIKE?
>
> - "Always be: bigger, stronger, wiser, and kind.
> - Whenever possible: follow my child's need.
> - Whenever necessary: take charge."[7]

Their honest imperfection can become a teaching tool—presenting an opportunity to love unconditionally, apologize, forgive, and learn from mistakes.[5]

So, friend—let's get real! Free yourself to simply love your baby, strive to be a good enough mama (accepting you have multiple roles in life, not just mother), and expect imperfection.[6] When imperfection happens, let it grow you. Mothering has a steep learning curve—at all stages of your child's life. Be kind to yourself, be realistic, and share your story with trusted people. When feeling guilty, ask yourself whether it's founded, and if so, learn from your mistakes. If you're struggling in this process, consider meeting with a mental health professional to explore motherhood expectations, shame, and perfectionism. Together, we can make this motherhood trek!

Digging Deeper

Phew! What a relief that our baby's growth, development, and healthy attachment don't hinge on our perfection! In fact, being a good enough parent is just what babies and children need to prepare for life. Let's reflect for a moment and consider: Has guilt or shame taken root in your life? If so, let's lighten this burden and practice some self-kindness, shall we? For the activity below, grab a piece of paper and something to write with.

» Jot down what you've felt guilty about lately.

» Star the ones you most often feel guilty about.

» Circle the ones you learned something from.

» Cross out any that stem from unrealistic motherhood expectations.

» Put a heart next to one for which you'd like to extend more grace to yourself this coming week.

Notes

MONTH 4

Baby

- Becomes much more interactive.
- Notices objects have names.
- Sees objects with both eyes together (binocular vision) and watches moving objects.
- Babbles and blows bubbles.
- Sits and stands (with support) and rolls (from tummy to side).
- Likes rolling balls, playing with hands, and facing forward when held.

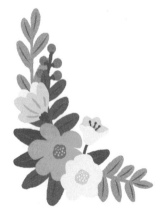

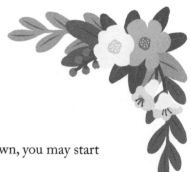

Mama

- Now that things might be settling down, you may start enjoying motherhood more.
- Likely, you are still tired.
- Your sex life may be improving, though if breastfeeding, you may notice vaginal dryness due to low estrogen levels.
  - Try a vaginal lubricant to slip 'n slide.
- Your recent pregnancy may still be evident in your pelvic floor, urinary incontinence, and the looser skin around your belly.
  - Be gracious with yourself while healing.
- If you are still above your prepregnancy weight, which is common, try using six months as your goal for getting back to your baseline.

WEEK 13

Stop the Clock!

I made my last leaning tower of outgrown baby clothes and placed it, not in Pisa, but at the edge of our bed. Countless other textured towers of folded cotton onesies, shirts, and pants piled next to one another are ready to be placed into our familiar cardboard boxes, since—who knows?—maybe one day there will be a baby number two.

Where did the time go? I can hardly remember. All this sleep deprivation has certainly squashed my recall abilities and given me the memory of a mosquito.

Setting the stacks neatly in the box, I was overcome with a sense of accomplishment and pride. We did it! Outgrown clothes mean we've done something right! We kept our baby alive for three entire months.

But almost as soon as the joy arrived, a somber realization hit. She will never fit into those itsy-bitsy items again. The little hand mittens, the tiny socks that are always missing, and the Gerber onesies. Those days are gone.

Moreover, our sweet pea is becoming more independent. She's already exerting her three-month will against ours. To make matters worse, Dan is counting down the days when she's six months old and he can offer her spoonfuls of her first pureed foods. Thank God a baby's digestive system is not ready for solid food much earlier; otherwise, I might have a heart attack.

Just stop the clock, will you?! I'm not ready for her to breastfeed less, stop nestling against me, or to sleep in the crib that is now *a whole four feet* away. I realize the goal is to raise a resilient and independent child, but when they warned it goes by fast, I didn't think it would be *this* fast. What's next, her going off to college?

The Real Superheroes

With Mother's Day around the bend, I'm compelled to reflect on the amazing qualities of mothers and mother figures. I think about my own wonderful mom and the mentors of many kinds I've had over the years who (with wisdom) encouraged, loved, and challenged me—over cups of coffee, during long walks, and amid laughter. I suppose it took becoming a mother myself, and getting a backstage view of the role, for me to really celebrate them. *Ladies and gentlemen, let's give it up for mamas of all kinds!* How do they do it?

I was never much into reading comic books, but I couldn't help but think of the superhero cartoons and movies I watched growing up. These classic superheroes could shoot lightning, spin webs, turn invisible, or grow claws. We'd sit at the edge of our seats and munch on popcorn while rooting for these superhumans as they leaped from skyscraper to skyscraper, traveled to other galaxies in a flash, or held aloft a busload of people with more ease than a waiter with my favorite entrée.

They lived common yet extraordinary lives for a cause—in the name of justice, peace, and love—and prevailed over the supervillains who snagged their capes, singed their mustaches, and ran out of ammo. And yet, if I were to nominate a superhero of all time, it would not be any of these popular ones. Rather, I would choose one with far more sophisticated powers: the *real* Wonder Woman.

She has eyes on the back of her head and stands on legs like two pillars that serve as a refuge for her children. Her abdomen doubles as a vacation rental and her breasts can shoot a magical, life-sustaining elixir. Her voice lulls the restless and the hurting, her love is fathomless, and her eyes are keen, watching over her young. We often don't recognize her as one of *them*, but that's only because she's camouflaged herself in an invisible cloak of humility.

Whoever said superheroes don't really exist?

Our mothers are everywhere.

⋙ LET'S TALK ABOUT IT ⋘

Remembering Mama's Healthcare Needs

Okay, you superhero, you, today we're going to chat about keeping up with your own healthcare needs. The life of a wonder woman is a busy and demanding one, and regular well-woman visits and periodic health screenings will help make sure her needs are met. Being proactive is the name of the game!

Well-woman visits

Firstly you may be wondering what a **well-woman visit** is. Good question! People sometimes will refer to it as an *annual, check-up,* or even *pap*. It's much like the well-child check-up your baby gets but is an insurance-covered visit tailored to a woman's unique needs.[1] So, this means you'll want to schedule this visit with your women's health or primary care provider about every one to two years, *even if you are doing well*.[2,3] Of course, if you're noticing health problems, you'll want to schedule a visit sooner, even if you're busily racing around saving the world.

The purpose of a well-woman visit is to address your questions or concerns, as well as to cover a smorgasbord of wellness topics. Depending on your unique situation, these subjects can include birth control, preconception counseling, STI checks, substance use, mental health, weight problems, vaccines to protect against things like human papillomavirus (HPV), intimate partner violence, and personal or family history of breast or ovarian cancer. If you have a lot going on, your healthcare provider will likely ask you to schedule a follow-up visit since it can be difficult to fit everything into one.

It's important to realize you may not get a pap smear or physical exam at every well-woman appointment. In fact, much of your visit may be a conversation with your healthcare provider, after a blood pressure and weight check. Make sure you note whether these measurements are normal, and if not, ask what transformative lifestyle changes are recommended. Since research studies haven't clearly shown the benefit of routine pelvic exams in healthy women without symptoms, you and your provider can discuss when you'd like a pelvic exam.[4,5] Schedule a physical exam if you are having a physical problem or if you're due for a screening test—a "red flag" test to see if you have an increased chance for a health problem, despite feeling well. Some years, this will also include labs to check blood sugar and cholesterol levels.[6]

Pap smears

The recommended screening tests given at your well-woman visit will vary based on your age and health. For example, the pap smear, which screens for cervical cancer, usually is recommended starting at age 21 (sometimes sooner) and is generally done every one to five years.[7-10] How often you get one depends on your past pap smear results and the particular type of test you're getting; a **cytology** test looks at your cells; *high-risk HPV* checks for certain types of viruses; and a **cotest** includes both of these.[7-10] That's right, this means you'll have some well-woman visits where you won't need a pap, though you may still have a vulvar exam.

As always, please speak up *prior* to your physical exam if you're nervous, have experienced sexual trauma, or had bad pelvic exam experiences. I know it's hard, but giving the heads-up prompts a clinician to slow down and work attentively together with you so you can have a much better experience.

While your healthcare provider should know what tests you are due for and when, be sure to keep track of them yourself. If needed, this can ease the transition between healthcare providers or facilities.

Breast cancer screening

To wrap up, let's cover a few notes about breast cancer screening, namely mammograms and in-office breast exams. It may be surprising that various national organizations have different opinions about whether or how often healthcare providers should give you breast exams when you don't have symptoms—like lumps, pain, nipple discharge—or increased risk for cancer based on your personal or family history. The same also goes for mammograms. Although recommendations vary, these screens typically start as early as age 40 and may start even sooner, depending on your personal or family health history.[11] So, bottom line? Have a conversation with your healthcare provider about a screening program that's right for you and determine whether genetic counseling could be helpful.

⟫⟫⟩ ✿ ✿ ✿ ⟨⟨⟨

Genetic counselors help people determine their risk for disease or cancers based on personal and family history. They talk about testing options and make recommendations based on test results.

And that, my friend, completes our whirlwind tour of well-woman visits. Be sure to stay on top of scheduling these so you can stay on top of your world. If you have medical problems, prioritize your daily self-care needs and appointments—it's what makes wonder-woman living possible!

Digging Deeper

Now that we've talked about well-woman visits and the importance of staying on top of your medical needs, let's get organized. Use these prompts below to get you started.

» Do you have any health problems? Are your symptoms under control? What do you need to take good care of yourself? Is your next follow-up scheduled? Do you need medication refills? Reach out to your healthcare provider as needed.

» Do you have any health problems that need to be addressed? If so, schedule an appointment.

» If you had gestational diabetes, be sure your blood sugar is checked every one-to-three years since you have a higher chance for developing type 2 diabetes.

» If you had preeclampsia, keep an eye on your blood pressure throughout your life since you have a higher chance of developing chronic high blood pressure.

WEEK 14

Safe Haven

Mommies are just big little girls.
—ANONYMOUS

At some point, every mama wishes her life were simpler and responsibilities lighter. This is exactly where I've found myself the past few days. For me, all I want to be is a little girl again—when my siblings and I shaped make-believe pastries in the sandbox or kept snails and grass clippings in jam jars. When I tried on for size my mother's favorite evening gowns, and so I tried on womanhood, but could hang it back up in the closet when I chose.

I long for my mother to brush my hair, hold my hand, make dinner, and sing me a lullaby. I want to curl up next to her and have her just hold me. Whenever my mother was near, there was no need to worry—not even the fiery dragons conjured by my mind's eye could harm me.

Oh, to be safe in her arms again and to feel like everything is going to be all right.

Legacy

Legacy (noun): a gift by will,
especially of money or other personal property
—MERRIAM-WEBSTER DICTIONARY[1]

When I consider the day in, day outs, the humdrum to-dos that fill each hour, I wonder if I'm living life well enough. It can feel so . . . unimpressive. My life is simply feeding, burping, and wiping a certain tiny bottom all day long. Is this how it's supposed to be? Will it always be like this?

I look around our apartment, which I can never keep clean, and think about the meals that rarely get cooked. I don't think I'm cut out for this good housewife gig. I'm ready for something different—some excitement and opportunity to help the world around me—but oh, *yeah*. When could I possibly fit that in?

Meshi, your life is so *fulfilled*, remember?

Will I ever have time to make a real impact in the world? Do I still have time to build a legacy, or have I missed my chance?

I pulled up a chair at the kitchen table and sat there, statuesque, thinking and thinking—with an intensity like my father's as he, a physics professor, contemplates the world through numbers. Except he usually paces the floor around his office like a hungry lion, ever poised to make a calculated pounce.

And then, in the quiet moment of contemplation, it hit me— I already have a legacy!

What?!

Yes, that's right! I already did it. I have a *real*, legitimate, living, breathing legacy—my baby. She is my focus, God's gift to me, and my gift to the world. My unique and beautiful contribution who is valuable beyond measure. She is my "gift by will," and the best part? She can carry on this legacy of giving.

I got up from the table, relieved by the bright dawn of revelation. Sure, my house is still a mess, but now it looks less like a hurricane and more like an artist's studio—colorful and unkept, just like when they, too, have something great in the making. Yes, my day may look ordinary, but each seemingly mundane moment serves to build and bolster her, my legacy. And so, each moment is sacred.

⤜ LET'S TALK ABOUT IT ⤛

Expectations and Advice

So, you've got this incredible gift—your soft and round legacy—in your arms. A special, one-of-a-kind human with no one else just like her!

She will develop at her own pace and have her own individual strengths, interests, personality, challenges, and special needs. She is *not* her sibling, neighbor, cousin, or family friend. And she's not you, or her father. As such, in time you'll notice some of her qualities will resonate with you, while others will perhaps seem foreign. She's spectacularly different! Isn't that beautiful?

While as a parent you are working to nurture, encourage, challenge, and love her—that she might blossom, thrive, and find her passions—it won't take long before the comparisons game will try to sneak up and douse that spark of individuality. How does your baby match up with other babies? Is she rolling, crawling, sitting, or sleeping through the night yet like the others? As a toddler, has she started talking or is she now potty-trained? As an older child, is she reading or playing competitive sports?

Breathe!

Please know you don't need to participate in this game if you don't want to. The great news is that raising a child is not meant to be a race or a competition. It's a slow, methodical process, tailored to her needs and those of your family. Watch attentively as your precious child's development slowly unfolds, and when a comment tempts you to join the competitive parenting track, take a step back, relax, and free yourself from the pressure to engage.

Let her play with stuffed animals, chase bugs, fly kites, find rocks, pet animals, hunt squirrels, climb trees, and pile sticks. Let her run through fields, roll down grassy hills, picnic under the open sky, build sandcastles, and stargaze.

Give yourself permission to be the keeper and protector of your baby's childhood. Savor these fleeting moments and preserve your child's ability to playfully explore her world. She only gets one childhood, so let it be. When she's older, try your darndest to avoid micromanaging or hovering. Freedom—to safely explore, fall, and experience life's natural consequences—is key to forging strong, resilient, and independent humans.

Advice

Of course, finding balance between freedom and direction may not always be easy, especially given how much advice people give. Have you noticed how they love coming to your "rescue," educating you on what your baby "really needs" and how you should parent? Sure, most of the time they mean well, but this can quickly get irritating and overwhelming. It's also easy to feel like you're flunking out of parenting school, which is simply not true.

Feel free to ignore most advice you hear. No, you don't have to obey your mother-in-law, even if she's tall and wears scary red lipstick. Rather, when you have questions, turn to one or two trusted people (which may include a healthcare provider) and never ignore your gut instinct. Though you may be tempted to shrug off your intuition, listen to yourself when something just doesn't seem right. Mama, you know your baby better than anyone else—she was inside of you for 10 months before the world caught its first glimpse. Sure, parenting take practice and time, but you're amazing. With support and wisdom, you can totally do it!

Digging Deeper

Getting to 14 weeks postpartum is such an incredible accomplishment! Yay, you! During this time, you've had such an opportunity to discover. Reflect for a moment and take a nice long look at this amazing human you just created. Let wonder and awe fill your heart as you admire your legacy.

What is he or she like? What have you noticed about him or her so far? Try to list off some qualities and jot them down here or in another treasured place, like a baby book. In a few years, have fun looking back and seeing how your baby has grown and changed, noting the ways your child's character and persona were already visible in his or her newborn self.

WEEK 15

Summer Again

Click. I fastened the baby carrier around my waist, set my curious blue-eyed little babe inside, and heeded the sunshine's invitation for a meander around the neighborhood. She *should* be good for another half hour before her next feeding, right?

Guess we're about to find out.

As she and I walked the sidewalks with her face peering out, I quickly realized this was no ordinary day around town. Across the way, a high school senior hurried by, tripping over his long graduation gown, tassel swaying. Up ahead, a lover strolled down the block with a dozen red roses clutched in hand, and once we turned the corner, we spied a pair of pigtails bouncing after the ice cream truck.

See that? Summer has come once again! It always does. Outside of our apartment, bees swarm around our blushing raspberries, and inside? Well, *there* we're piling our life back into those familiar moving boxes.

I can't believe it's been an entire year since our move to Cupertino. The transition that once felt like such a rude interruption to my life has turned out to be a warm and welcomed pause. We're leaving not just a cramped apartment but also a life that has been both simple and full.

What has felt like a place so far from home has now become just that—home. It's a place where Dan and I, and our baby, are just the three of us—together and alone. It's where my body inflated and then deflated like a balloon, where our little girl first smiled, laughed, and rolled over, and where she discovered her toes and the exquisite tastiness of her sweater.

An Upside-Down World

Intrigued by my little one's fascination with the upside-down world, I decided it was high time I took a look for myself. After all, she's frequently lying on my lap, scooching to the end just so she can dangle her head back and get a good look at what's below—I mean, *above*. What's so interesting? Is it far superior to the sights I know so well?

Since it's tricky to find a lap big enough to recreate her exact scenario, I figured lying on the ground would suffice. There we go. Nice and comfy. It's so good to lie down. I think I'll close my eyes, just for a moment . . . Oh no you don't! Wake up! This is no time for sleep.

So, what does the world look like through my baby's eyes?

Let's see what we have here. Well, tables and chairs stick to ceilings. *That's new.* People prefer to hang by their feet than stand. Short people magically become tall. I can see why she hasn't tired of the sight. It's actually quite fascinating.

It's as if I've stepped into Wonderland, experiencing Alice's intriguing discoveries, free of charge. I didn't even need to throw on a crisp apron, run after a time-obsessed rabbit, or tumble down a *looooonnnngggg* hole. Here in my very own home, roots and foundations have become the crowning glory of all objects, forgotten parts of life are now remembered, priorities reshuffled.

I let my gaze frolic through these novel sights and then stuffed a pillow under my head to better soak in the whole world, seams and all. I have no need to play croquet with a flamingo or say hello to a Cheshire cat because motherhood, in many ways, has turned my own upside-down world right side up.

⤷⤷⤷ LET'S TALK ABOUT IT ⤶⤶⤶

Consider This

Can you believe it? Here we are at the last "Let's Talk About It"! At first, I thought a collage focused on the theme of *mother* would be great, but somehow I have an inkling that you might not get the chance to flip through magazines, then clip out, thoughtfully place, and glue items on a piece of paper. Glue is sticky, life is messy, and you're more likely to have a decorated baby by the end of it. So, let's table this idea and, instead, pick something more realistic.

Here are sentence prompts for reflection. Feel free to apply them to pregnancy, childbirth, or mothering. You can even pace yourself and pitch each as a question of the day. Perhaps you can think about them in the shower or some other place where you can catch a couple of quiet minutes amid the rush of life. There are no right or wrong responses, so no need to censor your answers, my friend. Are you ready?

Memories and reflection

- A favorite memory of this journey is _____
- I was surprised when _____
- An embarrassing moment that I'll never forget is when _____
- During this journey, I learned that I _____
- Things went better than expected when _____
- My partner or friends surprised me when _____
- These days, I find beauty in _____
- It's hard to _____
- One thing I miss about myself (or my partner) is _____

Baby and parenting

- My baby and I love to _____
- My baby reminds me of _____
- If I could give my baby a superpower, it would be _____
- If I could give my baby a certain experience, it would be _____
- Parenthood is _____

Hopes and anticipation

- If I won the lottery, I would _____
- If I could pass on one thing about myself to my baby, it would be _____
- If I could have four hours to myself, I would _____
- I wish _____
- I can hardly wait for _____
- I hope my partner (or loved one) _____

Digging Deeper

For added fun, use this activity for relationship-building. With your partner or another loved one, select a few intriguing questions to talk about. You're bound to hear something surprising. Sit back, enjoy the process, and let it grow you!

AFTERWORD

As I write this last entry, dear mama, I think back on how far we've come together. Can you remember all the way back to the beginning when you just found out you were pregnant? You had so many thoughts and emotions, and probably a never-ending string of questions. Not too much later, you began to watch your body blossom and to see changes both within and around you. And look at you now! After having patiently (or semi-patiently) grown *and* delivered your own precious milk monster, here you are on the other side, figuring out what it means to mother your little legacy.

You may be too sleep-deprived to realize it, but getting this far definitely deserves an honorary moment of silence. *Yes, pause.* You're incredible! You've been encountering all sorts of surprises and uncertainties since the beginning of pregnancy, and now you are here—like the wild California flower in the crag, surviving amidst the hardness! You waddled, got your sass on, cried, laughed, worried, made tough decisions, and had numerous blood pressure and weight checks. Some of you mamas went through even more with complicated pregnancies and tougher deliveries. Some are still in the trenches, battling breastfeeding challenges, colicky babies, sleepless nights, relationship problems, or mental health or physical challenges. And yet, you are here, making it through day by day.

Remember, you are your baby's mother, not by chance. You are incredible! Sacrificial. Tough. You may not feel like one, but indeed, you are a Mother Atlas. No, I didn't say you were perfect (who is?) or didn't have things to learn (who doesn't?), but you are doing what you can. That definitely warrants a free round-trip ticket to Fiji, a full night of sleep, or a year's subscription of . . . diapers? Okay, maybe for now, treat yourself to a shower, rejuvenate yourself with a nice walk, or enjoy a nourishing, tasty treat.

When trying to sum up motherhood, I frequently think back on what a patient told me, long before I ever got pregnant. It was one of those sacred moments—the kind I live for—that catch me by surprise and make me pause to take it all in. This time, the sprinkle of insight came from a seasoned mother a generation before me: "Once you have a child," she said, "it's as if suddenly you start living in color."

I tucked her wisdom deep within and now think I must agree. There are constantly new dimensions appearing in this full-color-spectrum living—much like a kaleidoscope, I suppose. Although I can't say all aspects are lovelier or easier, in many ways life is deeper, richer, more striking, and—heavens!—never dull.

As we both continue this wild adventure of motherhood, dear friend, I wish you safe travels, courage, stamina, and countless rest stops. May you have meaningful friendships, plenty of laundry detergent, and opportunities for ongoing laughter, growth, and self-discovery. In our moments of self-doubt, may we wonder at how far we've come and how—just as a caterpillar is programmed to become a spectacular butterfly—so, too, within our womanly fibers, we have the natural capacity to be good mothers. Of course, it takes some figuring out. But through practice, learning from mistakes, prioritizing our own self-care, and investing in a supportive community, we can do it—together.

Let's stay in touch!

ACKNOWLEDGMENTS

After finally finishing this book and reflecting on how the manuscript and I both evolved over the past 11 years of writing and revising, I am at a loss for words. Surprising, right? I think back on all the people who encouraged me along the way, who helped me cling to my vision, and who believed I would, one day, be able to see it through—thank you. Without my family and friends, I would have surely given up countless times, whenever I squinted into the horizon, wondering when my finished project would appear.

Thank you—

To my parents, Márti and Paul, who daily encouraged me to keep writing until the end, even when I got tired of it all. Papi, I tamed the beast! Mami, I finally climbed the mountain.

To my sister, Lili, who suggested I add references to my memoir. Thanks a lot! I hope this does the trick.

To my husband, Dan, and my three lovely little legacies, who have given me the grace and space to plod along this journey. Dan, though it wasn't easy—the book is done! Your dream came true! Thank you for cheering me on in the process, for taking the kids swimming and on ski trips while I wrote, for tolerating a distracted wife, doing extra loads of laundry, and for waiting six months for me to finally mend your biking shorts. To my girls, I counted to 100 and not just 75, and finished the book to help women—now, let's go play!

To my incredible, talented, wonderful editor, project manager, and now friend, Rachel Richardson, without whom I couldn't have done this work: Thank you for your encouragement, optimism, perseverance, talent, creativity, good ideas, countless texts, and hours of your life. You not only helped me improve as a writer but also wisely reorganized the book, edited, smoothed my transitions, and convinced me to write a "Let's Talk About It" for *every* week (*Phew!*). We did it—we conquered the appendix and captured the fireflies. Eternal thanks!

To my wonderful, patient, and creative artists, who made this book beautiful and fun to read. Christa Pierce, for the awesome cover, milestone page borders, back stretches (A-3b), and breastfeeding positions (A-5d). Rafaela Perasinic, for the monthly fetal development images, pelvic floor illustrations (A-3c), postpartum flower bouquet, and labor positions (A-4b). Ariel Garcia, for the Pregnancy Roadmap (A-1), Healthy Weight Gain in Pregnancy and Where Does All the Weight Go (A-3f), Postpartum Care Plan (A-5a); Birth Control Options (A-5b), Tasty Snacks and Recipes (B-1e), My Pregnancy Plate (B-1g), When Things Don't Go as Planned (B-4i), Larkwell Press imprint logo, and line break icons.

To Carla Green, for helping me birth the book I've always envisioned. Thank you for your expertise, time, patience, guidance, and hard work!

Thank you, Jennifer Jas, for your meticulous proofreading, and to Heather Pendley for the detailed index.

To the many excellent and trusted healthcare professionals who provided feedback on selected sections: with your help, this book is now more robust and better tailored to meet women's needs. To the mental health consultants—Julie Jorgenson, LMFT; Livia Perry, FPMHNP-BC; and Erica Wright, LMFT—your expertise made these sections more relevant and useful! Thanks to Veronica Benjamin, RD, for the nutrition sections (week 7, 9; B-1a through B-1c); Michele Minero, LMFT, for Cultivating a Healthy Relationship with Your Body (B-4g); Kim Sterner, RN, CNM, NP, for labor sections (weeks 36, 38, 40; A-4a, A-4c through A-4g); Kathy Kates, FNP-BC, on pelvic floor health (week 31; A-3c); legal consultant Cynthia Calvert, for rights of working mothers (week 20, 25; A-3g); Ann Soliday Bench, MPH, RN, PHN, for substance use (B-4h); Karen Vikstrom, MS, CGC, for prenatal screening (week 10; A-3e); Veronica Jordan, MD, for developmental milestone sections; Elise Sullivan, MD, for Physical Changes that Affect Postpartum Sex (B-5e); Helen Spivak, MD, for When to Seek Medical Care (A-2); Michael Policar, MD, for Birth Control Options (A-5b); Chaplain Susan Cosio, MDiv, BCC, for Nurturing Your Spiritual Self (week 29) and for providing the clarity needed to write such a challenging section; and medical librarians Lindsey Gillespie, MLIS, AHIP, and Michelle Lieggi, MLS, AHIP, for patiently tracking down article after article.

Thanks, too, for all you dear women who shared your stories and allowed me to partner with you as a nurse practitioner. What an honor!

To Helen Spivak, MD, my mentor; Holly Fontenot, PhD, RN, WHNP-BC, my grad school nursing director; Rebecca Viloria, MD, my grad school preceptor; Julie Neff-Lipman, my undergrad writing professor; and Claudia Rengstorf, my inspirational friend—for each kindly wading through my very first draft and believing there was within it beauty and purpose worth pursuing.

And of course, most of all, to my loving God: my source of eternal strength, hope, and joy, who gave me a love for writing and the perseverance to carry on—even through pneumonia, a pandemic, and piles of dishes.

APPENDICES

APPENDIX A
A QUICK GUIDE TO PREGNANCY AND BEYOND

APPENDIX B
A HEALTHY YOU FOR A HEALTHY BABY

Appendix C

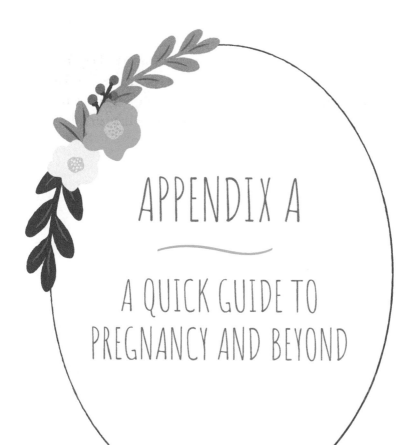

APPENDIX A

A QUICK GUIDE TO PREGNANCY AND BEYOND

1. PREGNANCY ROADMAP

Welcome, friend! Check out this general timeline to help plot your course through this exciting journey. While it's intended to help you plan and organize, just know, there may be slight variations based on your unique situation, needs, preferences, and place of prenatal care.

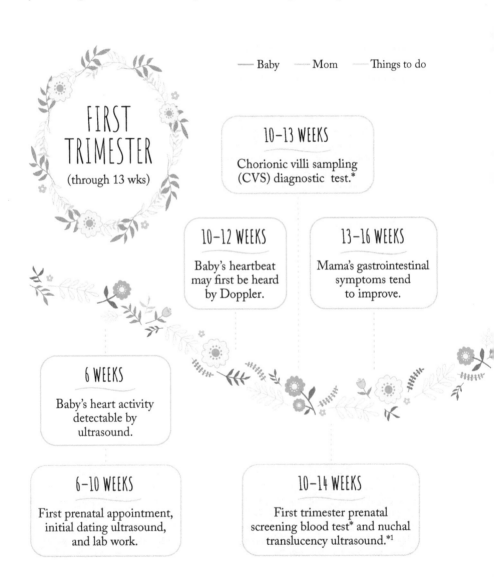

—— Baby ——— Mom ——— Things to do

FIRST TRIMESTER
(through 13 wks)

10–13 WEEKS
Chorionic villi sampling (CVS) diagnostic test.*

10–12 WEEKS
Baby's heartbeat may first be heard by Doppler.

13–16 WEEKS
Mama's gastrointestinal symptoms tend to improve.

6 WEEKS
Baby's heart activity detectable by ultrasound.

6–10 WEEKS
First prenatal appointment, initial dating ultrasound, and lab work.

10–14 WEEKS
First trimester prenatal screening blood test* and nuchal translucency ultrasound.*[1]

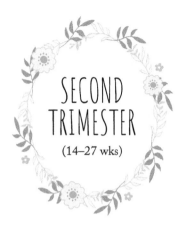

SECOND TRIMESTER

(14–27 wks)

TIMELINE NOTES

* Denotes optional prenatal screening and testing

First and Second Trimesters:
prenatal appointments generally every month.

23–25 WEEKS

Find classes to prepare for labor and newborn care.

18–21 WEEKS

Fetal anatomy ultrasound.[1]

26–28 WEEKS

Routine blood test checks mama for gestational diabetes, anemia, and more.[3-6]

14 WEEKS

Mama's energy starts improving.

18–21 WEEKS

Can feel baby's movements for the first time.

28 WEEKS

Start daily kick counts (unless recommended to do so earlier).

15–22 WEEKS

Second trimester "multiple markers" prenatal screening blood test*; amniocentesis diagnostic test.*[1]

24 WEEKS

Baby is viable!

24–28 WEEKS

If mama is RhD negative, get antibody screen blood test and Rho(D) immune globulin shot (unless the father of baby is also RhD negative).[6,10]

20 WEEKS

Lifting limits will incrementally decrease as you get closer to your due date.[2]

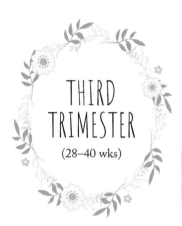

THIRD TRIMESTER
(28–40 wks)

36 WEEKS

Complete maternity leave paperwork.

36–37 WEEKS

Get screened for Group B *Streptococcus* (GBS) via a vaginal/rectal swab.[11-14]

30 WEEKS

Start planning maternity leave.

35 WEEKS

Belly is in full bloom! Great time to get those maternity photos.

37–38 WEEKS

Baby is early term.

27–36 WEEKS

Get Tdap vaccine (a combination vaccine that protects against whooping cough).[6-9]

39 WEEKS

Baby is full term! Scheduled Cesarean births occur, as well as some labor inductions.

TIMELINE NOTES

Third Trimester: prenatal appointments may be more frequent (such as every 2-3 weeks between weeks 28 and 36, and weekly from week 36 to delivery).

Anytime:
Optional cell-free DNA blood test can be done throughout pregnancy, as early as 9 weeks.[1]

If you're not immune to chickenpox or rubella, talk to your maternity care provider about getting the respective varicella or MMR vaccines.

An annual inactivated flu vaccine is recommended to protect against serious illness and is especially recommended if pregnant during flu season. It can be given anytime during pregnancy.[9,15,16]

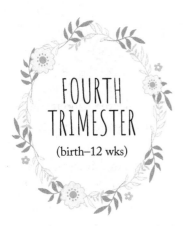

— Baby   — Mom   — Things to do

FOURTH TRIMESTER
(birth–12 wks)

From here on: Days are filled with joy, beauty, exhaustion, and challenges.

4–12 WEEKS
Take a follow-up glucose test if you had gestational diabetes.[4]

DAY 3–5
Mature milk comes in for most.

4 WEEKS
You may ovulate if not breastfeeding.

8 WEEKS
Lochia discharge normally ends now if it hasn't already.

1–2 WEEKS
"Baby blues" often occur. Consider mental wellness check-ins with a maternity care or mental health provider through the first year after birth.

6 WEEKS
Some body systems return to prepregnancy; many women start birth control.

TIMELINE NOTES

Fourth Trimester: postpartum visit will be based on your needs, perhaps 4–6 weeks after delivery, sooner if you had a Cesarean birth, or pregnancy or labor complications.[14]

2. WHEN TO SEEK PROFESSIONAL HELP

When to seek medical care

A good rule of thumb is to reach out when you're concerned about something or if something just doesn't seem quite right. Instead of wondering if everything is okay, be proactive!

What's the best way to seek care? It depends on the situation. Calling is best if it's urgent or if you'd like to talk to someone. Email is usually reserved for nonurgent situations, as it may take a day or two to hear back. And when it's an emergency, that's right—head to the emergency room or call 911.

Although it's impossible to write an exhaustive list on when to seek medical care, the following are some important situations in which to reach out.

Medical concerns

General symptoms
- Vaginal bleeding (though spotting can be normal, it's best to play it safe)
  - Specifically postpartum: reach out if you notice blood clots the size of golf balls (or larger), you soak a pad every hour, or have foul-smelling lochia
- Intense abdominal pain or cramps
- Pain in the right side of your abdomen
- Vision changes
- Severe headache or headache with new neurological symptoms (like numbness, trouble walking, slurred speech, or loss of vision or hearing)
- Dizziness
- Difficulty breathing or shortness of breath
- Uneven heart rate
- Calf pain or swelling
- Swelling of face, hands, or ankles
- Severe nausea, vomiting, or diarrhea

- Fever over 100°F or fever with neck stiffness
- Widespread itching, especially on palms and soles
- Hard and incredibly painful hemorrhoid
- Pain or burning during urination or trouble urinating
- Decreased or absent fetal movement or not meeting *kick counts* from 28 weeks on (or sooner, if recommended by your maternity care provider)
- Vaginal pain, irritation/itching, abnormal discharge, bumps or sores, odor, and/or painful sex

Potential labor (or preterm labor) symptoms
- Regular abdominal tightening or pain (in belly or back) for an hour, despite rest and hydration
- Pelvic pressure
- Leaking of fluid from your vagina (either a big gush or constant trickling)
- Bloody show (clear, pink, or blood-tinged, mucus-like vaginal discharge)

Breastfeeding concerns
- Baby with latching trouble
- Low milk supply
- Nipple pain/cracking
- Breast lump, pain, or redness
- Fever

When to seek mental health care

It's vital to seek mental health care when you need it. Check out B-4b for a detailed list of when to reach out, and B-4c for tips on finding a good fit for your care. Go ahead, mama, be courageous! Take your mental health needs seriously—you deserve it!

3. PREGNANCY TIPS

a. Getting Started

Ready for an amazing pregnancy journey? Prep yourself to start and finish well by checking out the following practical tips.

Listen to your body. Sleep when it sounds delicious. Yes, it may be *all* the time. It's as if mother nature is turning you into a sleeping beauty so your body is left alone to do its miraculous work.

Take a prenatal vitamin daily. It'll boost your diet with vitamins and minerals that support your body and your baby. For example: folic acid (vitamin B_9) reduces your risk for neural tube defects, vitamin D supports bone health, and iron helps red blood cells carry oxygen.

Folic acid (vitamin B_9). Make sure your prenatal vitamin has 400–800 mcg daily.[1-5] You'll need to take higher doses (4 mg) of a separate folic acid supplement if you've had a baby or close relative with neural tube defects or have other risk factors (like diabetes, digestive system absorption problems, prior surgery for obesity, or you take certain anti-seizure medications).[4,6-9] Some mamas may benefit from taking a different form of folate called 5-methyltetrahydrofolate (5-MTHF) instead.[8,10] Ask your maternity care provider to see if this is you.

Iron. The iron in your prenatal vitamin can make you more nauseous or constipated, so talk to your healthcare provider if you notice these effects. They may ask you to temporarily replace the prenatal vitamin with a simple gummy or folic acid vitamin.

> Most healthy women only need nutritious eating and a daily prenatal vitamin to meet their added vitamin and mineral requirements in pregnancy or while breastfeeding. If you have certain nutritional deficiencies or medical conditions, you may be asked to take additional or higher dose supplements, or a daily low-dose aspirin (81 mg).[11]

Contact your healthcare provider. Getting timely prenatal care is important. Did you know certain medical or mental health conditions (like diabetes, thyroid disorders, high blood pressure, certain mental health problems, eating disorders, or addictions) require special care from early on? Although the format of initial prenatal appointments varies, it's normal to get asked all sorts of questions. It's not meant to be an interrogation but an opportunity to get to know you, and for you and your maternity care provider to figure out how to best take care of you and your growing baby.

Questions usually include information about your last period, past pregnancies, your current/past medical and mental health problems, surgeries, current medications (also supplements and vitamins), possible environmental exposures (like chemicals at work or from travels), and genetic problems or birth defects as they relate to you, the father of the baby, or your family.

Let yourself be pampered. If the need arises, let yourself get pampered by an awesome team of professionals. These could include a genetic counselor, high-risk Ob-Gyn specialist (perinatologist), registered dietician, therapist, and/or addictions specialists. They're here to support you.

Keep taking your meds. It's *not* a good idea to suddenly stop prescription medications just because you're pregnant. Be sure to first talk with your healthcare provider. This especially goes for psychiatric medications (like antidepressants).

On the safe side, if you have any vaginal bleeding or severe abdominal pain, let your healthcare provider know. Some mild cramping and light spotting can be normal, but they'll want to make sure there is nothing else going on, like infection, miscarriage, or an *ectopic* pregnancy (when the fertilized egg is growing outside the uterus). For other times to seek medical care, see A-2.

WHAT'S WITH THESE LETTERS, ANYWAY?

In June of 2015, prescription drug labeling got a face-lift! Prior to this, pharmaceutical companies used letters—A, B, C, D, and X—to mark the degree of risk a medication posed to pregnant or lactating mamas.[12] Happily, this oversimplified lettering system was tossed in favor of more detailed descriptions, enabling women to more easily assess the risks and benefits.[13,14]

Thanks to the Pregnancy and Lactation Labeling Rule passed in 2014, new labels must detail the drug's impacts on pregnancy and lactation, as well as its potential reproductive implications.[12-14] Enjoy! Be aware, though, that medications approved prior to June 2001 only need to eliminate the letter classifications; they don't need to adhere to these new labeling requirements.[14]

Bottom line? When you consider taking a certain medication in pregnancy or while breastfeeding, forget the letters and ask your maternity care provider about the details available.

b. Managing Symptoms

The journey of pregnancy sure is an interesting one, full of surprises. As a continuation of "How to Survive Nausea, Vomiting, and Other Great Wonders" (week 6), here are tips to help you manage common physical symptoms of pregnancy—some of which may also pay you a visit after your babe's arrival. With most of these, there's not a single, one-size-fits-all solution, so go ahead and try a few options and see what works.[1]

Nausea and vomiting

Lifestyle ideas

- Get plenty of rest. Your nausea may worsen when you're exhausted.[2,3]
- Eat a small snack before getting up in the morning.[3]
- Don't skip meals. Eat a small snack or meal every 1.5–2 hours to avoid an empty stomach (which may trigger nausea).[2-4]

- Consume some protein each time you eat (e.g., nuts, seeds, dairy).[2-4]
- Don't eat and drink at the same time. Wait about 20–30 minutes between.[3]
- Avoid looking at, eating, or smelling foods or other things with strong odors. Sniffing a sliced lemon or orange may help.[3,4]
- Avoid fatty or spicy foods.[4]
- Try acupressure (e.g., motion sickness wristbands), acupuncture, or hypnosis.[3]
- Take your prenatal multivitamin after a meal.[2] Or, ask your maternity care provider about temporarily switching your prenatal vitamin to a folic acid supplement or a gummy vitamin. The iron in the prenatal can trigger nausea and will be more important after the first trimester.[3,4]

Trouble keeping fluids down? Try popsicles, ice chips, JELL-O, or smoothies.

Trouble keeping food down? Eat foods you can tolerate even if their nutritional value is low. Try liquid nutrition (like Ensure, BOOST, or Naked protein smoothies).

Got a terrible metallic or sour taste in your mouth? Try chewing gum or sucking on a hard candy to cover up the taste.[3]

Supplements and Medications

Ginger. The root of a flowering plant, ginger is known to reduce nausea and comes in a variety of forms—like teas, chews, or capsules. Note, the maximum daily dose is the equivalent to 1 gram of dried ginger root powder.[1,3,5]

Vitamin B$_6$ (pyridoxine). Can be used alone or with doxylamine. Take 25 mg every eight hours. You'll notice an improvement within a few days, though it's important to keep taking it to retain the effects. The maximum daily dose is 200 mg per day from all your dietary and supplement sources.[3,4]

Doxylamine succinate. This over-the-counter antihistamine is used as a first-line medication for nausea and vomiting. It works beautifully with vitamin B_6. Since it may make you a little sleepy, it's best taken at night.[4,6]

Prescriptions. There are also a handful of other medications your provider may prescribe to help you, which may come in liquid, sublingual, and suppository forms.[4] If needed, ask your maternity care provider about these alternatives. They can be lifesavers!

Excess salivation

Lifestyle ideas

Carry a water bottle or a small pill container with a pop-up lid with you. You can discretely spit in them throughout the day.[2,7]

Try drinking water or chewing gum to help deal with the excess spit.[7]

Medications

Medications or supplements to treat your nausea and vomiting may help this pregnancy symptom, too.[2,7]

Constipation and hemorrhoids

Lifestyle ideas

Fiber is your friend.[8,9] See B-1f for a list of great sources of fiber, which all contain helpful carbohydrates that your body can't digest but can use to move stool through your digestive tract. These *prebiotics* also help build a healthy gut and stabilize your blood sugar and hunger.

Consume about 29 g daily if pregnant or breastfeeding, and about 26 g otherwise.[10] A psyllium fiber supplement (like Metamucil) or a fiber bar are great ways of reaching your recommended fiber intake.[2] When consuming more fiber, you may notice more gas and bloating for a few weeks, but don't worry, it should resolve before long.

Stay well-hydrated, especially if you're increasing your fiber consumption.[2,9] Drink plenty of water throughout the day (8–12 c, or 64–96 oz, per day) and limit juices and sodas.[11] If your urine isn't light yellow or colorless, you probably need to drink more water. Though remember, your prenatal vitamin will turn your urine a psychedelic yellow color right after taking it.

Be active. Being physically active kicks your digestive system into gear! Aim for at least 30 minutes daily and break it up into 10- to 15-minute sessions if exhausted or limited on time (see B-2 to learn more).

Try probiotics.[12-16] Having a happy gastrointestinal (GI) tract and strong immune system hinges on having the right assortment of friendly GI microorganisms, like bacteria. You can find these live bacteria in kefir or live-cultured yogurt with *Lactobacillus* or *Bifidobacterium*; fermented foods, like sauerkraut, kimchi, or kombucha; or probiotic supplements (ask your maternity care provider or registered dietician for a recommendation).

Don't hold back. Girl, when you need to—go!

Soothe your hemorrhoid. Work to manage your constipation or diarrhea—it can make such a difference! For temporary relief of itching, discomfort, and mild pain, try warm baths, applying Tucks (or witch hazel) pads, or medicated hemorrhoid creams, ointments, wipes, or sprays, like those in the Preparation H lineup. For internal hemorrhoids, rectal suppositories offer more relief and can feel like heaven on earth, so ask your maternity care provider. Remember, long-term, daily use can damage your skin, so only use these occasionally.

Medications

Laxatives. In occasional moments of desperation, certain laxatives can help tremendously with constipation.[2,8,9] These are not created equal and work differently, so check in with your maternity care provider before trying any to avoid problems. Typically recommended options include a docusate sodium stool softener (like Colace) or polyethylene glycol (MiraLax).[17,18] Avoid products containing bismuth, castor oil, or mineral oil.[18]

Heartburn

Lifestyle ideas[2,19]

Avoid foods that cause symptoms, such as greasy, spicy, or acidic foods, and caffeinated or carbonated drinks.

Time your meals. Eat your day's last meal two to three hours before bedtime.

Sleep propped up so you're not lying flat in bed.

Medications

Antacids (calcium-, magnesium-, or aluminum-based ones) work well if you have mild heartburn and want quick relief.[2,19,20] Try Tums or Mylanta, though liquids may work better.[2,20] Avoid magnesium trisilicates or sodium bicarbonate–based antacids.[20]

Other medications.[2,19,20] If your over-the-counter antacid wears off too soon, talk to your maternity care provider. Other medications can prevent or relieve heartburn, such as histamine H2-receptor blockers (e.g., cimetidine, famotidine) and even proton-pump inhibitors (e.g., omeprazole and pantoprazole). The jury is still out on which is the best in pregnancy.[19]

Headaches

In pregnancy, headaches can get more or less frequent—let's hope you're in the latter group! Headaches can be caused by all sorts of things, ranging from hunger, low blood sugar, dehydration, inadequate sleep, neck problems, or sinusitis, to more serious conditions like infections, high blood pressure, preeclampsia, abuse, tumors, and stroke.[21-23] Most pregnant mamas, though, notice their migraines improve toward the end of the first trimester and also in the first six months of breastfeeding.[21-23] If you're experiencing debilitating headaches, be

> ⟫⟫ ❀ ❀ ❀ ⟪⟪
>
> Headaches sometimes warrant prompt medical attention. Check out A-2 for a list of symptoms to watch for.[22,23]

sure to keep reaching out to your maternity care provider until it's well controlled. You need to be able to function and enjoy your life!

Lifestyle ideas

Eat regularly throughout the day. Small, frequent, protein-rich snacks help stabilize your blood sugar (see B-1e & f for suggestions). See earlier tips on nausea and vomiting if those symptoms are making it hard for you to snack about every two hours.

Avoid dietary migraine triggers.[24] These often include chocolate, cheese (and dairy products), caffeine, cured meats, monosodium glutamate (MSG), and foods with strong smells.

Stay hydrated.[24] Adequate hydration can help with all sorts of things, even headaches! Aim for 8–12 c of water or non-caffeinated fluids throughout the day. Keep a water bottle with you.

Get your Zzs.[24] Sleep renews, while sleep deprivation makes everything worse and often leads to headaches. Prioritize getting to bed on time and aim for seven to nine hours a night (see B-3a for luxurious sleep tips).[25]

De-stress.[24] Although it's not always easy, try to rejuvenate yourself daily with rest, relaxation, meditation, spiritual practices, or physical activity—listen to what your body needs. Even 10–15 minutes a day can work wonders at rebalancing you!

Try acupuncture. Some people swear it helps prevent migraines, though you may need multiple sessions before you see a benefit.[26] Be sure to visit a professional who is well versed in pregnancy.

Medications

Acetaminophen (TYLENOL). This medication is a go-to for pain since it's considered to pose the lowest risk in pregnancy.[27] Ask your maternity care provider before using it and follow the label instructions for how often you can safely take it. To keep your liver happy, limit your use to 2,000 grams per 24 hours.

Others. In pregnancy, not all standard migraine medications are safe, so before you grab your go-to, please talk with your maternity care provider. For acute migraine treatment, metoclopramide (Reglan) or sumatriptan (Imitrex) may be recommended, while for prevention, a beta blocker medication (like propranolol) is often used.[21,22,27] Nonsteroidal anti-inflammatory drugs (NSAIDs) like ibuprofen or ketorolac are generally not recommended in pregnancy but may occasionally be used in the second trimester only.[22,27]

Back pain

As your beautiful belly grows and further curves your lower spine later in pregnancy, you may notice some back pain. Although back pain is common, it's best avoided when possible, right? Let's see if we can help you prevent it in the first place or feel better with the following tips. Since back pain can sometimes be caused by more serious conditions, play it safe. Seek medical advice if you've had back problems prior to pregnancy, your pain is so bad you can't easily move, or you develop other symptoms like leg weakness, inability to control bowel movements, or sudden onset or worsening of urinary leakage.

Lifestyle Ideas

Try a maternity belt. Different than a belly band, this is designed to offer extra support, off-loading some stress from your back. Try wearing this under your clothes during physical activity or if you're on your feet all day.

Find good shoes. Stash the favorite heels and flimsy flats and go for shoes with good support in pregnancy. Don't worry, they can still be cute. Believe it or not, what you wear really affects your back.

Stay active. Try to get about 30 minutes of physical activity daily (see B-2). You may need to adjust what you do depending on how your back feels while exercising. Swimming is a great option that takes the strain off your back muscles and can feel oh-so-nice!

Don't sit or stand all day. Keep your daily activity varied. If you have a desk job, get up and move around regularly, or better yet, ask for a height-adjustable desk so you can sit or stand as needed. Rather than standing all day, ask for a stool to sit on or a footstool upon which to rest a foot.

Bend with your knees, not your back. When it comes to picking things up or off the floor, keep your back straight and squat, as if sitting down in a chair.

Lift heavy objects with care. Hop on over to "Physical Activity in the Workplace" (in B-2b) for considerations specific to lifting objects while pregnant.

Pay attention. If you ignore your whimpering back, it will only get worse. Walk around, lie down, move, and stretch.

Massage. Treat yourself to a pregnancy massage focused on your lower back.

Ice/heat. Don't forget the relief you can get from using ice or heat. Try either for 15 minutes at a time and wrap the ice pack or heating pad in a towel to protect your skin and baby from the elements. Apply an ice pack when you need anti-inflammatory benefits, such as when you have a new injury or have sharp nerve pain (like sciatica). Apply heat to your back (and not on your belly) when you need to loosen tight muscles and increase blood flow to an injured area. Sometimes alternating ice with heat can make you feel like you won the lottery.

Stretch daily. Give your back a little care twice a day to loosen those tight muscles and relieve the tension. Try the illustrated stretches on the following pages.

Get a musculoskeletal assessment. An unhappy back can get much worse, quickly. If the prior suggestions are not doing the trick, talk to your healthcare provider for a referral to physical therapy or a musculoskeletal specialist, such as someone trained in sports medicine. A good assessment and tailored care and exercises can make a huge difference!

BACK STRETCHES

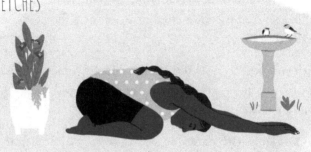

CHILD'S POSE

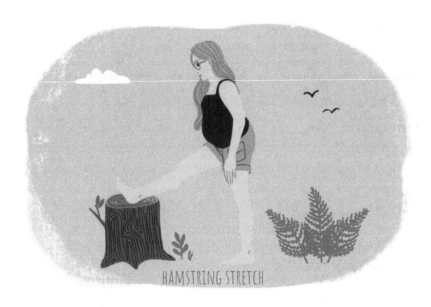

HAMSTRING STRETCH

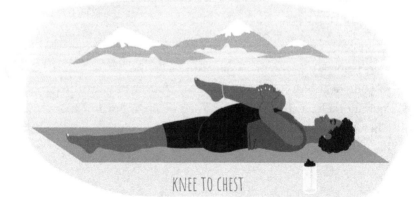

KNEE TO CHEST

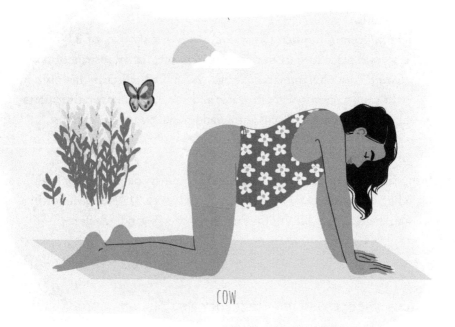

COW

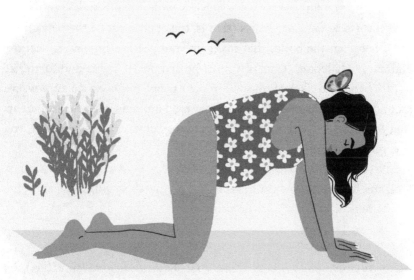

CAT

Medications

Generally, **acetaminophen** (TYLENOL), with a daily max of 2,000 mg, is a good place to start to relieve pain in pregnancy, instead of non-steroidal anti-inflammatory drugs (NSAIDs). Discuss this option with your maternity care provider and ask for a nonoperative sports medicine referral to discuss other additional treatment options.

Incontinence

Struggling with incontinence? You'll find a summary on pelvic floor health, including incontinence, in "Your Pelvic Floor" (week 31) and the following section, "Pelvic Floor Health for Pregnancy and Beyond" (A-3c).

c. Pelvic Floor Health for Pregnancy and Beyond

Welcome to your very own tour of your pelvis. Sit back and relax for a second and explore how wonderfully you are designed.

Aren't you beautiful?! Look how intricate your pelvis and pelvic floor are. I love how each hip bone is shaped like a half-heart. So fitting, isn't it? And did you know a woman's pelvis is wider than a male's, and it can have diverse *pelvic inlet* shapes (that is, the open space in the pelvis)?

Check out the bones that make up your pelvis—hip bones, sacrum, and *coccyx* (tailbone). Can you find the symphysis pubis and sacroiliac joints? See the basket of muscles in your pelvic floor? Some even weave around your vagina and anus. Consider for a moment all the components that form the pelvic girdle. These various structures are supporting you and your baby right now. Amazing!

Now that you have a clearer picture of the area, let's take a quick look at a few situations common in the perinatal period: stress and urge incontinence, and pelvic girdle pain.

Stress and urge urinary incontinence

Stress incontinence occurs when your *pelvic floor muscles* (*PFM*) are either weakened or too tight. This causes you to leak urine when you're involved in something that increases pressure (stress) on your

PELVIS

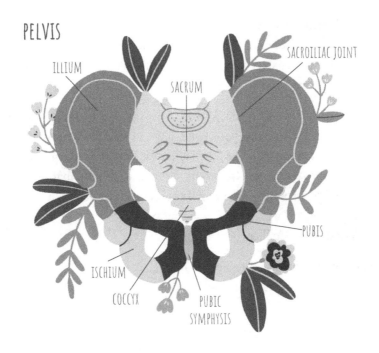

PELVIC FLOOR

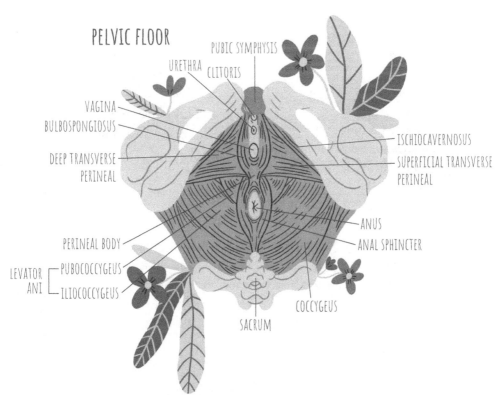

bladder, such as coughing, laughing, sneezing, jumping, or lifting. If you can relate, have your PFM evaluated by a pelvic floor physical therapist or maternity care provider to determine the cause of your incontinence and receive a unique treatment plan.[1,*]

Meanwhile, practice deep and cleansing (diaphragmatic) breathing, which will help relax your pelvic floor and ensure your bowel movements are regular.[†] The latter is important because constipation can aggravate symptoms (for more on this, see "Constipation and hemorrhoids" in A-3b). Other helpful lifestyle factors include maintaining a healthy weight and avoiding both cigarettes and bladder-irritant drinks (we'll cover those more next).[2]

Urge incontinence, on the other hand, occurs when your bladder contracts unexpectedly, prompting a sudden urge to urinate, causing you to unintentionally leak. These abnormal contractions can occur from irritants—such as coffee, tea, alcohol, carbonated drinks, and cigarettes—as well as from medical conditions, injury, or the natural pressure on your bladder from your blooming self.[1,2] These urges can be relieved through pelvic floor muscle work, bladder retraining, and deep breathing for 5–10 minutes daily.[1-4,‡] While not pregnant, some women may try medications, but these do have adverse side effects and don't tend to work as well.

> ### KEGEL TIP
>
> Don't forget to practice short contractions (or "quick flicks"), in addition to those longer squeezes. By doing so, you're priming your muscles to rescue you on a moment's notice.

If your maternity care provider or pelvic floor physical therapist has determined Kegels could help your symptoms, here is an awesome recipe for your own homemade pelvic floor muscles of steel.

---

* Kathy Kates, FNP-BC, personal communication, June 18, 2021
† Kates
‡ Kates

RECIPE | Emese's Recipe for Pelvic Floor Muscles of Steel

PREP TIME: Only a smidgen   COOKING TIME: Less than 5 min

NOTES:

To fully savor the benefits, make three times a week.

INGREDIENTS:

5 tbsp patience
½ tsp adventurous spirit
½ c commitment
¼ tsp time

DIRECTIONS FOR KEGELS:

1. Combine the first two ingredients.

2. Find the right muscles. While lying or sitting, put a finger in the vaginal opening. Try to squeeze around it. You should feel the muscles tighten. If not, sprinkle with patience and try again until you can. (Optional: Leave your finger in place during exercises to help verify you are using the right muscles.)

3. Whip in the commitment. Challenge yourself to 30 squeezes per day: 10 long holds and 20 quick ones, to strengthen both your "sprint" and "endurance" muscles. For maximum benefit, make sure you relax muscles entirely between squeezes, as if letting a marble roll out of you.

4. Sprinkle in time. Over the coming weeks, work up to holding the long squeezes 8–10 seconds every time.

Health benefits include: Stronger muscles to support pelvic organs and prevent urinary leakage, while likely making sex and orgasms more satisfying.[2,5]

Pelvic pain

Now that you've seen the bowl-shaped pelvis, you are hopefully more familiar with its components: your bones (hip, sacrum, and coccyx), three joints (symphysis pubis in the front, two sacroiliac joints in the back), and muscles. Combined, your pelvis holds your abdominal organs, bowels, bladder, and your glorious reproductive organs—oh, and your pelvic floor, of course.

Sometimes women can develop pain in the pelvis, such as symphysis pubis pain. This happens when changes in hormones, ligaments, and pelvic floor muscle strength make this joint either widen or move less, resulting in pain or popping at the joint, and possibly even pain in your inner thigh or vagina. If you experience this, be sure to connect with your maternity care provider and ask for a referral to a pelvic floor physical therapist.

In the meantime, try these:

- Wear a maternity belt.
- Keep your knees closer together.
- Stand with feet firmly planted.
- Take smaller steps as you walk.
- Avoid crossing your legs.
- Sleep with a pillow between your knees.

You'll feel better very soon, so hang in there! As always, if you're in severe pain, be sure to get immediate help.

d. Selecting a Maternity Care Provider and Practice

As we discussed in "Finding Good Prenatal Care" (week 8), selecting a single maternity care provider or a group of providers is one of the most important and exciting decisions you'll make in your pregnancy. Here's information about differences and similarities between various maternity care providers. Remember, these are just generalizations.

Types of providers

Midwives are trained to provide prenatal, labor, birth, and postpartum care to healthy women who are at low risk for developing pregnancy complications; they can provide gynecological care, as well as sometimes assist in surgeries. They believe pregnancy and birth are natural processes, best not hindered by unnecessary medical interventions. A *midwife* (literally meaning *with woman*) can work in a variety of settings like birth centers, clinics, and hospitals, and they can attend home births. Certified Nurse Midwives (*CNMs*), Certified Professional Midwives (*CPMs*), and Certified Midwives (*CMs*) have met nationally recognized standards for care. If a potential provider doesn't have one of these credentials, be sure to find out more about their training and experience.

Obstetricians (*Ob-Gyns*). Medically trained, board-certified Ob-Gyn physicians specialize in prenatal care, labor, birth, surgery, and gynecology. Their medical training focuses on caring for women with serious medical problems, pregnancy complications, and those at high risk for developing complications. You definitely want to be in their hands if you fall into this category. Ob-Gyns tend to work in Ob-Gyn practices or departments and deliver babies in hospitals. They also serve as consultants to other maternity care providers, as needed. *Perinatologists*, also called *maternal-fetal medicine (MFM) specialists*, are Ob-Gyns who complete additional years of training.

Family Physicians (*FPs*). Medically trained, board-certified FPs provide holistically focused medical care for families and people of all ages. Some provide prenatal care, attend births, and perform surgeries. Unless they've also completed an obstetrics fellowship, they usually care for low-risk pregnant women, and refer to Ob-Gyns if complications arise during pregnancy. Since they specialize in caring for your entire family, they can become the primary care provider for you and your baby after delivery.

Nurse Practitioners (*NPs*). Women's health nurse practitioners (*WHNP-BCs*) are board-certified NPs, or graduate-level-trained registered nurses (*RNs*), who specialize in providing women's healthcare across their lifespan. While they usually do not attend births, NPs provide prenatal and postpartum care to low-risk pregnant women in a variety of settings; they also provide gynecological care and sometimes assist in surgeries. You may also find a board-certified Family Nurse Practitioner (*FNP-BC*) working in a prenatal clinic. If complications arise, NPs will either collaborate with or refer you to an Ob-Gyn physician. Overall, nursing philosophy focuses on holistic care and disease prevention, as well as patient education, empowerment, and advocacy.

Physician Assistants (*PAs*). These nationally certified, state-licensed medical professionals work in a variety of healthcare settings, such as medical departments, hospitals, and health centers. Graduate-level-trained in the traditional, medical model view of health, they can diagnose and treat health conditions, prescribe medications, perform procedures, and assist in surgery. If complications arise, they will either collaborate with or refer you to an Ob-Gyn physician.

Considerations for picking a maternity care provider

Here are some additional aspects to think about as you select your provider or practice for prenatal and postpartum care:

Your physical health. Do you have any medical problems that would put your pregnancy at higher risk for complications? Examples include diabetes, high blood pressure, heart disease, and autoimmune conditions. If yes, you'll want to have an Ob-Gyn or fellowship-trained family physician involved in your care. Depending on how the maternity care practice is set up, you may still have the option of receiving some prenatal care from others as well.

Your mental health. If you currently have or previously struggled with certain mental health problems, it's incredibly helpful to find a maternity care and mental health provider specializing in perinatal mental health (see B-4c). In large, busy obstetric practices, you may wish to stick with one or two maternity care providers so you can build that trusting relationship and ensure your mental health needs are adequately addressed.

Your past experiences. Mamas who have gone through IVF, prior pregnancy losses, sexual abuse, or difficult or traumatizing birth experiences often need extra support. If this is you, I'm so sorry things have been hard. Please know there is hope for you to have a beautiful pregnancy and birth experience!

It's important for you to find a maternity care provider who compassionately partners with you, listens to your story, offers sensitive care, and strategizes with you on how to enhance your pregnancy and labor experience. Especially in the case of traumatic birth or sexual abuse, appropriate mental health care is vital so you can reach a place of healing (more on these circumstances in B-4i and B-5f).

Your personality. Are you a planner, a worrier, quietly reserved, or chatty and social? Would you enjoy working with someone who meets with you often and for longer visits or who keeps it short and sweet? Midwives, FPs, and NPs tend to favor longer visits, as they focus on holistic care and your experience of pregnancy, while Ob-Gyns may keep visits shorter and focused on your important medical concerns.

Your lifestyle. Do you have a flexible daily schedule or is your work or family life so busy that you don't know how you'll fit in prenatal visits? Some maternity care practices, such as larger healthcare systems, may open early, stay open later in the day, and give you creative ways of connecting with your healthcare team (e.g., email, and virtual or phone visits).

Your views on health. Is addressing health holistically through lifestyle and natural means important to you or not so much? Typically, midwives, FPs, and NPs focus more on this type of care. Do you want a provider who can also care for you and your family long after you have your baby? FPs and FNPs are trained to care for the whole family, as are PAs who work in family medicine.

Your pregnancy dreams. Sometimes specific pregnancy wishes can direct your search process. Do you have answers to the questions below? If you do, keep them in mind as you embark on your hunt.

- Do you have strong sentiments about what type of maternity care provider you're looking for (such as one who is a female or speaks certain languages)? Did you have a prior maternity care provider who you've worked with before and love?

- Is it important to you what type of setting you receive prenatal care in (like in an Ob-Gyn department, community center clinic, or small private practice)?

- Based on what you currently know about birth, are there some aspects about the labor experience that are important to you? For example, are you interested in a water birth? Or, if you've had a prior Cesarean birth, are you interested in finding a maternity care provider who can offer you the option of trying for a vaginal birth (see "Vaginal Births, Cesarean Births, and VBACs" in week 32)?

- Do you care where you deliver your baby (like at home, a birth center, or a hospital)?

Questions for your maternity care provider

To help you get to know your potential provider, you may wish to ask the office or maternity care provider some of these questions.

- Are they accepting new patients?
- Do they accept your insurance?
- What education does your maternity care provider have? How long has she or he been in practice?
- What is their philosophy of care?
- Who does your maternity care provider work with? Do they collaborate with a genetic counselor, nutritionist, mental health specialist, perinatologist, and other specialists as needed?
- Does the practice offer prenatal groups, classes, or postpartum support groups?

- Does your maternity care provider attend deliveries or only work in the clinic?
- Where do they attend deliveries?
- How many births have they attended? How many ended in a Cesarean birth?
- Will your midwife or physician be at your delivery or is it based on an "on call" schedule, which means, depending on the timing, other maternity care providers may attend the delivery instead? Are medical residents and nursing students involved?
- Do you have the option to meet with your potential maternity care provider before you make a final decision?

e. Prenatal Screening and Testing Options

Welcome to more information about prenatal screening, diagnostic tests, and genetic carrier screening. To begin with, you can give yourself a pat on the back for doing some research on this topic. Remember, it's normal to have questions because it's a complicated subject with big implications. Let's go a little deeper, expanding on "Prenatal Screening and Testing" (week 10), to help you decide where to go from here.

Birth defects: definition and causes

To recap, a *birth defect* is a physical or structural problem a baby develops while in the womb. Most major problems would develop in the first three months of pregnancy—when your baby's organs are developing and you're feeling quite subpar.[1,2] Not all abnormalities can be identified before birth, and those are instead discovered during a newborn screening, physical exam, or later.

While genetic abnormalities are a primary cause of birth defects, there are a plethora of external factors as well (yes, quite unhelpful for us professional worriers). Known external causes include diseases or illnesses (like diabetes, obesity, chicken pox, syphilis, rubella, and zika virus), supplements (like high vitamin A), drugs (medications, or recreational, like marijuana), cigarettes (and secondhand smoke), alcohol, work exposures (like chemicals or radiation), and environmental toxins (like pesticides or lead).[3,4]

Since exposure to environmental toxins can have such adverse repercussions, it's a good idea to pay attention, especially for the first 16 weeks when your baby's busy forming organs. During this time, and throughout pregnancy, what you eat, drink, inhale, and put on your skin could enter your body and possibly affect your baby.

⇘⇘⇘ ❀ ✿ ❀ ⇙⇙⇙

For more on environmental toxins and their sources, check out "Environmental Toxins" in A-3i.

To briefly summarize: although genetic variations typically cause about half of all birth defects, external exposures can also be at fault, and many times the exact cause is unclear.[3] It's possible that the abnormalities we see are caused by the interactions between two or more of these factors.

Prenatal screening

Of the three avenues available for learning more about possible birth defects—prenatal screening, genetic carrier screening, and diagnostic testing—the first two are noninvasive while the last is usually invasive. Of these categories, prenatal and genetic carrier screening determine if there is a *higher chance* of a birth defect, while diagnostic testing will show if there *is* an issue.

Tests that fall into the prenatal screening category include blood tests taken from your arm, like the integrated, quad screen, multiple markers, or cell-free DNA screens (which is also called **NIPT** or **NIPS**), as well as special ultrasounds of your baby (like a test called **nuchal translucency**).[5-7] It is important to realize, though, that the accuracy of detecting a problem is rarely 100% (more likely, 50%–99%) and varies by the specific condition being tested.[5,6] As always, if you're interested in testing, remember to ask what the test's **positive predictive value** is for you specifically—this refers to the chance that a positive test result is genuinely true (rather than a false positive).

A *low risk* test result means you can relax knowing your baby doesn't have an increased risk for those specific problems, while *high risk* means he or she has a higher chance of having a birth defect but may still be perfectly healthy. If the result is "high risk," you'd need follow-up diagnostic testing to know if there's truly a problem. In cases where the screening blood test shows a baby is at high risk for a chromosomal abnormality, you could also better estimate the risk with the much more accurate NIPT screening test before proceeding with an invasive test. Luckily, most women who receive a "high risk" test result go on to find out they do really have a healthy baby!

RECEIVING A TEST NOT PERFORMED RESULT[5,6]

Sometimes, the cell-free DNA test result can't be generated. Don't freak out! This doesn't automatically mean there's something wrong. For example, this may occur if the test was done too early or if you are a plus-size mama, are Black or South Asian, conceived through IVF, are carrying twins, or are on low-molecular-weight heparin (LMWH). Chat with your maternity care provider about next steps, which may be repeating the blood test or consulting with an Ob-Gyn specialist.

Prenatal diagnostic testing

While prenatal screening is a noninvasive indicator that will suggest the likelihood of an issue, prenatal diagnostic testing is (usually) invasive but also more conclusive: it truly verifies either the presence or absence of a condition. Depending on the condition that's being tested for, the diagnostic testing may be as simple as getting a more sensitive (level 2) ultrasound or may require a more involved, direct analysis of your baby's DNA. How wonderful to have these options!

There are several creative (albeit invasive) ways specialists can collect your baby's cells and analyze your child's DNA directly. Cells may be collected with a needle from: (1) your placenta, in a test called *chorionic villi sampling* (*CVS*), which occurs between 10 and 13 weeks gestational age (GA); (2) the amniotic fluid that surrounds your baby, in a test called *amniocentesis* (or *amnio*), which is typically performed between 15 and 20 weeks GA; or (3) your baby's blood, collected through the umbilical cord, in a procedure called *fetal blood sampling*, after 18 weeks GA.[8] Remember, with the amnio and CVS procedures, there's a small miscarriage risk (i.e., 0.1%–0.3%, or 1 miscarriage for every 333–1,000 procedures), while the fetal blood sampling involves an even higher risk (i.e., 1%–3%, or 1 to 3 miscarriages for every 100 procedures).[8,9]

Some women opt for invasive testing only if their prenatal screening results were abnormal, while others proactively choose it (perhaps when various other factors are increasing their baby's risk for certain conditions). These factors could include the mama being over age 35, the parents having had another child with genetic problems, or either parent with a family history of certain inherited conditions.

Now a little word for all of you beautiful, more "mature" women who will be at least 35 years old when you deliver: you don't automatically need to feel like a granny just because of the *advanced maternal age* label, and though you may choose to do so, you don't automatically need to choose invasive testing either.

You may be interested in opting for the *cell-free DNA* (NIPT or NIPS) screening blood test. This noninvasive test involves analyzing a blood sample for chromosomal abnormalities like trisomy 21 (Down syndrome) or trisomy 18 (Edwards syndrome), with a detection rate of 98%–99%.[5,6] As mamas get older, certain chromosomal abnormalities such as these occur more often. For example, your risk of any chromosomal abnormality at age thirty-three is 1 in 208; while at age thirty-five it's 1 in 132; at age thirty-seven it's 1 in 83; and at age forty it's 1 in 40.

Genetic carrier screening

Genetic carrier screenings analyze blood samples (taken from the arm) to check for variations of genes that are linked to specific disorders. Think of *genes* as the instructions within your cells that tell them how to function and grow. They're made up of DNA, are stored in structures called chromosomes, and your baby inherits them from you and the father. When this instruction set gets "rewritten" (through a gene change), it can cause alterations in how the body functions and grows. Scientists have been able to uncover many gene variations that are directly linked to certain physical issues and can determine (through these carrier screens) whether a person's genes have these anomalies.

Typically, all pregnant mamas are offered genetic screening for cystic fibrosis and spinal muscular atrophy.[10-14] Depending on ethnicity, some couples may also be offered sickle cell, thalassemia, or Ashkenazi Jewish screening.[10,11,14] As the number of possible tests increases and the technology becomes more available, couples have started to choose screening for many other rare conditions.

If you do find out that you're a genetic carrier for a particular disorder, don't freak out! Since your baby inherits one of every gene from you and one from the father, your maternity care provider will recommend he also get that blood test done. If he's not a carrier for that condition, the worst-case scenario is your baby will be a carrier for the disorder, like you (so if you're stressing out, remember you didn't even know you were a carrier until now). If the father of your baby is a carrier (or isn't able to get tested), a genetic counselor can help you understand the potential ways your baby may be affected.

Next steps

Since the types of prenatal tests are rapidly changing, check in with your maternity care provider or genetic counselor to receive an updated list of what's available to you. Some of them depend on how far along your pregnancy is and are therefore time sensitive, so mark your calendar to be sure you meet the deadlines (more on this in A-1). Remember, no test can identify every single problem known to humankind, and some newer or fancy tests may not be covered by your insurance.

So, let's pause for a moment. Are you feeling a tad bit overwhelmed after hearing the rundown of all your prenatal testing and screening options? That's totally normal! Check in with yourself and consider these questions:

- Would your baby's health change your plans for continuing your pregnancy?
- Would knowing ahead of time about your baby's health help you become equipped for meeting his or her special needs?

If you aren't sure what to choose and need more information than what your maternity care provider can offer, be sure to ask for a referral to a genetic counselor whose specialized knowledge may give you the tools you need to determine your route.

And then, after you've tracked down your options and chosen the one(s) you think will be the best fit for your circumstance, treat yourself to a nice nap or movie and remember—just by making an informed decision, you are being a caring mama.

f. Weight Gain Recommendations

At some point in pregnancy, it is common to have questions about weight gain. This may especially be true if this is your first pregnancy or if you didn't think much about it in a prior pregnancy and eventually found yourself 60 pounds above where you started. Since weight gain has many implications for pregnancy, your baby, and life beyond delivery, let's go over some basics here.

Firstly, rest assured, it is possible to gain a healthy amount in pregnancy and then lose it in about six months after birthing that adorableness inside of you. Although dieting is not recommended in pregnancy, careful eating and daily physical activity (see B-1) are splendid ways to achieve the desired weight gain goals. And yes, your energy should return early in the second trimester to help make this possible!

So what is a healthy weight gain in pregnancy?

There are two primary factors influencing your weight gain goals: (1) your prepregnancy weight, and (2) the number of babies you're carrying.[1]

Specifically, the *prepregnancy weight* considers your weight as it compares to your height (and no, wearing heels doesn't count). This type of weight classification, called **Body Mass Index** (**BMI**), is determined in a simple calculation: *kg/m2* (where *kg* is your weight in kilograms and *m* is your height in meters). The following chart outlines the typical goals for mamas carrying one or two babies, considering whether they began pregnancy underweight, normal, overweight, or obese as determined by their BMI.

Healthy Weight Gain in Pregnancy

>>>>>>>>>>>>>>>>>>>>>>> GOALS IN POUNDS <<<<<<<<<<<<<<<<<<<<<<<

Weight Before Pregnancy	For One Baby			For Twins
	Total	Total 1st Trimester	Weekly Average (2nd and 3rd Trimester)	Total
Underweight[a]	28-40		1	Variable
Normal[b]	25-35	1-4.5		37-54
Overweight[c]	15-25		0.5	31-50
Obese[d]	11-20			25-42

Note: These are Institute of Medicine recommendations for adults or teens (who had their very first period at least two years ago).[1] BMI: [a]less than 18.5; [b]18.5–24.9; [c]25–29.9; [d]30 or more.

Why does this weight gain matter?

Although globally, more mamas are gaining above the recommended amounts, many may not know that too much or too little weight gain is unhealthy for their babies.[2,3] By gaining too much weight, your baby can grow too big, leading to pregnancy and delivery complications, as well as potential health problems later in life.[1,4-6] By gaining too little, your baby may not get enough nutrients for growth and have a low birth weight, which can cause other health concerns.[1,4-6] So, let's set your future up for health and wellness by being proactive.

Where does all the weight go?

Before you get too nervous about your weight gain goal, remember: the weight gets distributed all over you and your baby, and includes the amniotic fluid, as well as your growing uterus, breasts, and placenta. Check out the illustration on the next page for a general breakdown of the distribution.[7]

g. Tips for Working While Pregnant

Welcome! Here you will find tips for mothers in the workforce (some might say "working mother," but let's be honest, since to be a mother *is* to be working, that's a bit redundant). Glad you're taking a moment to investigate your options for staying healthy while working and for keeping your little one safe and healthy, too. As one of the many employed women in the country, you've likely got quite a bit on your mind, so let's get straight to it, shall we?

Work accommodations

When seeking work accommodations, you're asking for reasonable and temporary work modifications so you *can* keep working.[1] It doesn't mean you're looking to go out on disability or leave, and it also doesn't mean you're trying to quit your job.[2]

To get these established with your employer, you must make your needs known. If you don't want to pee your pants or hurt your back

Where does all the weight go?

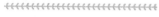

- Baby: 7.5 lbs
- Amniotic fluid: 2 lbs
- Blood volume/fluids: 7 lbs
- Fat/protein/nutrients: 8 lbs
- Uterus: 2 lbs
- Breasts: 2 lbs
- Placenta: 1.5 lbs

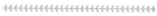

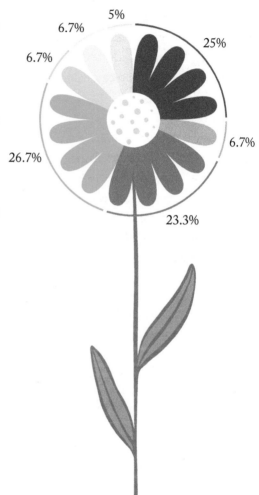

FUN FACT

The baby, placenta, and amniotic fluid account for about 35% of your total weight gain.[1]

from heavy lifting, then don't suffer in silence. Speak with your boss, and ask your maternity care provider to write you a "work accommodations" letter that you can give your employer. In fact, refer your maternity care provider to www.pregnantatwork.org, a resource that provides easy tips for writing an effective letter. A good letter can make such a positive impact, while a bad one can lead to more complications. Also, don't be surprised if there's some negotiating as you and your boss come up with what works.[1]

If you're unsure what accommodations you're legally entitled to (aren't we all?), call the free, legal hotlines like Center for WorkLife Law or A Better Balance. The federal Pregnancy Discrimination Act and Americans with Disabilities Act can legally support your case, as can your individual state's laws.[1,2] Unfortunately, in some states and circumstances, your boss is not obligated to grant you work accommodations, which is why those hotlines are super handy.

> If your boss says or does something that may be discriminatory or illegal, check out Center for WorkLife Law or A Better Balance (noted in appendix C) to access free, legal help for pregnant mamas like you.

To empower you further, let's review a few more facts: For most employees, it is illegal for your boss to fire you or not promote you, and for potential employers to not hire you just because of your pregnancy.[1,2] It may also be illegal for your boss to change your job responsibilities if you're able to perform them just fine, or require you to take leave if there isn't an available accommodation; this depends on state laws, where you work, and your job circumstances.[2,3] It may also be illegal for your employer to retaliate against you because you're asking about your rights or for accommodation.

Leave

Going on leave, on the other hand, is a situation where you don't work, such as for medical or health reasons. Jobs may be protected for some women during this time (meaning you won't lose it while you're out). Leave is time limited, may be unpaid or partially paid, and carries the possibility of termination if you're not ready to return to work after it ends.[2]

If you want to keep working while you're pregnant and you can do your job, as a general rule, your employer can't force you to take leave![2,3] In fact, it's best to *not* go out on leave unless you really need to, since it could be using precious time that you would have otherwise been able to spend with your little bundle. Also, it's a good idea to check into your leave eligibility before requesting it. If leave is not an option and a woman requests it, she could end up losing her job because the request prompts the boss to worry she is unsafe to work.[1,2]

The federal **Family Medical Leave Act** (**FMLA**) provides unpaid leave for up to 12 weeks for some lucky moms and dads who qualify; this time can be used for prenatal visits, baby bonding, or recovery from childbirth.[4] The good news is the state in which you live may also have additional leave laws that could give you added protection, time, and maybe even pay. For example, some states—including California, New York, and Massachusetts—have their own paid (*yes, paid!*) family and medical leave laws.[5-7] *What a concept.* Do some research and find out what you're eligible for by asking your employer, your maternity care provider, or checking out the resources mentioned here. Find out how much job-protected leave and how much paid leave you're entitled to— they may not be the same!

For more on this topic, check out "Planning Your Maternity Leave" (week 25).

h. Baby Naming

Okay, let's face it. Most mamas won't want to call their baby "peanut" forever. If you're ready to find that special name, here are items to consider.

Everyone's approach is unique. Only a handful of people always knew they'd call their firstborn Johnna Ellie (or John Elliott, depending). If that's not you, don't stress it.

Be patient. Finding a name is typically a process. Since names can carry great meaning and even shape a child's identity, it is good to take your time with it.

Embrace the adventure. Names can evoke all sorts of feelings in us, often related to our experiences. What a great opportunity to learn about yourself, your partner, friends, and family! While discussing options, you may uncover all sorts of hidden history, such as the time Joe Rummerfunk gave your partner a black eye after orchestra practice, or how Valentina was your aunt's best friend with whom she jumped rope every day after class in the third grade.

Make a list. Seeing all your top contenders, and those added at the spark of imagination, will make you look and feel incredibly organized.

Don't get physical. Try not to smack your partner if he or she hates every single name on your list. It's not worth it, and it won't help.

Go with your gut instinct. If you *try* to love a name but it's just not working, move on. It's that simple.

Don't forget to take the nickname test. If trusted kids in middle or high school say the name rhymes with or sounds like *zit*, *dummy*, or *booger* (to name a few), think again.

Give yourself space. You can have a few favorite names and then decide once you spend time with your little one after birth. If you're desperate, you can still rely on *pebble*, *acorn*, or (of course) *baby* for a while.

Know your county laws. You may have more time to decide on a baby name than you think. And, of course, if you later decide *Spud* reminds

> While the exact process varies by state, often the first step for a name change is to contact the court for the county your baby was born in to determine the next steps. Remember, once a name has been legally changed, you'll want to update associated paperwork (like a social security card).

you too much of a vegetable, you can always begin the process to legally change it.

Remember, picking a name isn't about pleasing people. Some people will *not* like your *amazingly awesome* chosen name. Yes, this should be impossible. But don't worry, they'll get used to it eventually, because who can resist your cute baby?

Optional extras

Consider the heritage. Names can carry a meaning or tell a story, reflect cultural heritage, or even facilitate assimilation into another society. They can honor a beloved family member or carry on a cherished family name (like your maiden name).

Choose your spelling. Names can sound familiar, but then pull a fast one on society with a crazy spelling no one could ever guess (like a-i-b-h-i for *Abbey*, or a-b-c-d-e for *Absidy*). Just please spell it in a way that your kid will remember.

Embrace your inner poet. Names can even showcase your alliteration skills—like your twins, Laney and Lucas, and your dog, Lennox. Now if you go this route, be extra patient with everyone around. It may take a while for us to not call your son by your dog's name.

i. Nesting Tips

Ready to start creating your nest? Awesome! Read on for essential baby gear and tips, as well as a list of safe materials that are great for baby and for the environment.

Baby-gear checklist

Car seat. Be sure to buy this new so it's in shipshape to protect your little one. There are as many types as there are flavors of ice cream. Infant car seats are convenient because they snap out of a base and voilà!

You're carrying your baby while running errands. Many of these are also stroller compatible.

Diapers. These are usually sized by baby weight ranges. Using the right size will help keep those blowouts ("poop parties") to a minimum. Many types exist, so feel free to use one type or a combination to fit your life. Simply readjust as you go.

How many? Plan on about 70–84 diapers a week for an infant, then less as they age.

Cloth. These are reusable, great for the environment, and need to be laundered (either at home or through a diaper service). Though it adds extra work for parents, these are healthier for baby and can be resold when no longer needed.

Disposable. Besides regular versions, these include types for sensitive skin, nighttime, and biodegradable options. These are convenient but cost about $70–$80/month. Plus, they are a significant contributor to landfills and many contain harmful chemicals.[1,2]

Clothes. Think about what season your little one will be born in. In general, your baby will be thrilled lounging around in PJs and onesies all day. They dislike outfit changes, so prepare to layer when needed.

Try used clothing! It's better for the environment and the budget. Be sure zippers work and buttons/snaps are well secured.

Look for items that zip, snap, or button in the front—these are way easier to use. Think twice about clothes that are secured in the back. It's not for the faint of heart! Make diaper changes a cinch with onesies or pants that have snaps between the legs.

Plan on a few newborn-sized items (5 PJs, 3 or 4 soft pants, and 4 or 5 long- and short-sleeved bodysuits).

Think ahead. Have the three- to six-month-sized clothes ready (6–8 long- and short-sleeved bodysuits, 6–10 one-piece outfits, 4–6 stretch pants). Your little one will grow into those in a blink!

For the cold months, try pants or PJs with feet to avoid losing one of each sock and bootie. Don't forget 2 or 3 sweaters, 1 or 2 hats, and a jacket.

Special occasions. Do you need a cute outfit for newborn photos or a special holiday or event? Most likely, zero- to three-months will be the right size if within a couple of months of birth.

Feeding accessories

Burp cloths. This is one of the few items where you really can never have too many. Have at least 5 or 6. Pre-folded cotton cloth diapers work great for this (for DIY, sew cute fabric on one side).

Bottles/nipples. Many types and sizes are available. Purchase 1 or 2 regular types initially and see if your baby's a fan. At first, use a 4–5 oz bottle with a slow flow nipple (marketed as a *Level 1* or *Stage 1*). As your baby gets bigger, you may use a larger bottle with a faster flowing nipple (8 oz, *Level 2* or greater). Glass or stainless bottles minimize chemical exposures.

Formula. Since most babies won't need formula, you only need to purchase it ahead of time if you've decided to not breastfeed. Your baby's healthcare provider or your lactation consultant may recommend that you supplement breastmilk with a certain type of formula. Many types exist, each with differing ingredients and formulations. Stores often carry powder, concentrate, and ready-to-feed versions.

Breast pump. Check with your insurance to see if a double electric pump (which can pump both breasts simultaneously) is a covered benefit for you—often it is! Although it's easier to have an electric pump, a manual one can be quite convenient while on the run. Not all pumps are created equal, so ask a trusted lactation consultant for a recommendation if needed. If you are working, try a hands-free breast pump bra—use the phone or computer, or even commute while pumping for an incredible time-saver. And don't forget accessories: three or four 4 oz bottles to pump into, milk storage bags, and possibly a drying rack for pump parts.

Sleeping space. When it comes to sleeping, safety is your primary consideration. The American Academy of Pediatrics recommends room sharing (baby sleeping close to your bed but on a separate space) for at least six months, preferably a year.[3]

Safe options include an infant- or portable crib, play yard, or bassinet.[3] All you need is a fitted sheet on the bottom, two to three baby swaddles, and voilà! You're ready to rumble. Remember that bumpers, blankets, or toys in the crib are no-nos due to suffocation risk.[3]

Bed sharing can be unsafe for your baby and is not recommended by the American Academy of Pediatrics.[3]

Storage. To keep items safely stowed when not needed, use shelving, bins, and under-the-bed space to store clothes, toys, and supplies.

Changing pad and table. You'll want a waist-level space where you can secure a changing pad. This way you can make eye contact with your baby during diaper changes and save your back at the same time. Beautiful! You can even put the pad on a bed (as long as you don't leave your baby unattended) and feel free to stash the pad under a couch or dresser when done.

Stroller and baby carrier. Having a way to explore the world with your baby is a blast. It's even more fun when you have hands free to wipe the sweat off your brow or drink your coffee.

Check out the **strollers** designed to carry you through all sorts of terrain. Make sure you find one that easily folds up, fits in your trunk, and can fit on a bus and through grocery store entrances.

As for **carriers**, again, there are so many. Work to find one that your baby enjoys and doesn't hurt your back. Look for a baby carrying group near you to try on styles and to learn how to customize them to your body. Your baby will love being close to you as much as possible.

Comfy rocker. You will be holding, rocking, feeding, and soothing your baby in all sorts of positions for months. Find something you like. Your feet will thank you for an ottoman—especially during the long nights. A yoga ball can also be a great place for you to sit and bounce your crying baby.

Bath-time accessories. Your baby won't need frequent baths, but when you opt for bath time, think safety first! Wet babies are slipperier than fish, so try an infant bathtub or cushion (designed to fit in a sink or tub). Avoid bath seats since they tip over easily. Use a non-toxic baby shampoo/soap and try bath toys when your baby's old enough to sit (around six months).

Medical/personal care supplies. These include wipes (for diaper changes), hairbrush, nail clipper/file, gentle laundry detergent, thermometer (various types, including digital and rectal versions), nasal aspirator (snot sucker), infant pain reliever, and diaper rash cream.

Playtime. Your baby's first toy will be you (your voice and touch)! You may consider placing a mobile over the crib or changing station, purchasing teething toys, a play yard, and board books for the months to come.

Miscellaneous items. Baby monitor (audio, with or without video), nightlight, white noise machine, diaper pail, diaper bag.

Environmental toxins

While it's impossible to avoid all toxins, we can still try to minimize our exposure by scanning ingredient lists (and if there are none, by calling the manufacturer). Also, while we'd like to think items marked *natural* or *gentle* mean *safe*, this is *not* always the case. Do a little more investigation to find out if it's truly safe for your little one. To avoid long-term health problems, stay clear of items that contain any of the following ingredients.

Environmental Toxins	
Toxic Ingredient	**Often Found In**
Bisphenol A (BPA) and possibly other bisphenol products	Hard, clear plastic products (like bottles, sippy cups, food packaging), metal food cans[4]
Dioxins	Personal care products, foods, disposable diapers[5,6]
Formaldehyde	Pressed wood, car exhaust, personal care products (like baby bath soaps, lotion, nail polish)[7]
Flame retardants (FRs)	Furniture, mattresses, nap mats, clothes, electronics[5]
Lead	Lead-based paint and dust (often in older homes), plumbing materials, contaminated soil, painted or vinyl toys, ceramics, furniture, toy jewelry[8]
Phthalates/polyvinyl chloride (PVC) plastic	Recyclable items (with codes 3, 6, and 7), plastic bags, food packaging, toy dolls, teething toys, rubber duckies, shower curtains[9,10]
Per- and polyfluoroalkyl substances (PFAS)	Nonstick cookware, fast food/take-out wrappers[11]
Volatile organic compounds (VOC)	Certain paints and engineered products, air freshener, flooring, carpet, pressed wood, varnishes, finishes[12]

Safe items to consider

- Solid wood furniture
- Nontoxic toys made of wood, cotton, wool, and polyester[13]
- Certified organic, nontoxic baby products (like shampoo and soap)
- Stainless steel, bamboo, silicone, heat/shatterproof glass bottles and tableware
- Paint that is zero- or no-VOC
- FR-free baby mattresses and nap mats[13]
- Waterproof mattress covers made of polyethylene or wool[14]

Tips

- If you can, minimize using plastics, and if you must use them, opt for BPA- and PVC-free.
- The Environmental Working Group has a fantastic website (www.ewg.org) where you can look up toxicity ratings for many personal care products (baby items, household cleaning agents, makeup, sunscreen, etc.).

And after all this, I hope you take a moment to stand in awe of yourself. In fact, take a deep breath and blow it out. It's not easy to build a nest thoughtfully. However, if you take the time now to find the few quality and safe baby products you need, you'll know you're building a little world that nurtures all your baby's various needs.

j. Twenty Ways to Pass the Time Before Birth

Wow, you've made it to week 38! Does it feel like forever before your little one's arrival? Don't worry; before you know it, your baby will be here! In the meantime, here are some ideas for how to pass the time.

Plump up your parenting library. Not only will you feel more prepared, but you'll also have quick go-to references when needed. For example, gather resources on the ins and outs of caring for your baby, understanding baby behavior, and breastfeeding. (See my website for some ideas.)

Take a few last maternity pictures. You won't stop looking at them later.

Get ready for newborn pictures. Select a couple of outfits for your little one and yourself. You may want yours less fitted since it will take a while for your belly to return to its former self.

Take care of yourself. Rest, but keep moving, since labor and mothering are active processes that require strength.

If you are still working, it's time to wrap things up. Make sure you complete and file your maternity leave paperwork with your employer and/or state.

Find your baby a healthcare provider. Within a few days after delivery, your baby will be getting his or her first check-up with a family physician, pediatrician, nurse practitioner, or physician's assistant. A pediatrician will be a valuable resource if your baby has medical problems or is preterm.

Install the car seat. This may feel like rocket science if this is your first time or if years have passed since you installed one. Check out your local fire station or hospitals for free help.

Spend time with your partner, family, and friends. It will be a while until you have time to think about anyone other than your baby or how much you need sleep.

Splurge on cute lounging clothes. You'll be working hard once your baby arrives, so pamper yourself with a little comfort and cuteness—it will help you feel better.

Prioritize self-love. Need a haircut or highlight? Do your eyebrows need waxing? Today's the day—it will seem like a monumental task later.

Make mommyhood prettier. Buy some under-eye concealer and dry shampoo. Although you may not always care, you'll have days when you'll want to spice things up.

Stock up. Stuff your freezer full of prepared foods and stock your fridge with healthy snacks (see "Tasty Snacks and Recipes" in B-1e for more ideas). You can even make a snack drawer with foods that will nourish you. Trust me, taking the time now will save you from prowling around the house later, looking for something to devour—especially if you're breastfeeding.

Make a contact list. Who do you want to update when your baby arrives?

Identify your postpartum support. Every mama needs support, especially for the first few months. The time has come to complete your postpartum care plan (A-5a) if you haven't already.

Buy or make thank-you cards. Catch up on ones needing to be sent or have them ready to go for after delivery.

A time to remember. If you haven't already, write your baby a keepsake letter. What are your wishes for your little one's life? Also, how will you want to mark your baby's milestones or first months of life? Great options include a calendar, journal, media/technology, or weekly baby photos with stickers (or check out other ideas in "Pregnancy and Baby Keepsakes," week 21).

Make a belly cast. Why not? Use your belly for creating art!

Journal. What will you miss and never miss about pregnancy? What are you looking forward to?

Perineal massage. Don't forget to continue your perineal massage most days of the week. This is especially important if this is your first vaginal delivery. (See A-4f for details.)

Have sex. It's bound to be an experience, and who knows, it might even help you go into labor.[1-3] Of course, ignore this one if you've been advised against sex in pregnancy.

4. BIRTHING TIPS

a. Preparing for Labor

Every baby has his own birth story with its own personality, rhythm, and timeline. These stories are full of intrigue and mystery because these little people never think to share their birth plans with their mommies in advance. Though the exact day will bring surprises, there are some things we can do to prepare. In this section, you'll learn about the stages of labor, contractions, pushing, and what comes after.

Prepare with a childbirth class and labor videos. Consider it a "must" if this is your first baby, you haven't seen childbirth before, or you have a partner who hasn't. While sometimes we wing it on school exams or even work presentations, labor deserves some reverence and preparation. The more aware you both are of what normal labor is like, the more equipped you are to handle that big day and its important decisions. Ask your maternity care provider for class recommendations.

Find your cheerleader. Having the right support person during labor is key! He or she could help you have a shorter labor, avoid a Cesarean birth, need less pain medication, and make you more satisfied with labor.[1-3] Pick at least one person to be there with you. It's especially luxurious if you can find support in addition to your partner. An awesome **doula** can be a lifesaver! If this is not an option, ask a trusted friend or family member to serve you, support you, and encourage you—not just kick back and observe. Make sure this person is familiar with labor (has taken a class or has personal experience), is great at empowering you, and knows what you expect of him or her.

Okay, where's the starting line? The process of going into labor looks different for every woman. Some women start labor with contractions, while for others, it begins with their bag of water breaking. Some need artificial hormones or other methods to get labor started (known as *induction*). Most labors are long (though generally shorter than 24 hours), but there are those that could be a new Olympic sport—speed birthing. Usually, first babies give you the longest labors, with subsequent ones being a few hours shorter.[4]

What is labor like and how will you handle it? Such a common question! Check out the stages in the following paragraphs, and remember, if this is not your first baby, this birth could feel very different than your last—for the better. You may be fitter, older, wiser, stronger, or better prepared for labor and another baby. What's more, some women do say labor wasn't nearly as bad as they had anticipated!

So how do we experience contractions, and what do they feel like? Contractions are actually an undercover gift, designed to serve you and to help you meet your baby. They help soften, thin, and open your cervix, as well as move your baby down through your birth canal. The thinning of your cervix is also called *effacement* (measured from 0% to 100%), while the opening up of your cervix is called *dilation* (measured from 0 cm to 10 cm). So, welcome contractions—be accepting and relax, remembering that each one is tucked between two moments of rest.

Contractions can feel like all sorts of things: belly pain, cramps, achiness, shooting or throbbing pain, or pressing.[5] You may even feel the sensation in your back, hips, and inner thighs. They usually come and go, for hours to days, at a slower pace in the beginning (with 15–45 minutes of rest in between each contraction) and then become regular and more frequent (with around 3–5 minutes of rest in between). This longer, slower part of labor is called *early (latent) labor.*[4] If you wonder how you'll get through the sensations, remember, women have done this for centuries in huts, forests, homes, and even elevators and taxis. You have more strength in you than you realize!

Active labor is a term used to indicate your body means business— you've dilated to about six centimeters, and contractions are getting stronger, longer, and closer together.[4] The *transition phase*, from around 7 to 10 centimeters dilation, is the shortest and most intense part of labor. At this point, your contractions will come 2–3 minutes apart, lasting 60–90 seconds. My dear friend, you may feel tired and restless, may have some nausea and vomiting, and could experience a range of intense emotions, sometimes even doubt about getting through labor. When you are here, remember—you are almost to the finish line! It's hard because you're almost done! Once you make it to 10 centimeters, you've made it through the *first stage of labor* (more on the other two stages to follow).

Comforting your body during labor without medications. Of the many options available to help get you through, the best is to find a good person who can support you throughout labor. Other, non-medication options include various labor positions, massage, using a rocking chair, taking a warm bath or shower, aromatherapy, reassurance, relaxation, hypnosis, guided imagery, or even transcutaneous electrical nerve stimulation (**TENS**).[2,6,7]

Pain-relieving medications include nitrous oxide (laughing gas) administered through inhalation, narcotics administered through IV or injections, and localized pain medications injected via epidurals or spinals.[8] All medications have potential side effects to you and your baby, so talk through these with your maternity care provider. For example, although **epidurals** are the most effective form of pain

MAKING THE MOST OF INDUCTIONS

Inductions are methods to initiate uterine contractions prior to going into labor on your own. If you do end up getting induced and have always dreamed of having a "natural" labor, be encouraged. You can still have many elements of what you were hoping for, with a few minor changes. Your birth can still be beautiful, and without pain medications, if you so choose. Bring all the goodies you still planned for, like the flowers, battery-operated candles, music, massage oil, and yoga ball. Just go with it. You've got a baby to meet!

relief, they generally make your labor about two hours longer, can decrease your blood pressure, and may increase your risk of getting a fever or having a delivery with instruments (like vacuum or forceps) or through Cesarean birth.[1,4,8,9]

Pushing. Once you're fully dilated to 10 cm, you'll get the green light to push. (This stage from 10 cm to giving birth is called the *second stage of labor*.[4]) If you don't have an epidural, push when you have the urge. It pretty much feels like you're trying to poop out your baby. If you have an epidural, it might be harder to figure out when to push exactly, since the medication dulls the sensations. It typically adds about an extra 15 minutes of pushing.[9] In either case, pushing can be hard work, though some people find it feels wonderfully relieving.

First-time moms without epidurals will push off and on for a few hours (a median of about one hour), while most women without epidurals who gave birth before will push their dumplings out in about 20 minutes.[4] While you'll likely be tired at this stage, keep it up. You'll be rewarded by seeing your little wonder soon. Right as your baby's head is coming out (called *crowning*), the attending physician or midwife will probably have you give little pushes or ask you to pause to minimize tearing around your vagina. Usually, within 15–30 minutes of your baby's entrance into the world, you'll deliver your placenta (the *third stage of labor*), which may cause brief cramping.

After delivery. You did it! If, immediately after birth, your baby looks well, they'll offer to place him on your chest and give you a chance to see if he really has your chin. This is a precious time to be together— protect it! If he starts moving his little face around, looking for a lost nipple, help him find it. No worries if breastfeeding doesn't happen right away. The nurse, maternity care provider, or lactation consultant will help you figure out how this works sometime shortly after birth unless medical reasons prevent it or you've decided to formula feed.

b. Illustrated Labor Positions

Here's the scoop: There are countless awesome labor positions to try on the big day. To get you started, check out the following two pages and surf the web for many more. Wondering which is best? You'll know in the moment by what feels right.

c. Decreasing Your Risk for Cesarean Birth

By now, you're probably not surprised to hear that *how* you have your baby matters. Earlier we chatted about the pros and cons of vaginal and Cesarean births, and here you'll find some awesome tips for decreasing your chance of unnecessary Cesarean birth during labor. These are adapted from the Childbirth Connection website.[1]

Use labor support. Having continuous support during labor can make all the difference. While it can be special to have a partner or family member with you, having the expertise of a trained birth attendant (a *doula*) can be invaluable.[2,3] For a description of a doula's role, see "Preparing for Labor" in A-4a.

Know your options when your baby is not head down. Sometimes our dumplings can try to pull a fast one on us in the last month by being *breech* (butt or feet down) or *transverse* (side-lying). In many places, this would be a reason for a Cesarean birth. If you find yourself in this situation, ask to try having your baby manually turned to the head-down position with a process called **External Cephalic Version (ECV)**. It may work!

Avoid an unnecessary labor induction. Getting induced means medications or other methods are used to get your labor started. While sometimes this is necessary, other times it's not. Be sure to ask questions if it's offered to you. For some women, labor induction can make a Cesarean birth more likely, especially among first-time moms and those whose cervix is not ready (ripe) enough for labor.

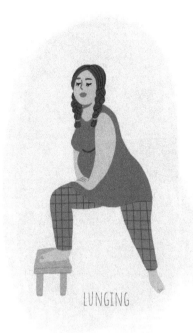

LUNGING

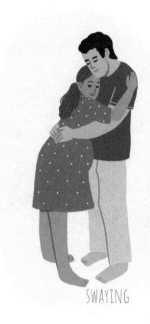

SWAYING

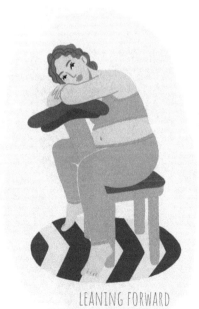

LEANING FORWARD

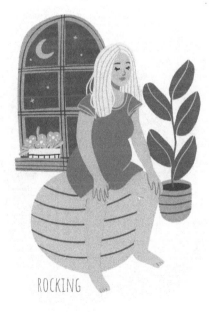

ROCKING

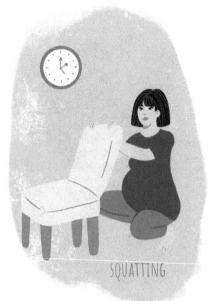

SQUATTING

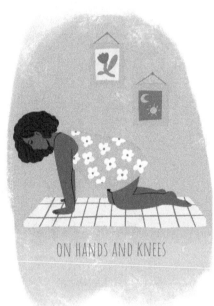

ON HANDS AND KNEES

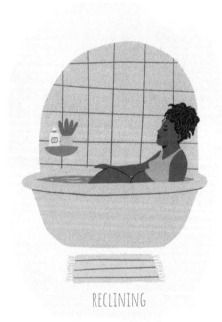

RECLINING

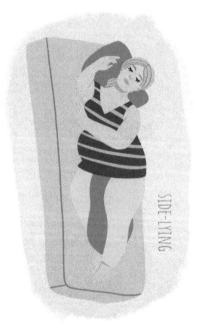

SIDE-LYING

Move during labor. Moving and staying upright during labor helps your baby more successfully shift downward into your pelvis.

Show up in active labor. It's best to show up to labor and delivery when in *active labor* instead of very early on (when you're in *latent labor*), unless advised otherwise. In active labor, your contractions are regular and strong enough to have dilated your cervix to six centimeters. Of course, if you live farther away or have fast labors, this may not be an option. As always, be in communication with the labor and delivery nurses to hear their recommendations.

Go for intermittent monitoring. Instead of always having a monitor on to track your baby's heart rate, ask for periodic monitoring instead. This is done at regular intervals according to professional guidelines, is safe for mamas without specific medical or pregnancy complications, and decreases your chance for associated Cesarean birth, or deliveries with vacuum or forceps, as compared to continuous monitoring.[4-6] You'll also be less restricted by the monitor and have more freedom to labor in positions and ways that comfort you.[4,6]

d. How to Improve Your Cesarean Birth Experience

For those of you mamas who have a Cesarean birth, here are some tips (adapted from the Childbirth Connection website) to help it go well during surgery and after.[1] Some of these are items to enhance a planned Cesarean birth experience, while others can even help in the event of an emergency Cesarean birth.

Schedule it right. If it's possible, have your Cesarean birth after 39 weeks, when your baby is older and more developed. Your baby needs this time to be ready for life outside of the womb.

Chew gum after surgery. Not only can it be refreshing, but it can also get your digestive system working faster after surgery. You'll feel so much better!

Decrease your chance of blood clots. When in the hospital bed, ask for special compression devices, which can promote blood flow in your legs. And as soon as you can, slowly get that beautiful body of yours out of bed and walk.

Make memories. Talk to your maternity care provider about your delivery hopes. If interested, find out about video and photo policies during delivery and whether the opaque drape hung between your chest and your belly can be lowered as your baby's being born.

Practice early skin-to-skin. Once your little dumpling is born, ask to have him or her put on your chest right away so you can get a whiff of your adorable newborn, as well as promote bonding and breastfeeding.

Call in the reinforcements. If breastfeeding, you may need extra support from lactation consultants. Don't be shy—that's what they're for. Also, when at home, ask for help around the house to allow you much-needed recovery time! After surgery, your recovery will include limiting lifting, and it will take at least six weeks for your skin incision and deeper tissues to heal.

e. Prepping Your Support

As we've mentioned earlier (A-4a), having the right support person(s) with you during labor can make a world of difference. To help you reap all those glorious benefits, let's get your nonprofessional support person(s) primed for the big day. Ask them to read this section carefully. You may also wish to peek at the remaining labor-related gems in A-4 if you haven't already.

To support person(s)

Explore. It's natural to be both honored to attend and nervous about the labor process. To equip yourself for the important day, use prenatal appointments or labor classes to address your lingering questions.

Also, as questions arise during labor, seek answers from your labor and delivery nurse, midwife, or attending physician.

Take care of yourself. Be sure to take 12–24 hours' worth of food, snacks, and water for yourself. You'll need the energy! For tips on what to bring to the hospital, peruse the checklist in A-4h.

Know her wishes. Prior to labor, ask mama what's important to her during labor. Listen carefully and write them down so you remember (more on this in A-4g). Although labor is full of surprises, the goal is to see if some of her dreams can be realized.

Be proactive. Prior to labor, compile labor support resources, such as labor position ideas (A-4b), things to say (more on this to follow), and comfort options (like walking, massage, warm bath or shower, aromatherapy, music, relaxation exercises, a yoga ball, and so on). Having these ideas easily accessible allows you to suggest various comfort measures quickly. Trust me, these can be easy to forget in the moment.

Don't take it personally. Remember, while in labor, mama may not always like your suggestions. That's okay. Please don't take it personally—even if she yells at you. Let it roll off and offer her something else on your list for comfort. She's working hard, and her needs will constantly change. Go with it.

Be present and encouraging. While it can be hard to see mama going through so much, stay positive, encouraging, and engaged during labor. Join her by freeing yourself from distractions like TV or electronics. She needs you!

Avoid pity. Pitying a laboring mama only disempowers her. Labor is a normal process, and she was made for this. She is strong and can do this! Remind her.

Use words of affirmation. Supportive words can keep a mama going big-time! She likely will be battling inner doubts about whether she can do this. So, use these truths liberally unless she tells you to shut up. Keep your voice calm and your tone low—it helps her relax.

- "You are strong."
- "You are doing it. Keep it up."
- "This is hard, but not too hard."
- "I believe in you."
- "Soon, you are going to meet your baby."
- "You're amazing. Look at what you're accomplishing!"
- "You are opening like a flower."
- "That contraction is gone now. Here is your chance to rest. Breathe. Relax."
- "Pain is power; pain is progress."
- "You can do it, one contraction at a time."

Advocate. When she needs help, be sure to let the nurse, midwife, or physician know. It's your job to make sure her needs are met. She won't be able to advocate for herself in labor as well as you can.

Ask for help. Most of the time, labor is not so much a sprint as a marathon. Be sure to ask for help from a doula or nurse if you feel overwhelmed, need ideas on how to comfort mama, or need a break to recharge (eat, rest, and pee). It's okay to take a breather, just make sure mama always has good support. During pushing, give yourself permission to be at mama's head, or outside of the room, and not watch the actual birth if that's your preference.

Ask for a warm blanket. After labor, mamas love warm blankets. Make sure she gets to snuggle in one shortly after the baby's debut.

Expect ups and downs. There are lots of emotions after a baby's birth! Please reassure her and keep tabs on how she's doing both mentally and physically. Her body will continue to undergo change in the weeks following delivery, so keep those affirmations coming and advocate for her needs.

Pay attention. Consider yourself her personal bouncer and be aware of her energy level. While she may enjoy seeing some visitors, having too many or too often will be exhausting. For more on mental health after childbirth, check out the postpartum section of B-4a and "Coping with Your Beautiful Mess" (week 1 postpartum).

f. Perineal Massage

Your *perineum* is the muscle and tissue between your vulva and anus. Sometimes, this area can tear and be painful for months after childbirth, which is—of course—no fun. The good news is perineal "massage" reduces your chance of postpartum pain, tearing, and even the likelihood of needing an *episiotomy* (a surgical cut in the perineum to make more room for the baby).[1] Although it's a bit unclear how helpful it is if you've already had a vaginal delivery, it's very effective if it will be your first, and there's certainly no harm in doing it even if this will not be your first vaginal delivery. In either case, strive for 5–10 minutes a day, for a few days a week, from 35 weeks on.

For the massage

With clean hands, start by putting some vaginal lubricant or vegetable oil on your (or your partner's) thumb or finger.

Lie down and, with your legs apart, insert the finger into the vaginal opening about an inch. This may cause some discomfort.

Next, thinking of your vaginal opening (*introitus*) like a clock with the 12 pointed toward the sky, press and slide the finger from 3:00 to 9:00, back and forth. The pressure will be similar to the burning during pushing.

Try to practice relaxation during discomfort. Initially, you may only tolerate a minute, but over time, it will get easier. Although it's tempting to skip out on this when you're tired and not in the mood—remember all the awesome benefits you can get if you invest the time.

g. Birth Plan (Wish List)

Most of us plan birthday parties, trips, and weddings, so it makes sense to plan another important event like childbirth, right? Although everyone's childbirth experience is full of surprises, there is wisdom in collecting your thoughts about your preferences beforehand.

A birth plan is often a one- to two-page written checklist, allowing you to clearly articulate your wishes for labor, birthing, and the moments after birth. Yes, mama, it's tempting to think of it as an order form, but unfortunately, filling one out isn't a guarantee all will go according to plan. Rather, think of it as a wish list that allows your support person and staff to be aware of your care preferences. As much as possible, they will work to honor your wishes and integrate them into your care. Of course, you can change your mind about various preferences—even when you're in the thick of it.

To get started, ask your maternity care provider for a birth plan form, or find a template online. Be sure to review it with your support person, share it with your maternity care provider at a prenatal appointment, and toss a copy into your hospital bag (so you can share it with your labor and delivery nurses). To get the creative juices flowing, here are common questions to consider.

Birth plan questions

General
- Who do you want with you during labor?
- Do you want to limit the number of healthcare providers in your room? If the hospital is a teaching facility, are you comfortable with nursing and medical students in your room?
- Are there specific cultural or religious considerations you want the staff to know about?
- Do you have any specific traditions you'd like to observe after your baby's born?
- Would you like the lights dimmed?

Labor

- Do you want to move around during labor? What positions do you want to labor in?
- What sort of comfort measures do you want to try? (See A-4a for some options.)
- Do you want to be offered pain medications if you're uncomfortable? If so, what kind? Do you want to have an epidural, and if so, would you like it as soon as possible?
- Do you prefer continuous or intermittent fetal monitoring?
- Can the nurse place a saline lock (i.e., a capped, saline-filled IV catheter) in your arm vein for in case you need IV medications or fluids?

Pushing

- Would you like your support person in the delivery room with you? If so, where do you want him/her to stand when the baby's head appears in the vaginal opening (*crowning*)?
- Would you like a mirror during delivery to watch your baby's birth?
- Do you want to reach down to feel your baby's head as he or she's crowning?

Immediately after birth and where you deliver

- Do you want delayed cord clamping?
- Who do you want to cut the cord?
- Do you want to hold your baby uninterrupted, skin-to-skin, for the first hour after birth?
- How do you plan to feed your baby? Would you like a visit with a lactation consultant?
- Do you want your baby to be with you all the time?
- If your baby needs to be taken for a medical intervention, who would you like to accompany your baby, if possible?
- Would you like staff to talk with you before giving your baby any formula, fluids, or a pacifier?
- Prior to any procedure or administering any recommended medications to your baby, would you like staff to explain the rationale, pros, and cons?

- If having a boy, do you want your son circumcised?
- Do you plan to have your baby's cord blood banked or donated?

DELAYED CORD CLAMPING, PLEASE!

Waiting a bit on the umbilical cord's clamping allows your baby to naturally get more blood on board! Recommended wait times vary: the American College of Obstetricians and Gynecologists suggests at least 30–60 seconds after birth, while the American College of Nurse-Midwives recommends at least 3–5 minutes for term infants.[1-3]

In just a few minutes, your baby gets an extra 80–100 ml of blood, which means extra iron, hemoglobin, and immune and stem cells to support his health and development for months to come.[1] The list of benefits for preterm babies is even longer![1,2]

h. Hospital Bag Checklist

There's so much to think about when it comes to packing your hospital bag. Consider the following checklist to help you get organized and ready for your big day!

For Mama

Basics
- Directions to the hospital or birthing center
- Wallet with ID and insurance card
- Birth plan (if you have one)

Memory-making
- Phone with charger
- Camera
- Video camera

Pampering
- Robe
- Slippers
- Nonskid socks

Clothes
- Baggy, loose-waisted pants or skirt
- 2 or 3 shirts with easy access to front (for skin-to-skin and/or breastfeeding). Try nursing tanks or shirts, or others with a front zipper or buttons.
- Second-rate panties (since you'll bleed after delivery)

Nourishment for early labor and after
- Salty options: tortilla chips, crackers
- Fruit: pineapple, apple, orange
- Calories: granola bar, dark chocolate/sea salt almonds, nuts
- Liquids: smoothies or juice, and water

Refreshment
- Hairbrush
- Toothbrush
- Soap
- Lotion
- Razor
- Makeup
- Jewelry

Nipple love for breastfeeding
- Nursing bra or tank
- Nursing pads
- Medical-grade lanolin (unless you are allergic to wool)
- Nipple shield if you have flat or inverted nipples

Labor support
- Birthing ball or nonskid yoga ball
- Music
- Aromatherapy

- Massage oil
- Pictures of labor positions
- Encouraging quotes/verses/pictures

Sharing the big news!
- List of people to contact after birth (e.g., email, phone, etc.)

For support person (and family)

Change of clothes
- Make sure they're comfy: appropriate for helping the laboring mama and then relaxing afterward

Swimsuit
- Great if you help the laboring mama with a shower or bath

Toiletries
- Toothbrush
- Toothpaste
- Razor
- Comb/brush
- Deodorant
- Shampoo
- Conditioner

Nourishment
- Snacks easy to grab during labor
- Water bottle(s)

Essentials/accessories
- Wallet
- ID
- Phone with charger
- Camera

For baby

- Car seat
- Diaper bag
- Clothes
  - ○ Onesies (including a newborn and 0–3 sized)
  - ○ Sleeper/PJs
  - ○ Hat
  - ○ Jacket/snowsuit (if cold)
- Newborn-sized diapers (3 or 4)
- Diaper wipes, diaper rash cream
- Burp cloths (1 or 2)

In general, keep one or two changes of clothes with you in case of blowout poops and spit-ups.

Notes

5. POSTPARTUM TIPS

a. Postpartum Care Plan

Let's prepare for your postpartum adventure! Join me as we consider various aspects of postpartum life, such as rest, meals, mental health, child care, baby wellness, and feeding support.

These tips are adapted from DONA International's "Postpartum Plan for the ___ Family" and Postpartum Support Virginia's "The Realistic Postpartum Plan for the ___ Family."[1,2] The mental health notes are based on Dr. Bennett's "Surveying the Elements of a Postpartum Plan."[3]

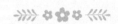

By the way, there are full-page PDF downloads of this content (with room to write) available at my author website. Also, feel free to work on this in sections and involve your partner or loved ones.

Getting rest

This is the secret to enjoying and finding strength for the early newborn weeks! Although it's not always possible, aim for at least five hours of uninterrupted nighttime sleep to help you function and promote your mental wellness. Useful strategies include finding nighttime help, splitting up the nighttime duties, going to bed when your little one does, and (of course) napping.

So, who can help watch your baby while you rest? Think about your community, including family, friends, neighbors, babysitters, coworkers, gym buddies, doulas, and your faith community.

THE REST SQUAD

- Write down each person's name, contact info, and availability.
- Can they "move in" if needed?

WAYS TO GET REST WHILE OFF BABY DUTY

- During part of the night, ____ feeds the baby (either breastmilk or formula) with a bottle. (To maintain milk supply, mama can still pump every two to three hours.)
- Sleep with earplugs or a sound machine
- For part of the night, at least, sleep in a room separate from the resident night owl
- Hire a babysitter, nanny, or postpartum doula to give respite during the day or night
- Other ideas: _____

Getting fed

Make life easier by giving your body the fuel it needs. This is especially important for the first two months when it seems you're climbing Machu Picchu. Stock up on freezer meals, fill up the pantry with nonperishables, and find grocery stores and restaurants that deliver.

Think about who can help prepare freezer meals before and after your little one arrives. A good way to spread out the home-cooked or ordered meals is to create a Mealtrain.com sign-up. Be sure to let people know if you have meal preferences or dietary restrictions.

Try to limit processed foods—you won't get the same health and energy benefits as with real foods. Drink plenty of water, while limiting sodas, juices, and energy drinks.

THE PLAN FOR EATING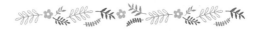

The goal is to have food prepared and/or delivered for the first ____ weeks postpartum. To help prepare, list each of the following:

- Meals that will be prepared and frozen *before the big day*
- People who can bring nutritious meals *postpartum*

- Restaurants with tasty/nutritious menus *(Note delivery/take-out options)*
- Grocery stores that deliver

Caring for your mental health

Mamas and partners *both* need time to care for their mental wellness. Remember, the postpartum period is a time when parents are more vulnerable to perinatal mood and anxiety disorders (PMADs). If you're struggling with mental health problems or have encountered such problems postpartum, it's wise to be plugged in with good mental health care.

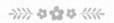

To more fully enjoy these special yet demanding days, aim for at least a smidgen of time for daily self-care. Keep tabs on how you're doing, and get timely, professional help when needed.

Since each day is a new day, your mental health needs may vary from one to the next. Check in with yourself and communicate your daily needs to your partner/support people. For quick "check-ins" throughout the day, consider using a mental wellness scale of 1 to 10 (1 = doing poorly, 10 = feeling optimal). If you're not even sure what you need, opt for going outside, taking a shower, sleeping, eating a nutritious snack, connecting with a friend, reading, or watching TV.

THE MENTAL WELLNESS PLAN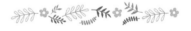

List each of the following:

- Activities or routines that boost my mental wellness
- Warning signs that indicate I'm not doing well *(Share this with your trusted support people.)*
- Knowledgeable professionals who support my mental health *(Name and contact info)*
- Additional mental wellness support organizations/groups *(Online and in person)*

IN CASE OF EMERGENCY

Dial 911, go to the nearest emergency room,
or dial 988, the Suicide & Crisis Lifeline.

FILL IN THE BLANKS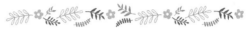

Postpartum, I plan to proactively check in about my mental health with my maternity care or mental health provider at ___ weeks after delivery. *(Discuss this with your provider.)*

If I'm struggling with my mental health, the first person I (or my main support person) will contact is: _____.

LET'S REFLECT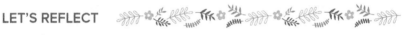

- What are your concerns, fears, and dreams for the postpartum period?
- If you've struggled with postpartum mental health problems before, what helped and what didn't?
- If in a relationship: What activities and "breathers" help us connect and strengthen our relationship? *(Consider these questions separately, chat about your answers together, and star the ones you'd like to prioritize.)*

Finding community

Having help with your baby offers you a break and a chance to connect with others while also expanding your little one's horizons. While parenting/baby groups can begin anytime postpartum, some fun baby classes (like swimming) can start as early as six months.

In terms of child care, the hardest aspect is finding people you trust. Think about close friends and family members and consider asking trusted people for names of babysitters or daycares they like. Other options include asking a stay-at-home mama for help (or swap), finding a nanny, or getting recommendations from mom/baby group leaders, your faith community's nursery coordinators, local colleges, or online caregiving companies (like Care.com).

PERINATAL MENTAL HEALTH RESOURCES

- Postpartum Support International: Postpartum.net
- Postpartum Men: Fatheringtogether.org, Bootcampfornewdads.org
- Postpartum Progress: Postpartumprogress.com

THE SUPPORTIVE VILLAGE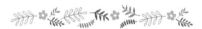

List the following groups:

- People who can provide child care (Contact info, availability, hourly wage)
- People to call when in a child-care bind
- Daycare options (Including in-home, child-care centers, Headstart, etc.)
- In-person or virtual parent/baby groups
- Friends, family, neighbors, and coworkers who have young babies

Wellness for baby

Once your baby's born, you'll have plenty of questions about your newborn's health and well-being. This is a great time to ask your maternity care provider about the process of finding a healthcare provider for your baby. Do the research to learn who might be a good fit. Remember, you can always switch later if needed.

For more on finding a good caregiver, see A-5e.

Breastfeeding and bottle feeding take practice. While it may end up being one of your favorite bonding moments with your baby, initially, there's a steep learning curve. Having knowledgeable, up-to-date support is a lifesaver. Consider contacting lactation consultants (even if formula feeding!), postpartum doulas, and healthcare providers, and be sure to ask for local and online resource recommendations.

WELLNESS AND FEEDING RESOURCES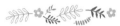

List each of the following:

- Healthcare provider options for baby (Note how to get help after office hours.)
- Local resources, both personal and professional, to help me feed my baby (Think lactation consultants, postpartum doulas, healthcare providers, nonprofits, etc.)
- Supportive people I can call for up-to-date info and recommendations for feeding

---

LACTATION AND DOULA RESOURCES

Lactation Support

- International Lactation Consultant Association: Ilca.org
- The Fed Is Best Foundation: Fedisbest.org
- United States Lactation Consultant Association (USLCA): Uslca.org
- WIC breastfeeding support: Wicbreastfeeding.fns.usda.gov

Postpartum Doulas

- DONA International: Dona.org
- Childbirth and Postpartum Professional Association: Cappa.net

---

b. Birth Control Options

Welcome, glad you're here! Picking a good birth control method helps you space your pregnancies and gives your body a much-needed breather from growing humans. As such, it can profoundly impact your quality of life and future pregnancies. This section will offer a potpourri of practical information to help you get started.

Remember, whichever method you choose is entirely up to you—and choosing a nonpermanent method means you can switch to a different option anytime. Ready to get started?

See the bigger picture. Birth control methods are not all created equal. In fact, they can be grouped into three categories according to effectiveness. A graphic at the end of this section highlights the options available, ranking them according to effectiveness with typical use. Many methods available today are more convenient and effective than the plain old little pill and can have additional perks you may simply love.

Discover the extra benefits. When deciding, explore what you are looking for in a method.[*]

- Want something super effective and convenient?
- Looking for something nonhormonal?
- Do you want to have monthly periods, lighter periods, or none at all?
- Do you need help avoiding premenstrual symptoms (PMS) or reducing acne, ovarian cysts, or risk for ovarian cancer?
- Do you want to prevent STIs?

A good maternity care provider should be able to help you address your questions and concerns, go over pros and cons, and let you know if there are any methods that are not recommended based on your medical history.

---

[*] Christine Dehlendorf, personal communication, February 15, 2019

Note the effectiveness—either for temporary or permanent methods.

For **temporary**, or *nonpermanent* methods, the top-of-the-line options are the T-shaped intrauterine devices (IUDs) and the match-sized implant that goes under the skin of your arm. Yes, they can last for years, be removed anytime, and are pros at helping you space pregnancies.[1-3] Other nonpermanent options are less effective, though of course they can work well, and using some method is always better than none.

All **permanent options**—a variety of surgical procedures—fall into this over 99% effective category.[1] This option is for those who are certain they're done having children, since these methods are meant to be permanent; while some could possibly be reversed, there is no guarantee the reversion would be successful. If a permanent method interests you, talk with your maternity care provider about your options, which may include tubal ligation, salpingectomy—or even a vasectomy for him. Yes, he can still be macho without his boys wreaking havoc!

As for timing, your surgery can be done during your hospital stay, your Cesarean birth, or even later on at your discretion. Be sure to ask how early you need to sign the consent form for the procedure, and remember, as with all consent forms, even if you've signed it, you can still change your mind at the last minute.

Know your hormonal options. These include some IUDs, the implant, pills (either the combined hormonal or progestin-only), the patch, vaginal ring, and Depo-Provera shot.[1] If it contains estrogen, you'll need to wait to use it until your risk for blood clots returns to baseline (at least three weeks after delivery, but sometimes longer depending on your medical history).[4]

Although hormonal methods don't always affect women's moods, some women find improvements while others notice depressive symptoms, irritability, anxiety, or mood swings.[5-9] Unfortunately, since it's hard to predict how you'll feel on a certain method, it's often trial and error. You may feel better on certain types of progestin hormones.

Know your nonhormonal options. These include the copper IUD and the temporary option called lactational amenorrhea, which we'll cover in a moment.[1] Condoms and diaphragms are less effective options but also hormone-free.[1] Remember, condoms only work if you use them every time.

Tracking only your periods with an application or calendar (the *rhythm method*) may help you stay in tune with your body, but it's *not* a very reliable form of birth control on its own. On the other hand, some of you science-minded women (who have regular periods and are in monogamous relationships) may like the **Fertility Awareness Method (FAM)**. The most effective type (the *Symptothermal Method*) is a combined method that can be over 99% effective with perfect use and 98% with typical use.[10] This method involves keeping tabs on your cervical mucus and cervical position, as well as your basal body temperature.[1,10] It requires diligently charting and assessing your body *daily*, and for it to be effective, you must learn the details and nuances of this method before use.

Know your invisible options (the ones you can keep private). These include the IUDs and the Depo-Provera shot. The implant is something that goes under the skin of your arm, but it can be felt through your skin, if pressure is applied right to that area.

Remember birth control, even if breastfeeding. Birth control methods, including estrogen-containing ones, are considered safe during breastfeeding.[1,4,11,12,†] However, some women still prefer to use nonhormonal methods so their baby is only exposed to their natural hormones.

Know how lactational amenorrhea (LAM) works. This is a fantastic *temporary* birth control for those of you planning to exclusively

---

† Michael Policar, MD, personal communication, February 26, 2019

breastfeed.[13] It's 98% effective, but here's the catch—*three* things must always be true for this to work as birth control: (1) your baby must be six months old or younger, (2) you must be *only* breastfeeding your baby (not supplementing with formula), and (3) you must *not* have had a period (any bleeding for two days or longer).[13] On the day when one of these is no longer true, this option ceases to be as effective! Be proactive and have another birth control method lined up.

Consider your mental health. If you are one of the many ladies struggling with mental health conditions like depression, anxiety, or bipolar, it's especially important to pick an effective and convenient method of birth control. If you're on psychiatric medication, consult your maternity care and mental health providers to ensure the birth control is compatible with your medication and that neither interferes with the effectiveness of the other.[4,7,9]

Newer antidepressants, like sertraline (ZOLOFT), fluoxetine (Prozac) or citalopram (Celexa), for example, will not interfere with birth control effectiveness, but certain anti-seizure medications like lamotrigine or topiramate may.[4,7] Be cautious with using the Depo-Provera shot because it's designed to stay in your body for months—which means it lasts that long, even if you don't love it. All other methods can be easily stopped or removed, if needed.

Use emergency contraception when needed. If you find yourself having had unprotected sex, no need to just cross your fingers. Remember emergency contraception—like Plan B (levonorgestrel), Ella (ulipristal acetate), or especially the copper Paragard IUD—can greatly reduce your chance of getting pregnant.

For best results, use one as soon as possible, though they can be effective up to 120 hours (5 days) later.[1,14] Ask your healthcare provider or local pharmacist to learn more. Plan B, available since 2009, has been over the counter since 2013.[15]

BIRTH CONTROL OPTIONS [1, 14, 16-20]

		OPTION	EFFECTIVENESS & TYPE	
TOP OF THE LINE If birth control were a pick-up line: *"I just lost my phone number. Is it okay to have yours instead?"*		Implant (Nexplanon)	1 ■	
		Intrauterine Device (IUD)	<1	▲ (copper) ■
		Sterilization	<1 ▲ ♀ ♂	
		Lactational Amenorrhea Method (LAM)	<2 ▲	
PRETTY DARN GOOD If birth control were a pick-up line: *"Do you believe in love at first sight, or should I walk by again?"*		Shot (Depo-Provera)	4 ■	
		Pill	7 ● ■	
		Patch (Xulane and Twirla)	7 ●	
		Ring (NuvaRing and Annovera)	7 ●	
CERTAINLY BETTER THAN NOTHING! If birth control were a pick-up line: *"If you were a fruit, you'd be a fine apple."*		Condom	13 ▲ ♂ 21 ▲ ♀ Internal	
		Diaphragm	17 ▲	
		Sponge	17 ▲	
		Withdrawal	20 ▲	
		Spermicide	21 ▲	
		Fertility Awareness Method	2-23 ▲	

● Combined hormonal ★   ■ Progestin only   ▲ Nonhormonal

LASTS⁺	NOTES
≤3 yrs	Placed in arm. Lasts 5 years.‡
≤10 yrs ≤3-8 yrs Varies by IUD	Placed in uterus ▲ Paragard lasts 12 years ‡ ■ Mirena and Liletta last 8 years; + Klylena, 5; and Skyla, 3‡
Forever	♀ Many methods exist ♂ Vasectomy, effective after 3 months
≤6 mos postpartum	*Temporary.* Must meet criteria to work well (see prior content)
13 wks	Two types, one given in clinic, one self-administered at home. Lasts up to 15 weeks. ‡
28 d cycle	Take daily ■ Doesn't have sugar pills. If >3 hours late, use backup method for 2 days.
28 d cycle	Apply weekly
28 d cycle	Placed in vagina A new NuvaRing is inserted monthly. Annovera is reusable for 13 cycles.
Single use	Use each time with sex
≤24 hrs	Use each time with sex. May (re)start use 6 weeks postpartum. Needs (re)fitting to ensure proper size. Effectiveness is based on use with spermicidal cream or jelly.
≤24 hrs	Use each time with sex
N/A	May (re)start use 6 weeks postpartum
Single use	
N/A	Track daily. The Symptothermal Method is most effective; others are less.

Effectiveness:
% of women with unintended pregnancy during the first year of "typical" (real world) use.

Without birth control, 85 out of 100 sexually active women will get pregnant in one year.

Be proactive: use condoms to protect yourself against STIs.

Remember emergency contraception!

★ Contains estrogen *and* progestin hormones

+ FDA-approved duration

‡ Research-based duration

c. Bonding with Baby

There are many wonderful ways to bond with your special little one. Below you'll find a list of ideas for building your loving relationship. Keep your eyes peeled—even in a few short weeks, your connection may deepen and your baby will become much more interactive!

Feed. Regardless of whether this involves breastmilk, formula, or both, use this time to snuggle, stroke her soft skin, sing, and look at this amazing baby YOU made! Don't let electronics distract you from this precious time. These moments are fleeting.

Hold. Using a baby carrier magically allows you to have arms free. Now you can eat, drink some water, or go on walks. There are so many baby carriers—no need to use one that hurts your back or shoulders. In fact, if you can, alternate between different ones so you don't over-stress one area of your body.

Make eye contact. Don't be surprised if you feel the sudden urge to make funny faces or odd sounds. Go with it and have fun.

Use your voice. Talk and sing to your baby. Yes, *already*. This is how they learn language. Find some soothing music. Soon you'll even be able to read a book to your little one.

Enjoy skin-to-skin. Put your unclothed babe on your bare chest. Leaving the diaper is not a bad idea, and if needed, drape a blanket over his back. This is super comforting for both you and your baby and is a great activity for both parents. Your body heat does a fabulous job regulating both his temperature and blood sugar.

Have bath time. Give your baby a bath (no, not a shower at this young age). To make sure the water temperature is just right, run it along the inside of your wrist. It should be comfortably warm. In a few months, bath toys can be a blast. Remember, keep the water level low, and never leave your baby unattended, even if only for a second.

Try infant massage. Parents around the world have been using this beautiful practice for centuries. To get started, find a comfortable, warm space, set the tone by asking if your baby is ready for a massage, and then gently rub and stroke your baby while making gentle eye contact.[1,2] To avoid too much skin friction, use a little coconut oil or another cold-pressed, unscented fruit or veggie oil—these won't irritate the skin or cause issues if ingested.[2] Make sure your baby is not starving or too full, and if your baby's not enjoying it, try another time instead.[1,2]

Benefits of infant massage include fostering relaxation, stimulating brain development, improving immune function, and enhancing circulation.[1,2] Go ahead, look around for an infant massage class or a good book to learn more.

WHAT IS SKIN-TO-SKIN AND WHY DOES IT MATTER?

Skin-to-skin is when your naked baby lies on your bare chest, belly down. Often this is done right after birth, once your bundle of love is dried off. Your amazing body warms his, regulates his blood sugar and breathing, and soothes both of you; this special time builds your bond, and when done soon after birth, it can even kick-start breastfeeding.[3,4]

To make this a priority, go ahead and ask for early skin-to-skin and delay the first bath until 12 hours later to get more time to snuggle![3,4] Consider enjoying skin-to-skin often in your baby's early months and encouraging your partner or loved one to bond with your baby in this way.

d. Feeding Your Milk Monster

Feeding your little one is definitely a process, as well as a unique opportunity for you to slow down and live in the moment. To help you prepare, let's address what to expect along with some survival tips. Of course, if your baby is *preterm* (born before 37 weeks), the methods of nourishing your little one will change based on her unique needs. The NICU and pediatricians will help guide you in this process. Remember, full-term babies only get breastmilk or formula and no other liquids or foods until about six months.[1]

The early days. In the first 24 hours, you'll notice that your baby will be pretty mellow and sleepy. This is your chance to recuperate, take a deep breath, and stand in awe of this precious wonder you created! Your baby will feed eight or more times, off and on, in that first 24 hours since her tummy is only the size of a marble. By the second day, she will be more alert and ready to engage.

Timing feedings. Generally, plan on breastfeeding or giving your baby formula about every two to three hours around the clock *and* whenever she seems hungry (more on this to come). Yes, you'll be feeding your baby on-demand. No, this doesn't mean your baby will learn unhealthy eating habits. A few days after birth and each month, all babies have well-child checks with their healthcare provider. These appointments will help you know if feedings need to be adjusted and eventually, when you can stop waking your baby for night feeds.

> ### BREASTMILK STORAGE AND PREPARATION
>
> Check out "Proper Storage and Preparation of Breast Milk" on CDC.gov for guidelines.

Formula amount. If you're exclusively formula feeding your baby, typically in the first few days of life, you'll offer her 1–2 oz of formula every two to three hours.[2] You'll notice over the coming weeks to months, she may stretch feeds out to every three to four hours.[2] Usually at 12 months of age, you can start transitioning to cow's milk or unsweetened soy milk.[2]

Cluster feedings. In the first few months of life, your milk monster will likely have growth spurts. These occur at somewhat predictable times: around seven to ten days old; three and six weeks old; and three, six, and nine months old. You may notice your baby will want to feed constantly (*cluster feed*) for a few hours a day, sometimes soon after you just finished feeding her! Yes, go ahead and feed her once again, even though it's déjà vu. You may also notice cluster feedings if your baby was born early term or smaller for her age, or if she doesn't feel well.

Breastfeeding all the time is exhausting, but these growth spurts will pass within a few days, and frequent feedings will ramp up your milk supply. It's important to remember that cluster feeds don't mean you're not making enough milk. Let her feed as much as she wants, and don't worry, there's usually some milk left in your breast for her to enjoy.

Signs of hunger and fullness. You'll quickly become a pro at determining if your baby's hungry. Crying is the latest hunger sign and means "Pay attention to me now, I'm starving!" Have grace for yourself when this happens, and next time try to catch those earlier signs before her meltdown. Of course, crying can be for other reasons, too, so keep tabs on when she last fed and do some investigative work, as needed. Your baby may be full if she closes her mouth, turns her head away from your breast or bottle, and relaxes her hands.[3]

Counting wet and poopy diapers. This is generally a good way to estimate if your baby's getting enough milk.[4] It's not as precise as the weight checks your baby's healthcare provider or your lactation consultant will use, but it generally suf-fices. If you're breastfeeding, it's normal for your baby's poops (which are darkly colored when she is newborn) to turn to a transitional green color before eventually becoming mustard yellow and seedy.

> ## SIGNS OF HUNGER[3,11]
> - Rooting (turning her head as if trying to latch)
> - Sucking her hands
> - Clenching her hands
> - Moving her mouth

If you're new at this, try using newborn diapers, which change color when your baby pees. Check in with your baby's healthcare provider if your baby's not meeting the diaper counts highlighted here, since it could be a sign of dehydration.

Feeding positions. By now, you've probably seen all sorts of fancy positions for **breastfeeding**. It's a great idea to try out different options and see which ones work. Breastfeeding prop pillows can be a huge blessing by helping you stabilize your baby in a good position. While positions can aid the process, the most important goal is for you to learn how to have your baby *latch* correctly. This means her mouth attaches properly to your breast, *around* (and not *on*) your nipple.

If you're **bottle feeding**, cradle your baby in the crook of your arms and have her sit upright (not flat on her back like in the pretty commercials). This helps her drink slower, which prevents her from guzzling down too much, too quickly. Remember to pay attention to the speed at which your baby is drinking and avoid propping up the bottle as it can lead to many problems including choking and even ear infections.

> ## WET AND POOPY DIAPER GOALS[1]
> - **At 1-2 days old:** 1-2 wet and poopy diapers
> - **By 3-5 days old:** 3-5 wet and 3-4 poopy diapers
> - **By 3-7 days old:** 4-6 wet and 3-4 poopy diapers

Patience. It may seem like an eternity for your newborn to get full during breastfeeding or bottle feeds: around 20–40 minutes! What a love—she's trying to figure out this whole suck, swallow, breathe deal. Also, she can be a perfect little sleep monster, falling asleep *while* eating. Don't worry, she will get more efficient over time.

Save the day with burping. Don't forget the 10–15 minutes of burping during and after feeds. If you're breastfeeding, get a session in before switching breasts; if bottle feeding, aim for about every 2–3 oz. To rookies, it feels like a waste of time, but veterans know it's truly a time-saver. Without burping, painful air bubbles get trapped inside her belly, and she'll be sure to let you know. Use a burp cloth to avoid getting drenched from spit-up.

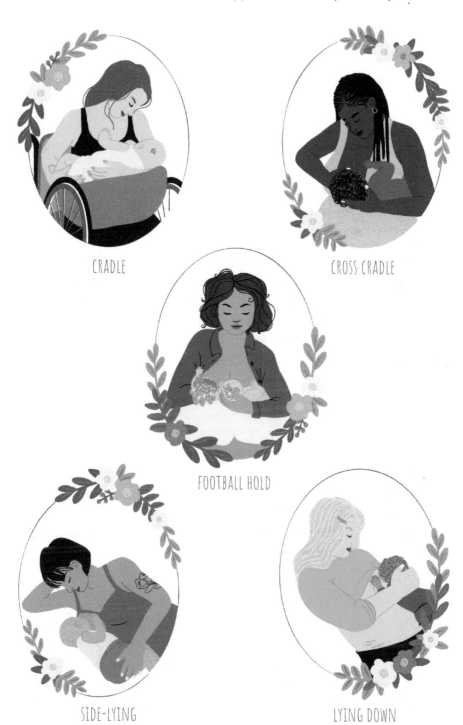

CRADLE

CROSS CRADLE

FOOTBALL HOLD

SIDE-LYING

LYING DOWN

Breastfeeding tips and support

While breastfeeding can be challenging early on, it should get easier! Be sure to thank your breasts for however much milk they are producing—every drop is a gift! (For more on the benefits for both you and your baby, see "Feeding Your Milk Monster" in week 28.)

Remember, happy breasts depend on your baby attaching to them (latching) properly. If needed, a lactation consultant can provide tips for this to help you avoid nipple or breast pain, plugged ducts, and even breast inflammation, called *mastitis*. Plus, it stimulates milk production and helps your little darling grow.

To keep your breasts content and healthy: breastfeed regularly to keep that beautiful milk flowing like a fountain; wear comfortable and varied styles of nursing bras or tanks, without underwires; limit constant pressure on your breasts from actions like nonstop baby-wearing; and strengthen your immune system with rest and nutritious foods. Although it's unclear which nipple care products are best for pain, it may help to apply expressed breastmilk or medical-grade lanolin.[5-8]

If you notice a tender lump or some redness, try applying a warm compress, massaging the area, and pointing your baby's chin toward that lump while feeding. If your symptoms don't improve after 24 hours or if you ever feel sick (with fever, chills, or body aches), call your maternity care provider or lactation consultant. These are common mastitis symptoms, which may require breastfeeding-compatible antibiotic treatment. Mama, you'll feel so much better with the right help!

Introducing the bottle to breastfed babies. This may take some time and coaxing since breastfeeding isn't just about the milk—it's about a relationship with you.[9] Ideally, someone other than you introduces the bottle *after* your little one is breastfeeding like a champ and is at least three to four weeks old.[9,10] The reason is, she will be more likely to accept the bottle from someone other than you. Plus, if you wait until she is breastfeeding well, which takes a little more time and work than navigating a nipple on a bottle, her skill will allow for continued breastfeeding, thereby protecting your milk supply.

If you're returning to work or school, a good time to try is about two weeks before showtime.[9] The good news is if your baby is older than six months, you may not even need to introduce the bottle, since she will be old enough to drink from a cup and will be starting on solid foods.[10] Ask your partner or caregiver to offer the bottle when your baby's happy, relaxed, and not famished.[10] Let your baby play with the bottle, and try again next time if she starts having a meltdown.[10] Your partner or caregiver can even try different holding positions, milk temperatures, and nipples and bottles. Sometimes, even wrapping your shirt on the bottle can help your baby enjoy your smell even if you're not there!

If after multiple attempts, your little one is still resisting the bottle, all is not lost. Check in with a lactation consultant or lactation support group for helpful ideas.

e. Child-Care Provider Tips

Finding the right child care is one of the most important decisions you'll make as a parent. After all, you're trusting another individual with your most precious possession! Although it's easy to get scared based on what you hear in the media, let me reassure you, the world is not all bad and there are still wonderful, loving, and trustworthy people out there who can be fantastic caregivers. It's just a matter of finding them and not settling until you find someone you're comfortable with. Join me as we review some important considerations as you embark on this journey.

Finding suitable child care

Know what to look for. When your baby is under the age of one, he especially needs a loving, patient, and warm caregiver who can keep him safe, as well as meet his emotional and physical needs. The caregiver also needs to be able to engage your little one in play, talking, learning, and reading books (plus all the extras if your baby has special needs). Someone who is insensitive, impatient, or who is distracted by the TV or smartphone all day is not the right person.

For older kids (toddlers and up), your caregiver needs stamina! He or she needs to be able to be loving, yet firm, organized, able to discipline (in a way in which you feel comfortable), teach your kids about healthy interactions and boundaries, and be able to answer the endless streams of "why" questions. Find someone whose worldview fits yours.

Find continuity. Continuity with a caregiver is ideal. Having a different person with your baby is hard for everyone. That being said, having one or more backup caregiver(s) is a fabulous idea in case your caregiver gets sick or dares to go on vacation.

Ask around. Get babysitter or nanny recommendations from family, friends, neighbors, coworkers, schools, parents at playgroups, and religious organizations with children's programs. Check out local in-home day cares or sitter websites. Consider nanny-sharing if you're working or going to school part-time. Background checks are a definite plus, and be sure to ask for a few references! It's incredibly helpful if they have experience taking care of children in your kids' age range.

Use an activity log. Ask your caregiver to keep a log of daily naps (or missed naps), feedings (time and amount), and general activities. Review this with them when you get home. You'll have a better sense of your baby's day, which will make for a more seamless transition back to you—and help you figure out what might be going on if your baby (or babysitter) is fussy.

Address your concerns. Listen to your gut when it comes to caregivers. Sometimes there can be a mismatch in your baby's and caregiver's personalities. Warning signs that you need to take a closer look at your caregiver include your baby being scared, upset, or crying whenever he sees the caregiver. Obviously, also give them the boot if your baby hasn't been well taken care of or kept safe.

Caregiver interview checklist

- What is his or her general philosophy to child care? (Is it congruent with yours and respectful of your wishes?) Does the caregiver also help with chores around the house?
- How much does the caregiver charge? Is there a minimum number of hours he or she requires per visit? Does his or her schedule work with yours?
- Is the caregiver experienced in taking care of young children who are your child(ren)'s age(s)?
- Can they give you a list of recent references for you to call?
  - When calling references, ask: How long have they known the caregiver? How old were their kids when taken care of by the caregiver? What did the caregiver's responsibilities involve? How were the family's general experiences with the caregiver (both kids and parents)? Do they recommend hiring the caregiver, or have any concerns?
- Is the caregiver current with infant/child CPR training (and possibly first aid)?
- Does the caregiver have a current driver's license and a good driving record?
- Is he or she up to date with relevant vaccines (like Tdap and the annual flu vaccine)?
- How did the caregiver interact with your baby/child(ren) at the interview?

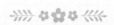

Arrange times when you, the caregiver, and your baby (and older children) can hang out together (in 1- to 2-hour chunks) to get a better sense of how that caregiver interacts. You can also ask for references and even use a nanny cam.

Caregiver training checklist

Nest orientation. Give the general layout of your living space and note, as applicable: baby-related essentials (baby clothes, laundry, baby care products, toys, first aid kit, burp cloths, bibs, pacifier, feeding supplies, stroller, baby carrier, car seat); other family members (such as pets); and mechanical sundries (like the car, dishwasher, washing machine/dryer, AC, security systems, etc.).

Activities. Do you have a general daily plan/schedule you'd like the caregiver to follow?

Feeding. Share how often baby generally gets hungry. Describe your baby's cues for being hungry or full. Give tips on burping and how to hold baby for feedings. Clarify if your caregiver should give a full or partial feeding if your baby is hungry when it's close to your return.

Preparing milk. Review how many ounces to warm/prepare at a time and the method for warming milk or preparing formula.

Milk storage. Leftover breastmilk goes in fridge for next time, and formula gets tossed.

Sleeping. Share how often your baby naps and describe his general sleep routines.

Outings/gatherings. Determine whether you are okay with (or would encourage) the caregiver to take your baby out of the house (like backyard or beyond) and share your preferences.

Diaper changes. Ask if your caregiver knows how to change boys and girls. If there are any special instructions needed for the types of diapers you use, let the caregiver know.

Review up-to-date sleeping recommendations. Put baby on his back to sleep, and note the importance of keeping crib free of blankets, pillows, and toys.

Special considerations. Does your baby have any special needs, allergies, or daily medications? If so, share these with your caregiver and even keep a note on the fridge with specifics.

Reaching you. When do you want to be contacted? If caregiver has a question or an urgent matter to discuss, what's the best way to reach you? Do you have any secondary contacts?

f. Tips for Returning to Work or School

Although there are many things we can "wing" in life, returning to work or school is not one of them! To help you prepare, we've discussed maternity leave ("Planning Your Maternity Leave," week 25), common experiences of going back ("Heading Back to Work or School," postpartum week 7), as well as tips for finding child care (A-5e). Here, we'll build on these by adding some insights into the logistics of your return. Enjoy!

General logistics

Work hours. If possible, ease slowly back into work or school! Can you work from home or have shorter or more flexible days?

Go to bed on time. Since you'll be getting up earlier in the morning (and likely during the night with your night owl), give yourself the glorious gift of more sleep.

Making your exit. Starting when your baby is around 6 months old, he may cry when you try to leave due to separation anxiety. This is normal and may reappear at 12–18 months when he starts to walk. The best thing to do is tell him you love him, and you'll be back soon (sneaking off is not a good idea). Give him a big hug and a kiss—and then leave, while your caregiver offers distractions (such as toys or a book). Try to avoid a long, dramatic goodbye. You'll be late, and it only makes it harder on both of you. Usually, babies and children stop crying soon after you're out of sight, and remember, you're actually teaching him that you're dependable.

Breastfeeding and pumping logistics

Introducing the bottle to breastfeeding babies. Check out "Feeding Your Milk Monster" in A-5d for details.

Building your breastmilk stash. Give yourself a few weeks to start building your milk stash in the freezer. Once or twice a day, pump after breastfeeding to collect whatever little you have left.[1] Don't worry, after a few days, your supply should start to increase. Be grateful for whatever your body does produce—it's so wonderful for your baby!

How much you need stored up depends on how long you'll be gone and the age of your milk monster. In general, he will drink 24–30 oz in a 24-hour period, feeding 2–4 oz at a time (60–120 ml), or about 12 oz total in nine hours.[1,2] Freeze milk in 1 and 2 oz quantities, storing it in bags or BPA-free containers. This way, your caregiver can mix and match bags based on your baby's hunger level. Always have a little extra in the freezer, and pump more on weekends, if your stash starts to run low.

Pumping while away to protect your milk supply. Though it's likely not high on your list of fun things to do, pumping is the best bet for protecting your milk supply. It can also be a great way for you to snatch 15–30 minutes of rest throughout the day. To prepare for pumping while at work or school, learn about your pumping rights by asking your supervisors or checking out the resources in appendix C.

Before the first day, be sure to talk to your work or school so they can help you find a safe and clean pumping space. You'll want to pump about every three to four hours to keep your milk supply up. (For example, pump at ten o'clock, lunchtime, and three.) Even pumping once a day is better than nothing. For you busy mamas, try a hands-free, battery-operated electric pump to help you multitask or pump while commuting.

Don't forget about your breasts. Plan your meetings around your pumping times. If you don't, your breasts *will* make their needs known by getting sore and engorged, or even leaking. This can even lead to *mastitis* (a breast inflammation and sometimes infection) or plugged ducts.

Getting your milk out. Just because your breasts are full of milk or you're in a hurry, it doesn't mean your milk will flow out like a fountain while pumping. You can turn that machine up on full crank, and you'll still barely get anything if you don't have a real letdown. While normally you'd have your cute baby to help you relax, it takes a little more effort to unwind while pumping. Try deep breathing and looking at pictures or videos of your baby. *Slow down, mama.*

Pumping supplies. Always have extra milk bags, batteries, nursing pads, and supplies in your car.

Don't get tangled up. Wear clothes that give you easy access to your breasts. Shirts with zippers and buttons are helpful, as are those specifically designed for breastfeeding. To pump in a regular dress will require you to strip everything off and pump practically naked. *Plan, mama.*

Snacks and hydration. You'll thank yourself if you packed extra snacks and water with your pump.

Something is better than nothing. If pumping feels impossible, please know breastfeeding your baby before and after work is still a wonderful option. Your body is so incredible that it will adjust its milk production to make this possible.

Notes

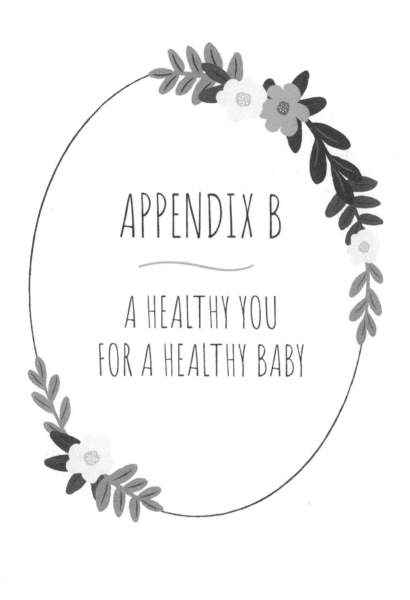

APPENDIX B

A HEALTHY YOU FOR A HEALTHY BABY

1. NUTRITION

Since *well and wisely* is the foundation for a flourishing life, the next few pages are designed to give you important and practical tips for this type of nourishment. While foods give us caloric energy to live and function, the truth is, they are not all created equal.

Revamp how you look at food. First off, rather than thinking about food as "naughty" or "nice," let's think of food as "nutrient-dense" or "nutrient-light."* In other words, is your food packed with nutrients or not? Examples of nutrient-rich foods are eggs or vegetables, and chicken or bean soups, while sodas, juices, and Twinkies fall into the nutrient-light world.[1,†]

The nutrients in question here include carbohydrates, proteins, and fats, plus vitamins (like vitamins C, D, and folic acid), minerals (like iron, calcium, and iodine), and antioxidants. Since foods can contain different combinations of these elements, eating a variety of foods daily helps you get a brilliant assortment of these compounds. This variety is key to nourishing and healing your body so that even in the face of harming factors like chronic stress, the right foods can rejuvenate and heal you on the microscopic level.

A great guideline: "Eat food. Not too much. Mostly plants."[2,3] Eat more veggies, fruits, and whole grains. Eat less meat and fewer processed foods, sodas, and juices. In doing so, you'll be more energetic and beautiful, live longer, and decrease your chance of getting diabetes, obesity, heart disease, and cancer.[4]

Consider the impact. Many of us don't realize that the food choices we make also greatly impact our environment. For example, 14.5% of our global greenhouse gas emissions come from livestock, especially beef.[5] Similarly, agricultural choices can lead to deforestation, water

---

* Veronica Benjamin, RD, personal communication, August 1, 2015
† Benjamin

problems (contamination and freshwater depletion), pollution, and even extinction of species.[4]

So, when *not* pregnant or breast-feeding, eat less meat (especially red meat) and dairy—it's better for your body and the environment. However, pregnancy is a great time to indulge in animal-based proteins since they are also rich in easily absorbable iron.

In general, fish is a great source of healthy fats (known as omega-3) and protein. Eating certain fish two to three times a week is fabulous if you can tolerate it (more on this in "Seafood Dos and Don'ts" in B-1a).

> ⁂
>
> ## "PROCESSED FOOD" RED FLAGS[2]
>
> - It's located in the middle aisles of the grocery store
> - It arrived through your car window
> - Our grandparents wouldn't recognize it
> - The ingredient list contains words a third grader can't pronounce
> - It has more than five ingredients
> - Contains "high-fructose corn syrup"

To make seafood choices that are good for the ocean and environment, check out Monterey Bay Aquarium's online consumer guide produced as part of their Seafood Watch Program.[6] The guide is customizable to your area and will help you make an informed decision on which types of seafood are safe and sustainable. And how awesome is it that by making informed decisions, you're cutting unsustainable fishing practices globally and leaving a better world for your baby's generation? You go, mama!

a. Eating for Two While Pregnant

Yes, eating nutritiously in pregnancy is an underappreciated art. To seek good nutrition while eating, meal planning, and prepping is to become a sort of culinary artist. Perhaps you've never thought too much about eating carefully or healthfully, but what a great opportunity to start doing that now—for both your sake and the wellness of your baby and family. Let your pregnancy launch you into becoming a better version of yourself!

First, toss the dieting. Before we jump into the fun part of mindful eating tips for pregnancy, let's review that pregnancy is *not* the time to diet or try to lose weight. While some diets may be okay for a time before pregnancy, weight loss drinks, supplements, and fad diets (like ketogenic, Paleo, Atkins, and hCG) are not recommended in pregnancy. Of course, this does not refer to customized diets recommended by ***registered dietitians*** (***RDs***)—diets that are specifically designed to control medical conditions, such as diabetes or celiac disease.

While pregnancy is not the time to be dieting, don't freak out if eating more nutritiously naturally leads to a little unintentional weight loss. That's okay. Likewise, if there is a month where you have a much larger than recommended weight jump, it's okay to try to slow your weight gain through more nutritious eating and increased physical activity. The main importance is that you don't take this time to try to lose weight. As always, moderation is the key. Keeping this focus means proactively preparing for a healthy weight postpartum.

Vegetarians and vegans. If you're a die-hard fan, it's okay to continue in pregnancy, but it will be extra important to eat a rich assortment of foods throughout your day. With these dietary restrictions, it's easier to be deficient in protein and important vitamins and minerals (like iron, vitamin B_{12}, zinc, and calcium) if you're not careful.[1,2] Good protein sources include beans, grains, nuts, nut butters, seeds, soy, tofu, green leafy veggies, and milk and egg products (depending on your restrictions).[1,‡] (See B-1f for more great nutrient sources.) Ask your maternity care provider or RD if you need any additional supplements beyond your daily prenatal vitamin.

---

‡ Veronica Benjamin, RD, personal communication, August 1, 2015

Mindful eating in pregnancy

Now for the fun part: tips and tricks! Many of these apply no matter what stage of life you're in. However, if you're still battling nausea and vomiting, have grace for yourself and come back to this later when you're feeling better.

Frequency

Eat regularly.[§] Try three meals and two small snacks in between, even if your appetite took a hike. Early in pregnancy, this can help you battle your nausea, and later it'll help you navigate your stomach filling quicker. Also, eating small, frequent meals ensures your baby is fed all day long (yay!) and will help you feel better (double yay!). It will also stabilize your blood sugar so you're less likely to be irritable as a grizzly bear, and less inclined toward dizziness and headaches.

Remember breakfast.[¶] It may be easy to forget this poor, underappreciated meal, but it is, in fact, the most important meal of the day— even if you feel like you're sleepwalking through it. Breakfast kickstarts your day with a blast of energy and helps you avoid overeating, a common mistake if your first meal is delayed too long. If you don't like "breakfast" foods, such as cereal or oatmeal, try less traditional foods, like a burrito or dinner leftovers.

Content

Pick the right foods: go for color .[3,**] Eat a rainbow at every meal (no, not Skittles, we're still talking about nutrient-rich food here). The more naturally colorful foods you have on your plate, the better! It's an easy way to tell that you're getting a variety of vitamins and minerals.

Prepare it well.[4] Explore the vast array of foods safe in pregnancy but avoid consuming unnecessary microscopic bugs and contaminants that could be harmful to you and your bambino. Minimize your risk

---

§   Benjamin
¶   Benjamin
** Veronica Benjamin, RD, personal communication, August 1, 2015

SEAFOOD DOS AND DON'TS[6]

Try salmon, tuna (non-albacore), shrimp, scallops, tilapia, cod, and haddock. Avoid shark, swordfish, tuna steaks, and tilefish.

by making sure meats, fish, and eggs are **well cooked**, and cheeses, dairy, and juices are **pasteurized**. While deli meats and hot dogs are not recommended (since they are processed foods), they are safer if first cooked to steaming hot. Why? Raw, undercooked, unwashed, and unpasteurized foods can harbor bacteria (like *Listeria*, *Salmonella*, and *Brucella*) as well as the parasite *Toxoplasma gondii*.

Minimize risky seafood.[4-6] Remember, try low-mercury fish when pregnant or breastfeeding. These tend to be smaller fish that are further down in the food chain, as opposed to massive predator fish that accumulate more mercury from their diets.

Quality

Eat clean: organic. What a great time to buy USDA-certified organic produce and meats—these tend to have fewer synthetic chemicals or substances (like pesticides or fertilizers).[7] To help you decide what's worth your money, check out the Environmental Working Group's annually updated list of "Dirty Dozen" and "Clean 15" in their "Shopper's Guide to Pesticides and Produce."[8] In the U.S., some of the most frequently pesticide-laden produce are potatoes, spinach, kale, cherry tomatoes, bell peppers, cucumbers, apples, strawberries, peaches, and grapes.[8]

TIP

Wash your produce with a vinegar solution made from 1 part distilled white vinegar and 3 to 4 parts water.

If you're lucky to have a local farmers market, you may hit the jackpot by finding a farmer who doesn't charge organic prices but still avoids spraying crops with the types of pesticides and fertilizers banned in organic farming. They may simply not be able to afford the official organic certification, so ask around.

Eat clean: well washed. Why eat pesticide and harmful microscopic bugs if you don't have to? Try either a vinegar-water rinse or scrubbing your produce with warm water and a little dish soap. Either can help you get some of the pesticide residue off. Peeling your conventional produce (like apples, pears, and cucumbers) will also help decrease some of your chemical exposure.

Drink plenty of water. Your body will thank you since it's 60% water, and it needs to get about 8–12 cups of water daily (64–96 ounces).[9] This amount helps your body function better, prevents urinary tract infections, and helps keep preterm contractions at bay. An easy way to make sure you're getting enough is to drink water (preferably filtered) when you're thirsty, and especially if your urine is not clear or has a stronger smell. Remember, increase your intake if it's hot outside or if you're exercising.

Avoid alcohol.[10,11] Unfortunately, there is no safe amount in pregnancy. Alcohol can cause *Fetal Alcohol Syndrome* (*FAS*), a condition where your baby develops lifelong brain damage and physical problems.

> ➤➤➤ ❁ ❁ ❁ ❬❬❬
> ## CONSIDERING A CUPPA?
> See B-3a for notes on teas that are safe in pregnancy.

Quantity

How many extra calories? Growing a baby may not require as many extra calories as you think. Get this—it's only an extra small snack a day, starting in the second trimester! On average, women need about 350 extra calories per day in the second trimester, and 450 in the third.[4,12] You'll need more calories starting the first trimester if you're underweight when starting pregnancy or are carrying more than one baby (an extra 300 calories for each baby you're carrying).[13]

If you hate math, you're in luck: most women don't need to count their calories during pregnancy to make sure they're getting enough nutrients. A good maternity care provider will be tracking your weight gain to gauge how well you're eating. Feel free to ask them if it's progressing at the right pace or consider using a pregnancy weight tracker app.

WHAT DOES 300 CALORIES LOOK LIKE?[††]

- Apple (or banana) plus 2 tbsp peanut butter
- Half an avocado and 10–15 crackers
- Pita bread plus 2–3 tbsp hummus
- Half cup dried fruits/nuts
- One cup low-fat yogurt and one cup strawberries

An RD can be a valuable resource.[‡‡] There are specific times when meeting with an RD is helpful since they can better estimate your nutritional intake and help tailor meal plans, as needed. Even if you already know "all the right things to do," RDs can often provide additional tools to help you make necessary changes. If you have any questions about whether you should consult with one, feel free to ask your maternity care provider.

In general, an RD visit is beneficial if you are carrying more than one baby, started pregnancy underweight or obese, have diabetes or dietary restrictions, have an eating disorder now or had one in the past, or are gaining weight too quickly or too slowly.

Watch portions. Eating healthy quantities of various nutrient-rich food is the secret to making sure you get enough of the nutrients needed during pregnancy. For nutrient guides, use the "My Pregnancy Plate" (B-1g) and "Nitty-Gritty Nutrition" (B-1f). For portion control, try serving food in smaller plates and bowls.

Remember your daily prenatal vitamin. Though it is not powerful enough to offset 24/7 nutrient-light eating, it's a great way to make sure your body gets some basic daily vitamins and minerals required during pregnancy and while breastfeeding.

[††] Veronica Benjamin, RD, personal communication, August 1, 2015
[‡‡] Benjamin

b. Choosing Healthier Options

While we all experience cravings for certain types of food, it's best to try experimenting with more nutrient-rich options instead of going for the nutrient-light ones, while keeping portion size in mind.

Need a crunch?[§§] Try one cup of popcorn or two rice cakes with almond butter, cucumber wedges or carrots with hummus, or frozen grapes.

Need a flavored drink? Try flavored mineral water, or add lime, lemon, or cucumber slices to cold (and preferably purified) water. Minimize juices and sodas since they are packed full of unnecessary sugar.

Need a sweet? Try a one-inch square of 70% dark chocolate with a tablespoon of peanut butter.

Need coffee? Enjoy a cup if necessary, limiting added syrups and sweeteners. Stick to no more than about 200 mg of caffeine per day.[1] Although large amounts of caffeine can feel like the magic bullet for living a busy life, don't overdo caffeine in pregnancy. Aside from the fact that it turns you into a peeing machine, it crosses the placenta and it's unknown how large amounts of caffeine impact your delicately developing baby.[1] It can also block absorption of certain vital nutrients (like iron) and may even make you moodier.

Want second helpings? Focus on veggies or salads.

Going out to eat? Try splitting a meal with someone, and rake in generosity points, or take half of it home for leftovers. In general, restaurant portion sizes are way more than even one pregnant person needs.

---

§§ Veronica Benjamin, RD, personal communication, August 1, 2015

c. Navigating Cravings and Food Aversions

Cravings[11]

When you get a craving, pause a moment before grabbing that amazing food that seems to promise you the world. First, check in with your body:

What's causing your craving? Is it hunger, a nutritional need, or maybe something else? Questions to ask yourself include: Are you hungry? When did you eat last? What sorts of foods have you eaten today? How do you feel emotionally?

If you are hungry and haven't eaten in a while, or have eaten nutrient-light foods, then go ahead and fix a snack, keeping its nutrients in mind. If, on the other hand, you've eaten recently and the craving might stem from depression, anxiety, or another emotion, check out an alternative.

Is there a pattern to your cravings? What sorts of foods have you craved and eaten lately?

Having a new craving or one for a nutrient-dense food? Go for it and enjoy! Try a smaller portion if it's not as nutrient-rich.

Craving a nutrient-light food? An occasional small splurge is fine. Savor and enjoy it!

Always craving nutrient-light foods, day in and day out? Try to find alternative foods so your baby and your body get more variety.

Craving foods when life gets tough? Look for ways to cope without food. For example, can you communicate with your partner, work to resolve whatever issue is worrying you, or pick up a new hobby? Or perhaps go on a walk, brush your teeth, or distract yourself (e.g., call a friend, look up baby names, learn to knit). Get creative and mix it up.

Is the craved food safe in pregnancy? Very few items are completely off-limits (on the "no-nos in pregnancy" list). However, if you crave

---

¶¶ Veronica Benjamin, RD, personal communication, August 1, 2015 nonfoods like clay, starch, chalk, or lots of ice, you may have *pica*. Tell your provider so they can check to see if you are low in iron and connect you with a registered dietician to help you. Don't eat nonfoods, even if they are tasty.

Food aversions***

Free yourself from guilt and do your best. If only a few foods sound bearable, go with those for now, freeing yourself from worrying about eating ultra-nutritiously. In early pregnancy, your baby's nutritional requirements are less than later in pregnancy, anyway. Try to eat small, frequent snacks to avoid losing weight, and keep hydrated.

Get creative. See if modifying the detested food helps. Is it better hot or cold? Does a different seasoning or sauce help? Is the egg better hard-boiled or scrambled?

d. After Childbirth

What we put in our bodies always matters, even after childbirth. Nutritious and mindful eating habits will nourish that exhausted body of yours and give you the needed energy to care for your baby, especially if you are breastfeeding. Since after delivery you barely have time to eat, let alone think of *what* you're eating, here are some survival tips!

Prepare grab-and-go items. Eat small, frequent snacks that are easy to grab, especially if you're breastfeeding (see snack list in B-1e for ideas). Make yourself a snack drawer (both at home and at work, if possible). Must-haves early on include freezer foods, prepared ultra-simple meals, and take-out. Yep, these are completely appropriate for the first few months, and will help you survive.

Say yes. Allow friends and family to shop, make you food, and order you take-out. Doubled meals means you can freeze some for later. Don't

---

*** Benjamin

even think about trying to pull a superwoman stunt and cooking for them. You'll pay for it later.

Take prenatal vitamins. Most maternity care providers will recommend you continue to take this daily, especially if you're breastfeeding. In fact, in your childbearing years, it's a great idea to take a daily prenatal vitamin or folic acid supplement in case you get pregnant again, though hopefully not before your baby's 12–24 months old.[1-4] (For more on birth spacing, flip to week 34.)

Breastfeeding

Producing milk takes energy. In fact, it's an extra 500 calories a day for each baby compared to your intake prior to pregnancy![5-7] (However, for the first six months, aim more for 300–450 calories a day, per baby, to allow for healthy postpartum weight loss.[5]) So, don't be surprised if you feel like you're starving all the time, even at night. Focus on nutritional eating as much as possible and know you don't need to drink milk to produce milk.

Listen to your body. Eat when you're hungry and stop when you're comfortably full. Again, most women don't need to calorie count.

Eat a variety of foods. Isn't it amazing that what you eat can change the way your breastmilk tastes? It's a way for you to help your baby to develop a palate for nutritious, cultural, or ethnic foods. The good news is babies generally can handle quite a variety of foods in moderation, but if you graze on one type of food all day, they may not be able to handle it as well.

Foods that can make breastfed babies fussy include beef, chicken, dairy, nuts, wheat, broccoli, onions, green peppers, tomatoes, and cow's milk (which is the most common food to cause problems).[8] If your baby gets a reaction (like gassy, fussy, or eczematous) every time after you eat a certain food, hold off on it for a few weeks or months and see if your baby feels better.[8] It may take a week or two for your system to clear it out and for you to see a happier baby. Don't give up too soon—you may still be on the right track!

Drink plenty of water.[9] Breastfeeding can easily make you parched. Do yourself a favor and have a large, BPA-free water bottle with you whenever you nurse. Don't sit down without it!

Keep alcohol to an occasional, preplanned treat. Alcohol gets into your breastmilk and can decrease your milk supply, so it's best to avoid it.[10] However, if you're yearning for a small glass (or standard drink), have it right after you breastfeed. Waiting at least two hours until the next breastfeeding or pumping session will give your body time to decrease the alcohol content in your milk.[5]

Coffee and caffeine. Moderate use while breastfeeding is reasonable, though there are variations in opinion on what this looks like. Most medical professionals suggest limiting it to under 200–300 mg of caffeine daily, with some postulating 300–500 mg daily might be safe.[7,11,12] Just know that if you do have over two cups of coffee a day, it may decrease your breastmilk's iron levels, potentially causing a mild iron deficiency anemia in your little one.[12]

Bottom line? If you're a coffee lover, limit your use to one-to-two cups a day, especially the first week after delivery or if your baby's preterm.[7,12] Although only a percentage of the caffeine you consume makes it into your breastmilk, it can take days for your baby to clear it out of his or her system.[11,12] This means days of a fussy and irritable baby who can't sleep long. Not fun!

e. Tasty Snacks and Recipes

Want to refresh your snack list while rejuvenating your body and palate? Check out these ideas for some fun, nutritious options.

Cold Combos

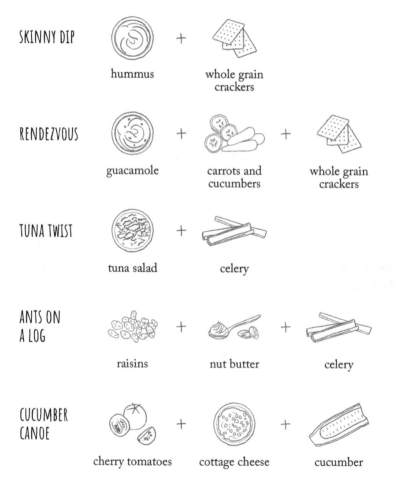

SKINNY DIP   hummus   +   whole grain crackers

RENDEZVOUS   guacamole   +   carrots and cucumbers   +   whole grain crackers

TUNA TWIST   tuna salad   +   celery

ANTS ON A LOG   raisins   +   nut butter   +   celery

CUCUMBER CANOE   cherry tomatoes   +   cottage cheese   +   cucumber

Super Sandwiches 🌿

For a twist: try toast, pita bread, or make it an open sandwich (one bread slice).

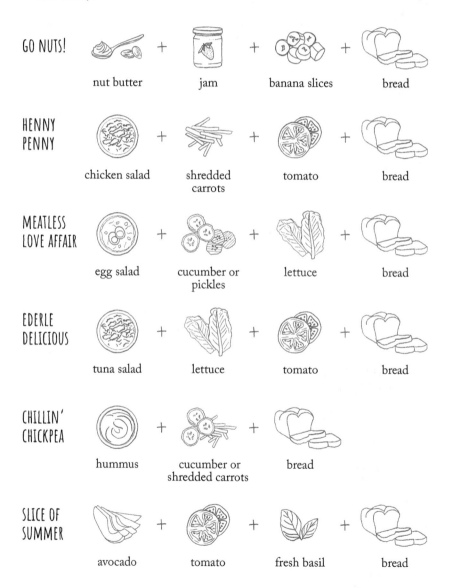

GO NUTS!
nut butter + jam + banana slices + bread

HENNY PENNY
chicken salad + shredded carrots + tomato + bread

MEATLESS LOVE AFFAIR
egg salad + cucumber or pickles + lettuce + bread

EDERLE DELICIOUS
tuna salad + lettuce + tomato + bread

CHILLIN' CHICKPEA
hummus + cucumber or shredded carrots + bread

SLICE OF SUMMER
avocado + tomato + fresh basil + bread

Fruit Frenzy

DANCING MAMA SMOOTHIE

 + + +

1 c fresh or frozen berries   1 banana or ½ avocado   1–2 handfuls of spinach or kale   water, or coconut or almond milk

Optional Mix-ins:

 + + +

1 tbsp nut butter   1 tbsp ground flaxseed   1 tbsp cocoa powder   handful of ice

MILKY WAY SMOOTHIE

 + +  +

1 c milk   1 banana   1 tbsp raw cocoa + 1 tbsp nut butter   handful of ice

YOU'VE GOT THIS! YOGURT BOWL

 + → Possible Toppings: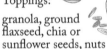

plain yogurt   honey or jam   granola, ground flaxseed, chia or sunflower seeds, nuts

---

STRONG START BREAKFAST BOWL	**RAINBOW SALAD**	**DYNAMIC DUO**
sliced fruit or berries	sliced seasonal fruit	string cheese
+	+	+
cottage cheese	put on a skewer	apple or pear slices

Delicious Desserts

COSMOS   +

dark chocolate   1 tbsp nut
square   butter

APPLE BLISS + + +

core an apple   stuff with nut butter   drizzle with   sprinkle of
                (or granola and a little honey or   cinnamon or
                butter or coconut oil)   maple syrup   nutmeg

 Add ¾ c water to bottom of baking dish.
Bake at 375° for 30–45 min or until soft.

Finger Food

---

hard-boiled   popcorn   nuts and   baby carrots
egg   raisins

snacking   quesadilla kale chips   roasted
peppers   chickpeas

RECIPE | **Peanut Butter POW! Balls**[1]

PREP TIME: 10 min   **COOKING TIME:** None

NOTES:

Store at room
temp for up
to three days
or in fridge
for one week.
For variety, try
adding pumpkin
or sunflower
seeds.

INGREDIENTS:

1 c peanut butter (or sunflower seed butter)
¼ c honey (or brown rice syrup)
2 tsp vanilla extract
1 ½ c rolled oats
½ c unsweetened shredded coconut
Pinch of iodized salt
⅓ c mini chocolate chips
2–4 tsp water (or additional vanilla extract)

DIRECTIONS:

1. In a medium mixing bowl, stir together the first three ingredients.

2. Stir in the oats, coconut, and salt until well combined and then add the chocolate chips. If the mixture doesn't hold well when pinched together, add the additional water or vanilla, a teaspoon at a time, as needed.

3. Form 1" balls using about one tablespoon of the mixture.

RECIPE | Healthy Oat & Blueberry Blender Muffins[2]

PREP TIME: 5 min   COOKING TIME: 15–20 min

NOTES:

Store in airtight container for up to three days.

INGREDIENTS:

2 c rolled oats
2 large ripe bananas
2 large eggs
1 c Greek yogurt (or regular plain)
3 tbsp honey
1 ½ tsp baking powder
1 ½ tsp baking soda
½ tsp vanilla extract
Pinch of salt
1 c blueberries, fresh or frozen

DIRECTIONS:

1. Preheat your oven to 390°F. Place muffin tin liners in a muffin tray and spray them with a little oil.

2. Put all the ingredients except the blueberries into a blender or food processor and blitz until combined. Stir in half the blueberries.

3. Pour the mixture into muffin liners, filling to three-quarters full. Top with the remaining blueberries.

4. Bake in the oven for between 15 to 20 minutes or until a toothpick comes out clean. Remove from the muffin pan and allow to cool on a wire rack.

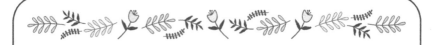

RECIPE | **Morning Glory Muffins**

PREP TIME: 15 min   COOKING TIME: 20 min

NOTES:

Batter will keep
two weeks in
your fridge!

INGREDIENTS:

2 c flour
2 tsp baking soda
2 tsp cinnamon
½ tsp salt
1 apple, grated
2 c carrots, grated
1 (8 oz) can crushed pineapple, drained
½ c raisins
½ c almonds (or walnuts or pecans),
    chopped
½ c coconut, shredded
3 eggs
1 c honey
½ c vegetable oil (or 1 c unsweetened
    applesauce)
1 tsp vanilla

DIRECTIONS:

1. Preheat your oven to 350°F.

2. Combine the dry ingredients in a large bowl and stir to combine.

3. Add the remaining ingredients and mix well.

4. Pour batter into muffin cups or greased muffin tin and bake for
   20 minutes.

5. Remove from the muffin pan and allow to cool on a wire rack.

HOW MUCH CAFFEINE IS IN MY DRINK?[2]

Caffeine content varies by coffee or tea type and brew strength, and, of course, the quantity served. Often, people brew coffee or tea stronger than the directions on the package and then consume more than eight ounces (a cup) of it.

The following are estimates based on 8 oz servings, though these beverages are often served in larger (12–20 oz) cups or bottles, so they would have a higher total caffeine content.

- Starbucks espresso* = 800 mg
- Coffee shop coffees = 47.5–180 mg
- Keurig pods = 75–160 mg
- Home brewed ground coffee = 100–106.5 mg
- Black tea (hot or iced) = 55–60 mg
- Green tea (hot or iced) = 35–58 mg
- Kombucha = typically 2.5–36 mg, but can get up to 60 mg
- Coffee shop decaf coffee = 12.5 mg
- Home brewed decaf coffee = 1.5–5.5 mg
- Hot cocoa = 1–3 mg
- Herbal tea (hot or iced) = 0 mg

*150 mg for 1.5 oz

f. Nitty-Gritty Nutrition

	Average Recommended Daily Nutrient Intake for Adults[1]			Good Natural Sources[2-9]
	Non-Pregnant	Pregnant	Lactating	
Fat-Soluble Vitamins				
Vitamin A (mcg)	700	770	1300	Liver, fish, meat, poultry, eggs, dairy, darkly colored fruits, leafy vegetables
Vitamin D (mcg)	600 IU			Sunlight, fatty fish (salmon, canned light tuna, canned sardine), fish liver oil, mushrooms, egg yolk, fortified milk, plant milks, cereals, orange juice
Vitamin E (mg)	15		19	Vegetable oils, unprocessed cereal grains, nuts, fruits, vegetables, meats
Vitamin K (mcg)*	90			Green vegetables (collards, spinach, salad greens, broccoli), brussels sprouts, cabbage, plant oils, margarine
Water-Soluble Vitamins				
Folate/folic acid (mg)	400	600	500	Enriched cereal grains, leafy vegetables (darkly colored), enriched and whole grain breads and bread products, fortified ready-to-eat cereals
Niacin (mg)	14	18	17	Meat, fish, poultry, breads and bread products (enriched and whole grain), fortified ready-to-eat cereals

	Average Recommended Daily Nutrient Intake for Adults[1]			Good Natural Sources[2-9]
	Non-Pregnant	Pregnant	Lactating	
Riboflavin (mg)	1.1	1.4	1.6	Organ meats, milk, bread products, fortified cereals
Thiamin/B$_1$ (mg)	1.1	1.4		Enriched, fortified, or whole-grain products, bread and bread products, mixed foods whose main ingredient is grain, ready-to-eat cereals
Vitamin B$_6$ (mg)	1.3	1.9	2	Fortified cereals, organ meats, fortified soy-based meat substitutes
Vitamin B$_{12}$ (mcg)	2.4	2.6	2.8	Fortified cereals, meat, fish, poultry
Vitamin C (mg)	75	85	120	Citrus fruits, tomatoes, tomato juice, potatoes, brussels sprouts, cauliflower, broccoli, strawberries, cabbage, spinach
Minerals				
Calcium (mg)*	1,000			Leafy greens, dairy, plant milks, tofu, tahini, canned sardines, canned bone-in salmon
Iodine (mcg)	150	220	290	Iodized salt, seafood (like fish, seaweed, shrimp), dairy
Iron (mg)	18	27	9	Enriched cereal grains, oyster, mussels, bison, beef, canned sardines, turkey, leafy greens, beans, prune juice, sesame seeds, cashews

	Average Recommended Daily Nutrient Intake for Adults[1]			Good Natural Sources[2-9]
	Non-Pregnant	Pregnant	Lactating	
Selenium (mcg)	55	60	70	Seafood, meat, poultry, eggs, dairy, bread, cereal, grain
Phosphorus (mg)	700			Dairy, grains, meats, poultry, fish, eggs, nuts, seeds, lentils, beans, peas, veggies
Other				
Choline (mg)*	425	450	550	Beef, egg (with yolk), soybean, chicken, red potatoes, cod, wheat germ
Carbohydrates (g)	130	175	210	Brown bread, bran, grains, oats, brown rice, pasta, beans, fruits, veggies
Fiber (g)*	25	28	29	Grains, beans, peas, lentils, chickpeas, veggies, fruit, almonds, pistachios, pine nuts, dates, seeds (pumpkin, chia, sunflower, flax)
Proteins and Amino Acids (g)	46	71		Meats, fish, tofu, beans, dairy, legumes, quinoa, nuts, seeds, soybeans, vegetables, grains

	Average Recommended Daily Nutrient Intake for Adults[1]			Good Natural Sources[2-9]
	Non-Pregnant	Pregnant	Lactating	
Fat (g)	Unknown			Olive oil, butter, flax seed or ground flax, nuts, avocado
				Omega-3 fatty acid, ALA sources: flaxseed, chia seeds, walnuts, soybean oil, canola oil
				Omega-3 fatty acid, DHA and EPA sources: fish (especially salmon, tuna, sardines, mackerel, trout), seafood, fish oil
Total Water (c)* (from all food and liquid sources combined)	11.5	12.75	16	Plain water, drinks, smoothies, foods, soups

Note: These are recommended (daily) dietary allowances (RDA) for women ages 18 and up. They estimate the amount most healthy women will need in a day to meet nutritional requirements. Your requirements may be different if you have certain conditions or health problems. Be sure to check with a healthcare provider or RD for a customized list tailored to your needs.

*Adequate intake (AI) used since RDA is not yet established. This is the minimum recommended daily amount for healthy individuals.

g. My Pregnancy Plate[1]

Choose large portions of a variety of non-starchy vegetables, such as leafy greens, broccoli, carrots, peppers, or cabbage.

Choose small amounts of healthy oils (olive and canola) for cooking or to flavor foods. Nuts, seeds, and avocados contain healthy fats.

Choose a variety of whole fruits. Limit juice and dried fruits.

Fruit is great for snacks and desserts, too.

Aim for at least 30 minutes of walking or another physical activity each day.

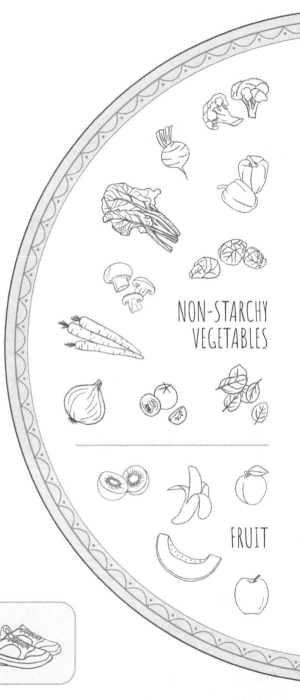

NON-STARCHY VEGETABLES

FRUIT

Choose 2 to 3 servings of nonfat or 1% milk or yogurt (cow, soy, or almond). A serving is 8 oz. Choose yogurt with less than 15 g of sugar per serving.

Drink mainly water, decaf tea, or decaf coffee and avoid sugary beverages.

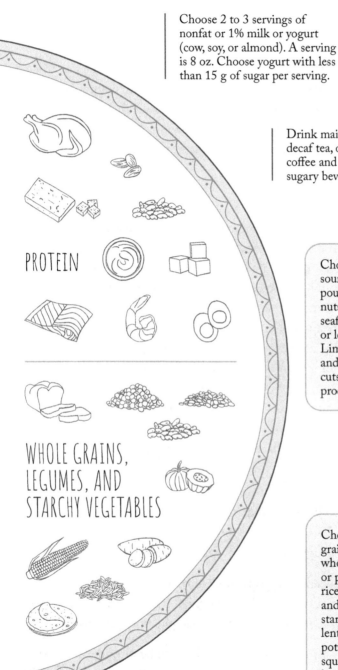

PROTEIN

Choose protein sources such as poultry, beans, nuts, low-mercury seafood, eggs, tofu, or low-fat cheese. Limit red meat and avoid cold cuts and other processed meats.

WHOLE GRAINS, LEGUMES, AND STARCHY VEGETABLES

Choose whole grains, such as whole wheat bread or pasta, brown rice, quinoa or oats, and other healthy starches like beans, lentils, sweet potatoes, or acorn squash. Limit white bread, white rice, and fried potatoes.

2. PHYSICAL ACTIVITY

Welcome, mama! Physical activity is a topic that often elicits a strong reaction in people. Some love the idea, since it's as natural to them as breathing, while others would rather deep-clean their toilet with a toothbrush. Regardless of which camp you're in, I hope what follows will be both informative and encouraging for you in this—incredibly beneficial—pursuit.

So, what are the benefits?

Glad you asked! For everyone, pregnant or not, physical activity decreases the chance of heart disease, stroke, type 2 diabetes, breast or colon cancer, and fall-related injuries.[1,2] Physical activity also improves mood, brain function, sleep, overall well-being, cholesterol, and blood pressure, promotes bone health, and decreases body fat.[1,2]

Yes, it's totally appropriate to stand in awe of these—they're truly impressive. As this illustrates, our bodies thrive when we move. Put another way, we simply miss out if we don't. That's why the medical gurus encourage us to be physically active most days of the week.

Keep reading, mama, for physical activity recommendations, as well as for some practical (down and dirty) pregnancy- and then postpartum-specific items to keep in mind.

a. General Activity Guidelines

To get started, you'll be relieved to hear that some physical activity is better than none. *Phew.* However, there is a minimum amount that has proven to benefit people greatly. Are you ready? Here it is!

Basics. For healthy adults (pregnant or not), medical professionals recommend at least two-and-a-half hours of moderately intense aerobic activity (*cardio*) throughout the week, plus strength training.[1,2]

Cardio. A tip-off that you're engaged in moderate-intensity cardio is if you can talk while doing it, but not sing. So, yes, try to belt out your favorite line and see what happens. Activities that usually do the trick include recreational swimming, water aerobics, hiking, power vinyasa yoga, dancing, and kayaking.

Strength training. Weight or resistance training twice weekly will promote the development of all those beautiful major muscle groups. This strength training makes you fitter, boosts your metabolism, keeps your bones and muscles strong, prevents injury, and improves brain function and mood.[1,2]

Beyond the basics. On the other hand, for those who enjoy (and are used to) *vigorous*-intensity cardio, the general goal is to do at least 1 hour and 15 minutes of it during the week instead of moderate-intensity cardio, or to do a combo of moderate and vigorous cardio.[1,2]

Vigorous cardio. A good way to tell you're reaching vigorous cardio levels is if you can only speak a few words at a time before you need to take a breath. The minimum recommended time for the vigorous category is shorter than the recommendation for moderately intense activity because your body is working way harder. Examples of vigorous cardio include jogging, running, lap swimming, step aerobics, kickboxing, uphill biking, or biking over 10 miles per hour.

Age matters. While these are the overall physical activity tips for the average healthy adult, it varies for those who are younger (kids between ages 6 and 17) and those who are older (such as your parents).[1] This younger group needs at least an hour of moderate-to-vigorous cardio *daily*, while older adults may need to customize their physical activity based on their health and abilities.

Now, as you read through these guidelines, you might have found yourself thinking that there's a bit of work involved in making an active lifestyle happen. After all, who has an extra couple of hours lying around every week just waiting to be filled? With all your other obligations and pressures, it can be hard to prioritize physical activity, and yes, it may take some figuring out. But just know—it's never too late to start. Not even when you're pregnant.

MODERATE-INTENSITY ACTIVITY	VIGOROUS-INTENSITY ACTIVITY
• Brisk walk (2.5–4 mph)	• Jogging or running
• Water aerobics	• Lap swimming
• Recreational swimming	• Biking (>10 mph)
• Active yoga	• Vigorous dancing
• Hiking	• Fitness classes

b. Move That Pregnant Bod

Since pregnancy is a unique time in a woman's life, it comes as no surprise that there are some pregnancy-specific considerations regarding when and how to be active. To begin, unless your maternity care provider has specifically advised you to avoid physical activity due to medical or pregnancy complications (like severe anemia, incompetent cervix or cerclage, or placenta previa after week 26), there is no need to cut it out of your life.[1,2]

Contrary to popular belief, physical exertion while pregnant actually has great benefits for both a mother and her baby. In fact, pregnancy is a fantastic time to be active. While pregnant, aim for about two-and-a-half hours of moderate intensity aerobic physical activity, sprinkled throughout the week.[1,3,4]

If you haven't been too active up until now, this is a wonderful time to develop healthy habits that you can continue into mommydom.[3] It will prepare you for an active life with your baby, filled with long walks, hide-and-seek, tag, and eventually all sorts of other adventures as he grows. It's what babies and kids are wired for.

If prioritizing movement hasn't been your thing, start slowly to increase your stamina. Try 15 minutes of walking, three times a week, gradually increasing to 30 minutes per day most days of the week.[1,3,4] Swimming, stationary biking, and even prenatal fitness classes are also great options. While pregnancy is not a time to dramatically increase your fitness level, it certainly is a great time to become more active.

If you exercised regularly before pregnancy (and of course, may have fallen off that bandwagon since becoming pregnant), be encouraged—you can generally maintain your moderate-to-vigorous fitness routine, assuming it's not too risky for pregnancy.[1] If you're a competitive athlete, work with a maternity care provider to monitor your activity more closely.[3]

Remember, your pregnant body is different now than it used to be. It has done all sorts of things behind your back to protect your baby while you're active (like increasing your heart rate and burning more calories).[1] As your belly gets bigger, you'll notice your balance changing and even an authentic pregnancy walk going on. Also, your knee and hip joints experience more force, and even your ligaments have grown laxer from estrogen and relaxin hormones (throughout your entire body, not just in your pelvis).[1,5] For these reasons, be careful going down stairs and avoid zipping up ladders. Honor your body, listen to it, and avoid overstretching or lifting heavy objects without care.

GREAT PHYSICAL ACTIVITY OPTIONS IN PREGNANCY[1,5]

- Walk
- Hike
- Jog/run
- Swim
- Water aerobics
- Prenatal yoga
- Dance
- Stationary bike
- Weight training

Skip contact sports or activities with fall risks—like boxing, soccer, basketball, single racquet sports, ice skating, downhill skiing, or snowboarding.

Pregnancy quick tips

Prioritize yourself. Your well-being and health are essential for pregnancy and mothering, so be sure to snatch time for yourself. This is not selfishness; it's wisdom. Both you and your baby (who also relies on you to be well) deserve it. It may be tempting to prioritize household chores, but if you go that route, you may never get around to self-care. Chores magically self-perpetuate.

Find something you enjoy. You're more likely to stick with it and can avoid torturing yourself unnecessarily. Remember to minimize your risk for falls, abdominal trauma, and joint stress.

Be realistic. A decrease in your performance level is totally normal.[1] You're growing a baby! Instead of monitoring your exercise intensity with heart rate (it's too variable in pregnancy), use the 1–10 perceived hardness scale.[1,5] Aim for a (moderate) 6–7 or a little higher if you're used to and shooting for vigorous activity.

Hydrate and don't overheat! Both air conditioning and cooler outdoor temperatures make exercise safer and more pleasant. This is especially true if you're getting a harder or longer workout (over 45 minutes).[1,5] Remember to hydrate plenty during *and* after your workouts, especially if you get stuck in a hot or humid situation.[1] Dehydration can lead to premature contractions—which is *not* on the pregnancy to-do list for anyone.

Nourish your body. Eat a snack after your workout, and certainly during, if it's a long one.[1]

Building that muscle. You can decrease your injury risk if you prioritize more repetitions over greater weight (e.g., lower weight at 14–16 reps per set, versus greater weight at 6–10 reps per set). Also, avoid lying on your back for long periods of time.[1]

Physical activity in the workplace

Now let's explore physical activity considerations for maintaining a healthy pregnancy while at work. Although the level of physical intensity required by each job can vary greatly, here are a few items to keep in mind.

If you have a desk job, or one that requires standing in place for long periods of time, make sure you walk around for a few minutes at least every two hours. Blood pumping through your veins is a lovely thing; it circulates blood to your baby (which delivers much-needed nutrients and oxygen), decreases your risk for blood clots, and can greatly reduce back pain and swollen ankles.

If you're stuck in meetings all day, try tracing favorite or most hated baby names in the air with your toes (discreetly, of course). If you're standing often, try alternately resting a foot on a step stool to ease the tension in your lower back. If you're standing all day, ask for a stool to sit on, since prolonged standing may hinder adequate circulation to your little one.

WARNING SIGNS TO STOP EXERCISING[1]

Use common sense! Stop if you have dizziness, headache, chest pain, muscle weakness, difficulty breathing, vaginal bleeding, amniotic fluid leakage, preterm labor, decreased fetal movement, or calf pain/swelling. In any of these instances, contact your maternity care provider immediately.

If you have a job that requires lifting, keep objects close to yourself, held securely with both hands, and squat when setting objects down instead of bending forward. Leaning forward sacrifices your back and can easily cause long-term injuries. You only have one back— protect it! From around 20 weeks on, avoid lifting heavier items above your head height or below your shin level, moving unbalanced (wobbly) items, and twisting your torso while carrying objects.[6]

In general, most healthy pregnant ladies who are less than 20 weeks along can lift 17–36 pounds occasionally, while from 20 weeks and on it's 17–26 pounds.[6] As you get further along in pregnancy, the weight restrictions increase, meaning lower weights as you get closer to your due date.[6] If you're lifting repetitively (more than three times a minute) and you're at least 20 weeks, the threshold drops to a maximum of 9–22 pounds per item, depending on frequency, item type, and the specific type of lifting motion.[6] Feel free to ask your maternity care provider for a personalized recommendation on weight lifting limits for you. They can even write you a "work accommodation" letter so you stay safe at work (see A-3g).

c. Activity Postpartum

Transitioning back into an active lifestyle after delivery looks different for every mama. While some women may feel like exercising a few days after delivery, many will wait a lot longer. So, quit the comparisons game and give yourself grace. Mommies need a lot of grace—and not just during pregnancy.

To begin, focus on easing back in. Soon after delivery is not the time to stress about meeting the standard goals for moderate- or vigorous-intensity cardio. Instead, be impressed you actually got out of the house fully clothed, no matter how stained your outfit may be. It's especially impressive if you had delivery complications or Cesarean birth. Again, in such cases, be sure to get your maternity care provider's blessing before stepping up your physical activity program.

For more tips on protecting your back in life and at work, check out A-3b.

Address expectations. Many mamas assume their bodies and physical stamina will bounce back immediately after having their baby. In their minds, it's like: *Baby is out, and bam, we're back in business. Mama gets her body and fitness back.* Well, my friend, please know that for most women, delivery is less of a turning point and more a step in the journey. From a purely physiological perspective, it takes about six weeks for many of the body's system functions to get back to their prepregnancy state.

Regardless of whether you had a Cesarean birth or vaginal birth, multiple factors mean it takes a few months for you to feel normal again.

Recovery after childbirth is especially a process if you had a Cesarean birth, which is major abdominal surgery. It will take *at least* six-to-eight weeks for your uterine incision, muscles, and skin to fully heal. Even if your scar has healed nicely, remember, layers deeper inside are still mending. If you overdo it, it will be painful, and it may even slow down the healing process. So, avoid lifting things heavier than your baby, and start with light physical activity like casual walks.

After six weeks, keep listening to your body during physical activity for several months to see how it feels. Any pain? If so, pull back on the intensity for now (and don't feel guilty about asking your maternity care provider for pain medication if needed). Then, after a few weeks, see how it feels to increase your physical activity intensity again, slowly. Remember, recovery time is different for every mama.

Finding time for physical activity is certainly one of the trickiest parts of mommyhood. While it's easy to become overwhelmed at the prospect of finding time without the aid of a magic wand—don't despair. There are still several options for sneaking in some vital movement when you feel up to it.

Ideas for increased activity include taking walks with your baby in a wrap or carrier, going on a run with your little one in a jogging stroller, joining a postpartum moms' stroller-based exercise class, finding a gym that provides child care, or using online workout videos at home. If you don't have an eager friend or relative begging to babysit, you may need to get creative. This could even mean making time right after you feed your little one, or when your partner or family gets back from work.

For breastfeeding mamas, great news—physical activity is safe while breastfeeding, and aerobic activity doesn't negatively impact milk production.[1] Even moderate weight loss because of physical activity is safe and shouldn't impact your baby's weight gain. It's good, though, to remember that your body continues to produce the relaxin hormone while you're breastfeeding, which means your ligaments will continue to be looser and your joints more vulnerable even though you gave birth. Continue to use caution and ease up if you need to.

Don't give up. Snatch any free minute in which you have motivation and energy. There will be days when this will be impossible, and that may be disappointing, but that's okay. Carry a healthy dose of wonder to see what the next day holds.

Postpartum quick tips

Celebrate your accomplishments, no matter how small they seem. Seriously, even if you only make it out of the house for 10 minutes before your baby vomits all over you, give yourself credit. You got out and tried to be active. Go clean up and see if you can try again— whether it's later that day or the next. Along this journey, don't forget to laugh. Many of the things you'll go through belong in a movie.

Walk like a queen. This is a prime time to remember what good posture looks like. It's so easy to maintain our pregnancy posture even after birth, because for many women, it's as if our core abdominal muscles went on holiday and never got an invite home. When possible, stand tall. Pull in your abs and bring your shoulders back and down, even while wearing a baby carrier or pushing a stroller. It's so easy to hunch forward all day long from all your sweet cuddles and carrying activities. But if the habit continues, before too long, your shoulders, back, and pelvic floor will start to complain.

Strengthen your core. Your core-stabilizing abdominal muscles often get weaker from pregnancy and childbirth. Time to show them some love and strengthen them. This will also help protect your back and benefit your pelvic floor. Go for it: try crunches, Pilates, and yoga, and consider a pelvic floor assessment by a physical therapist to get recommendations tailored for you! If they recommend Kegels, check out the fun "recipe" in A-3c.

While it's recommended to exercise your abs, you'll want to hold off on sit-ups and push-ups for at least six-to-eight weeks if you had a Cesarean birth, and also if you are among the many mamas with

diastasis recti (since these exercises can greatly extend the time it takes to heal these areas).

Addressing *diastasis recti.* This condition occurs when the stress on your abdominal muscles causes them to separate. It is common, can start during pregnancy, and still affects 39%–45% of women at six months postpartum.[2,3] If you have diastasis recti, be encouraged: there are resources for you. Physical therapy exercises can help, as well as surgery for more severe cases. Ask your maternity care provider for a referral. (To check if you have it, lie on your back with your knees bent, do a partial sit-up, and see if there's a soft bulge in your belly around your belly button.)

Swimmers, hold off on your trip to the pool until after you stop bleeding, which may take up to four-to-seven weeks after delivery.

Breastfeeding mamas, remember to feed your baby before exercising to avoid engorged breasts (they can be painful!).[1] Breastfeeding before you exercise can also decrease the acidity in your milk—a byproduct of lactic acid buildup that generally occurs with more intense activity. Last, be sure to wear a good, supportive sports bra and nursing pads before you waltz off to work out. In fact, do yourself a favor and keep extra nursing pads in your purse. At some point, they are almost guaranteed to fall into the toilet, and you'll be stuffing toilet paper in your bra to keep yourself from leaking through your shirt.

Recover. All those memorable sleepless nights may slow your muscle recovery after intense workouts. Honor and listen to your body and adjust your activity level as needed.

3. REST AND RELAXATION

a. Sleeping Tips for Pregnancy

As you continue traveling through pregnancy, you've probably noticed it's harder to get a refreshing night of sleep than before. Since many other pregnant mamas feel this way, here are tips dedicated to helping you rest.

Make rest your priority. It's super common for people to put everything else above sleep.[1]

Develop healthy sleep habits. Go to bed around the same time every day, and make sure your bedroom is quiet, dark, and cool (60°F–67°F).[2] Relax before bedtime and make your bed a haven for only sleep and sex.[2] Don't forget to turn off the computer and electronics at least 30 minutes before bed, since artificial lights wake you up.[3-5] If you have varying day and night shifts at work, ask your maternity care provider to write your employer a note asking for a consistent day or night shift—a much healthier option.

Be a pillow queen. The more pillows, the better. Try shoving a pillow under your belly or hips, between or under your legs. You can even try hugging a huge body pillow as you lie on your side. Though make sure you leave a sliver of room for your partner.

Change where you sleep. Of course, it's important for you to have a comfortable and supportive mattress, along with comfy bedsheets and blankets.[2] However, sometimes pregnancy calls for a little creativity. Don't underestimate the glorious sleep you can get in an armchair, recliner, or couch. Be open to life's unexpected blessings.

Nap. This can help you make up for some lost sleep. If you're working, close your office door, or find a break room, park bench, or even car-camp if it's cool enough. Even 20–30 little minutes can increase alertness and work performance. If napping interferes with your

COULD I HAVE SLEEP-DISORDERED BREATHING (SDB)?

SDB covers a range of breathing problems during sleep—such as obstructive sleep apnea and frequent and loud snoring, where the airway is partially or completely obstructed during sleep.[10,11] This not only leads to poor quality sleep but also various health and pregnancy complications.

So, be proactive. If you snore often, wake up gasping for air, or have extreme daytime sleepiness, ask your maternity care provider for a referral to a sleep medicine specialist for an evaluation. Restful sleep could be around the corner for you!

ability to fall asleep at night, try napping earlier in the day and for a shorter time.

Move! Daily physical activity is a must if you want to sleep.[2] Break a little sweat. Obviously, skip this step if your maternity care provider told you otherwise. In that case, try a weekly prenatal massage instead.

Have a cuppa! Feel like a queen with a sophisticated cup of tea a few times a week. Buying organic will limit your exposure to pesticides, while sticking to caffeine-free closer to bedtime will help you fall asleep easier.

Use medication if needed. Sometimes you just need a little momentum to fall asleep. Ask your maternity care provider about over-the-counter options like doxylamine (Unisom) or diphenhydramine (BENADRYL), or other suggestions that are considered safe in pregnancy. Remember, avoid substances or drugs like alcohol and marijuana, and limit caffeine later in the afternoon.

Explore essential oils.[6] Inhaling certain scents can be an effective and fun way to help with problems like sleep, anxiety, and morning sickness. While not all essential oils are safe in pregnancy or safe for everyone, in general, lavender (*Lavandula angustifolia*) and citrus (bergamot, lemon, neroli, and petitgrain) can be used in pregnancy. To find options personalized to your needs and health history, consult a clinical aromatherapist certified by the National Association for Holistic Aromatherapy (NAHA).

Manage leg cramps. To help decrease those painful leg cramps, try: (1) daily physical exercise, even if only mild intensity; (2) dorsiflexing your feet in the mornings and evenings, holding for about 20 seconds with each stretch; and (3) massaging the area.[7] If cramps continue frequently and are excruciating, check in with your maternity care provider for further evaluation. A magnesium supplement may do the trick.[7]

Manage restless leg syndrome. This unpleasant urge to move or shake your sexy-mama legs typically occurs during rest or inactivity, and especially in the evenings.[7,8] Since this can be caused by iron or folate

WHICH TEAS ARE SAFE IN PREGNANCY?

Pregnant mamas can sure love their tea, but often wonder if it's safe to continue drinking it. Many, but not all, herbs can be safely used in moderate amounts during pregnancy, meaning in two cups a day or less.[12] Some herbs can interact with medications, impact health conditions, or even cause pregnancy or health complications.[12,13] Look for your favorite tea in the categories below, and stick to those that are safe. As always, if you're unsure, it's wise to check in with your maternity care provider.

- **Likely safe** (with amount commonly found in foods): strawberry, blueberry, peppermint, cranberry, ginger, and red raspberry *fruit* (not *leaf*).[14-19]
- **Possibly safe** (with moderate or occasional use): green, oolong, and black (moderate use); echinacea (occasional use only); and red raspberry leaf (in appropriate amounts toward the end of pregnancy, under maternity care provider supervision).[19-23]
- **Unsafe/possibly unsafe** (with standard or even minimal use): chamomile, licorice, hibiscus, rose hip, passionflower, yerba mate, ephedra, and ginkgo).[12,24-32]
- **Unknown** (insufficient data): lemon balm and rooibos.[33,34]

deficiency, ask your maternity care provider to check these levels with labs.[8,9] You'll feel better if you try the leg cramp tips described above, and also warm baths, compression stockings, sleeping with a weighted blanket, and eliminating caffeine.[8] If you're smoking cigarettes, this is yet another reason to stop.[8]

Be real with your maternity care provider. If none of these tips are cutting it for you, you have a history of insomnia, or are having trouble falling asleep because of anxiety—let your maternity care provider know! There are other things that might help you, such as other sleep medicines, antianxiety medications, or even a referral to a mental health provider.

b. Sleeping Tips for Postpartum

Getting sleep as a parent, especially in the first few months, can be a rare delicacy. Rest assured, you will one day sleep again, though it'll take some time to figure out routines and sleeping arrangements that work for your baby and family. There's not a one-size-fits-all solution. Keep learning about your baby, share the nighttime duties whenever possible, and don't give up! Eventually, you'll find what works. Here are a few general considerations as you embark on this part of your parenting journey.

Catch the sleep wave. Think of sleepiness as an ocean wave.[1] If you time it right, the wave can carry your baby blissfully into dreamland. So, notice when she is giving you *I'm tired of this* cues (like being fussy, closing eyes, turning away) or *overstimulated* cues (like turning away from you or arching her back). In these moments, drop everything and attend to her needs.[2] You'll thank yourself for doing so, since it's much harder to get an overtired or overstimulated baby to sleep.

Time it right. Put your baby down to sleep when she is sleepy (but not entirely asleep) or when sleeping deeply. A lightly sleeping baby will wake right up as you set her down for the night. Closed eyes are exciting to see but not sufficient for a successful escape from your baby. Wait an extra 10 minutes and look for these clues: eye flutters, slowed breathing, and her arm falling limp when you raise it.

Share the love. There's nothing like mama getting at least a five-to-six-hour chunk of sleep! It's especially important if you struggle with mental health problems. So, break up the night in shifts or pick certain days for someone else to take charge, and try earplugs or a white noise machine when it's your turn to rest. Hiring a night nanny (two-to-four times a week) for a few months can also be luxurious. Just know if you're trying to maintain your milk supply, you'll still likely need to pump every few hours on your nights off.

BACK TO SLEEP

Until age one, put your baby down to sleep on her back on a firm, non-inclined surface.[5] Get this, by simply following this practice, and having your baby sleep in your bedroom with her own bed for at least the first six months, you cut the chance of sudden infant death syndrome (SIDS) in half![5,6]

Minimize nighttime stimulation. While talking to your baby and playing are so important for development, save those for daytime. Minimize stimulation during the night, unless you're trying to train up a night owl.

Swaddle. Wrapping your baby carefully in a swaddle may help her feel secure and fall asleep easier. Some babies don't like being swaddled at all, while others just prefer to have their arms out. Find out what your little one likes best. Just know, your baby's hips develop properly when she is able to splay her legs out like a little frog, so find swaddles with a sack or loose pouch around the legs.[3,4] Also, avoid swaddling too tight and for too long.[3,4] Swaddling can be used until your baby starts rolling—we don't want any face-plants![5]

Try overnight diapers. Sure, babies need frequent diaper changes, but you can limit this by using an overnight diaper. They're designed to last through the night and absorb so much more urine. If your baby poops, though, a diaper change will still be needed.

Use a nightlight. No need to blast a bright light in your faces when up at night. Instead, use a dim nightlight so it's easier to fall back asleep.

Try a noise machine. Noise machines can help both you and your baby sleep more soundly. It's like hanging a sound curtain around you with rain, waves, or heartbeat sounds. This is especially glorious if you're a light sleeper who's distracted by all the funny sounds your newborn makes while sleeping. Remember to be mindful of the volume to protect your baby's hearing.

Avoid aromatherapy. While aromatherapy can be soothing, it's best to generally avoid it around babies. The strong smells can be unsafe for them. Check with your baby's healthcare provider for more information about this.

Skip the bedding. Like you, babies don't like to be hot or cold while sleeping. To keep your baby comfortable, play around with the thermostat, PJs, and any sleep sack or swaddles you're using. For safety reasons, avoid blankets, pillows, and crib bumpers until she's a toddler.[5]

Use caution with meds that make you drowsy. When in charge of your little one's caregiving, you need to be ready to rumble and attend to your baby's every need. If you need to take a medicine that can make you drowsy, be sure to designate someone else for caregiving.

Soothe. Guess what? Soothing your baby also soothes you. Brush up on all the practical ways via "Soothing Baby and Regaining Your Cool" (postpartum week 2).

Sleep training. When sleeping is a disaster, training your child to sleep using a method from a book or a sleep trainer

> -»»» ✿ ✿ ✿ «««-
>
> Mama, if you can't fall sleep, even when your baby is sleeping, check in with your maternity care or mental health provider. This is especially important if you feel you can "go, go, go" on very little sleep without getting tired.

can seem to offer such hope. Though there can certainly be a place for this, wait until your little one is at least six months old to actively sleep train. Before this, infants are not developmentally ready.

c. Relaxation Tips for Pregnancy and Beyond

Relaxation is a gift for all of us humans, right? It's especially important to carve out time for this if you're stressed, struggle with your mental health, or if you are postpartum. Why? Because it nourishes your soul and restores your inner balance. If you're postpartum, rest assured, some items on this list will be more possible as your baby gets a little older.

- Take a luxurious shower/bath
- Get a massage
- Take a "sound bath" by playing or listening to music
- Meditate or pray
- Practice mindfulness
- Journal
- Do guided imagery—go to that favorite place
- Go on a walk, hike, or exercise
- Make an herb garden
- Read a book, blog, or magazine
- Watch a movie
- Draw or color
- Create
- Call a friend
- Go on a date
- Drink a yummy, nutrient-dense smoothie
- Order some take-out
- Sleep

4. MENTAL HEALTH

a. Mental Wellness in Pregnancy and Beyond

Since mental health is the foundation for living fully and parenting well, I'm thrilled you're here to spend more time on it. Put your feet up and feel free to grab a friend, partner, or family member to read this with you. The more the merrier.

General notes on mental health

Mental health is a state of emotional, psychological, and social wellness—a position from which you can take care of yourself, find purpose and fulfillment, form meaningful relationships, and cope with hardships. Yes, the definition is a bit more complex, but this will suffice here.[1-3] In essence, mental wellness is necessary for life and wholeness, and everyone deserves to enjoy it.

When we hear the phrase *mental wellness*, many of us think about the opposite: the oh-so-common realm of mental health problems. Did you know, about one in five U.S. adults and about one in seven youth (aged 12–17) live with a mental health disorder like depression, anxiety, or bipolar?[4,5] It spans all racial, cultural, and socioeconomic lines but is more common among females, adults aged 18–25, and those who identify with two races.[6]

Despite how common mental health problems are, only about half of those experiencing them are receiving treatment.[4] It's mind-boggling to think about what a common human experience this is and to consider how many millions of us are suffering needlessly.

To make matters worse, many cultures, families, and communities are so hush-hush about mental health they perpetuate the struggles by keeping it enshrouded in misconceptions. By doing this, we create a sort of Pandora's box that only causes ongoing—and unnecessary—pain and hardship for everyone.

It is only through finding the courage to talk about it that we remove the stigma and realize we are not alone. Only then do we gain insight into ourselves or our loved ones, beginning a wonderful journey of healing and freedom.

Perinatal considerations

During pregnancy and the *postpartum period* (the first year after delivery), certain mental health issues are grouped together under the label **perinatal mood and anxiety disorders** (**PMADs**). This category encompasses these disorders: anxiety, depression, obsessive-compulsive, post-traumatic-stress, bipolar, and the very rare but serious condition called psychosis (although infrequent, it's a postpartum emergency, so we'll talk about this one later). Theories on why we develop PMADs point to a range of factors including environmental, genetic, immunologic, social, spiritual, and even personal characteristics (such as a person being more sensitive to hormonal changes, like those who experience premenstrual syndrome or premenstrual dysphoric disorder).

In this perinatal season, PMADs are common either for the first time or as a recurrence. You are, in this time, like an orchid—beautiful, flourishing, and strong, though vulnerable. With all the factors at play, about 1 in 7 women and 1 in 11 men will experience depression sometime during pregnancy or within the first year of the baby's life.[7-10] Anxiety is also common among parents during this time and frequently, though not always, appears with depression.[10,11]

In pregnancy

Did you know your mental health impacts your pregnancy and baby? Think of it this way: your uterus is a unique ecosystem for your baby, sensitive to your life and surroundings. While studies are still underway to uncover how exactly mental health problems negatively impact our bodies' systems, preliminary evidence points to changes in hormone regulation, metabolism, immune system and placenta functions, and even DNA processes (*epigenetic changes*).[8,12-14]

Research has shown that untreated depression, stress, and anxiety increase the chance for certain pregnancy complications, like preterm birth and having a baby with a low birth weight.[12,13,15-20] When a mama is unwell, there is also a higher risk of behavioral, learning, and emotional problems among infants, children, and teens. While these problems are not eventualities, untreated mental health concerns make them more likely.[10,13,21-23]

Clearly, taking care of your mental health during pregnancy has many benefits that extend beyond you to those you love.

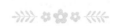

Of course, you may not experience PMADs, but it does happen often enough that it's worth paying attention to.

The great news is this—by actively supporting your mental well-being in pregnancy and by keeping close tabs on it, you may either prevent problems entirely or identify any problems sooner. You'll enjoy pregnancy more and be able to take better care of yourself—a fantastic way to set yourself up for wellness postpartum.[24]

So, on that note, let's wrap up our perinatal and pregnancy mental health considerations here, since we'll come back to postpartum considerations later on. For now, consider checking out the tips for nurturing your mental wellness and developing a postpartum care plan, in B-4f and A-5a.

In postpartum

Welcome to postpartum life—an exciting and exhausting time full of wonder and surprise. In "You and Your Baby-Centered World" (postpartum week 3) and "Postpartum Depression" (postpartum week 4), we discussed baby blues, postpartum depression (PPD), and anxiety. Here, we'll review general postpartum mental health considerations for parents. Are you ready?

First, you're not alone! PMADs are quite common postpartum, affecting up to about 1 in 7 women. Specifically in the first year postpartum, about 13%–25% of mothers and 8.5%–10% of fathers have depression, while 2%–18% of mamas and 5%–10% of fathers develop anxiety.[10,11,25,26] This is a lot of us! For some parents, this is a recurrence, while for others, it appears for the first time.[27] It may present as a single mental health problem or together with another, since certain ones often appear together—such as either anxiety or substance use with either depression or bipolar.[25] Keeping tabs on how you're doing is the way to go.

When your little dumpling is born, he is ready to soak up your love and cuddles. In your baby's early years of life especially, your baby's growth, development, and well-being are greatly influenced by how sensitively you interact with him and attend to his needs.[10] When experiencing emotional suffering, it is hard to parent well and be your best, even though you might be trying your hardest. With depression, for example, it is natural to become more withdrawn or angry, irritated, or just be less attuned to your baby's cues.[8,28] In moments like these, you and your baby miss out on wonderful times together.

Just as in pregnancy, your mental wellness has a significant effect on your baby and family. If mommy or partner is not well emotionally, your little one is impacted in profound ways. He may have delayed or lower mental, social, language, and emotional development, may have more behavioral problems, and may have increased challenges with mental health and substance use throughout his life.[29] Even fundamental aspects like your baby's sleep and feeding patterns can be negatively affected—which, in turn, directly impacts his brain development.[29]

The good news is—this doesn't have to be your story. So, when tempted to skip self-care, feeling guilty that it takes time away from your family, remind yourself that it is, in fact, your lifeline. When you are the best version of you, you are the best *you* for them.

Important considerations

If you already have a bipolar diagnosis, it's important to know that this postpartum season is when you have the highest chance for experiencing a recurrent bipolar episode.[25,27] Bipolar also significantly increases your chance of experiencing postpartum psychosis, which is a mental health emergency (more on this next).

Because your little one needs you to be well, be proactive and make sure you get enough nighttime sleep, exercise, and nutritious food.[30] If you're on a medication, take it daily, even if you're feeling stable. Also, pay attention to symptoms of depression (see postpartum week 4) as well as *mania*—characterized by extreme high spirits or irritability most days, racing thoughts, feeling rested with minimal sleep, or having poor judgment (like reckless driving, sexual risk-taking, or shopping sprees).[30,31] If you notice any of these, reach out for help without delay.

Psychosis is a psychiatric emergency. This is a dangerous mood disorder that, like others, is treatable! Although it's incredibly rare (so breathe!), it's good to be aware of what it is and isn't, since it can be misrepresented in the media. Are you with me?

Postpartum psychosis appears in the first month after delivery, usually within 3–10 days.[32] The greatest risk factors are if the woman has a personal or family history of bipolar disorder or postpartum psychosis.[32] Symptoms include disorientation, insomnia, paranoia, confusion, hallucinations (seeing, hearing, or feeling things that others don't), and bizarre behavior or thoughts (such as feeling the need to harm your baby or yourself).[30,32]

It's very rare for women to realize they are having these symptoms; they are more commonly noticed by others. Anyone with these symptoms needs immediate medical care, temporary hospitalization, and treatment. Loved ones, please know that until mama is well, she should never be left alone for safety reasons, and afterward, she may need to receive treatment for depression.[30] But with the right help and support, recovery is possible!

b. Self Check-in

Ready to be proactive about your mental health, but wondering where to start? Well, various organizations have created many paper- and technology-based surveys and trackers to help people stay on top of their mental wellness. For example, the Edinburgh Postnatal Depression Scale is a popular one used in pregnancy and postpartum and is available in multiple languages.

To get you started, check out the following pregnancy and postpartum tool by Postpartum Support International. Consider using it as a conversation aid with your maternity or primary care provider, or mental health professional; it's also a wonderful tool to use for personal check-ins every few months while pregnant and for the first year after delivery.[1] Go ahead, check it out and see if any apply to you.

Perinatal mental health discussion tool

- ☐ Feeling depressed or void of feeling
- ☐ Feelings of hopelessness
- ☐ Trouble concentrating
- ☐ Brain feels foggy
- ☐ Feeling anxious or panicky
- ☐ Feeling angry or irritable
- ☐ Dizziness or heart palpitations
- ☐ Extreme worry or fears (including for the health and safety of the baby)
- ☐ Scary and unwanted thoughts
- ☐ Feeling an urge to repeat certain behaviors to reduce anxiety
- ☐ Needing very little sleep while still functioning
- ☐ Flashbacks regarding the pregnancy and delivery
- ☐ Avoiding things related to the delivery
- ☐ Not able to sleep when baby sleeps
- ☐ Seeing images or hearing sounds that others cannot see/hear
- ☐ Lack of interest in the baby
- ☐ Thoughts of harming yourself or the baby

As you can see, if our mental health is suffering, our bodies give us all sorts of helpful clues to get our attention. Sometimes it's through emotional cues (like crying often, not enjoying the things we used to, or being irritable), while other times, it's through physical symptoms (like being nauseous or tired, or having heart palpitations or trouble concentrating). Of course, it's important to touch base with your healthcare provider since our physical symptoms may be caused by other medical conditions.

Not sure whether to reach out for professional help? If you're not doing well, aren't feeling like yourself, or are having trouble functioning, the time has come! It doesn't mean you are weak or that you did something wrong. PMADs are common and can happen to anyone, remember? The sooner you reach out for help, the quicker you'll be on the road to recovery. If you ignore your mental health needs, your problems will only multiply (like when postpartum depression, for example, turns into chronic depression).

If ever you are feeling so hopeless that you are seriously contemplating hurting yourself or others, get immediate help. Reach out to your loved ones, don't leave their sight, and get to a hospital or call 911 or 988 immediately. Your baby and family need you to be well! You are irreplaceable!

c. Find the Right Professional Help

If you've decided to reach out for professional help, congratulations for making that big decision! Well done for prioritizing you and your family. Yes, it's normal to be a little nervous, and if your sense of adventure is waning, you can always ask a trusted friend or family member(s) to help you take this next step. Remember, what you are going through is perfectly treatable, and all you've got to do is be willing to step out.

So where do you start? Which professional you reach out to will depend on where you live, your insurance, and your healthcare options. There are many ways to get plugged into mental health care. The most important thing is to begin somewhere and decide not to quit until you get the help you need.

You might first reach out to your maternity or primary care provider, or to a mental health provider directly. If any of the professionals don't take you seriously or you find pregnancy and postpartum mental health disorders are beyond the scope of their practice, don't get discouraged. Rather, ask for a referral or recommendation. Your insurance can also give you a list of covered professionals in your area, and appendix C lists some helpful organizations, as well. You might also decide to pay out of pocket for someone who is known to provide excellent care. It may be the best investment you ever make!

> REMEMBER
>
> You have some freedom: who you begin your mental health care journey with may or may not be the person you decide to work with long-term.

Find someone you like who is caring, attentive, and available. Your options for mental health specialists include psychiatrists (*MDs* or *DOs*), psychiatric nurse practitioners (*PMHNPs*), clinical psychologists (*LCPs*), licensed professional counselors (*LPCs*), marriage family therapists (*MFTs*), or licensed clinical social workers (*LCSWs*). While all of these listed here can diagnose mental health problems, only the first two can prescribe medications. Often, though, non-prescribing mental health professionals will collaborate with those who do.

To help you determine if a mental health professional is adequately trained in supporting families and women like you, consider using these screening questions suggested by Dr. Bennett and Dr. Indman:[1]

- What specific training have you received in perinatal mood and anxiety disorders?

- Do you belong to any organization dedicated to education about perinatal mood and anxiety disorders? (Per Bennett and Indman, reputable ones include Postpartum Support International, Marce Society, North American Society for Psychosocial Obstetrics and Gynecology.[1])
- What books do you recommend to women with prenatal or postpartum depression or anxiety?

If the professional doesn't seem to have much experience, but you really connect well, all is not lost—as long as your desired candidate is compassionate and open to learning about PMADs.[1]

Last, don't give up on finding help. Accessing mental health care may feel like you're being asked to navigate an obstacle course. While this can be frustrating and discouraging, don't give up. You deserve to be well! So, keep fighting for your health and asking for help. Though challenging, it is worth it.

While finding the care you deserve may be a far-from-perfect process, the truth is, there's lots of work being done in the mental health field to improve insurance coverage and reimbursement and expand the number of mental health professionals in a network. If you are still finding it difficult to navigate, reach out to your loved ones and see if they can help advocate for you. You may also check out Postpartum Support International (PSI), an excellent resource committed to helping women and families find the help that they need.

d. Diagnosis and Treatment

So you've found a mental health professional, but what are the next steps?

Your first meeting with the professional sets the foundation for your success and may be in person, by phone, or online. No need to feel intimidated—it's simply a conversation where you share your concerns and answer questions designed to help them help you. This information is vital for the professional to start piecing together what might be going on. How much you share is up to you, and please know that privacy laws are in place to help you feel safe to share.

To reach an accurate diagnosis, your provider will use an official diagnostic tool called the *Diagnostic and Statistical Manual of Mental Health Disorders.*[1] While at times a diagnosis can come pretty quickly, other times it can take longer to tease out. Take heart and be patient.

To reach a specific diagnosis, the clinician groups together certain behaviors and common reported experiences, just as we cluster stars together to see constellations in the night sky (as some psychologists have likened it to). You may not fit neatly into one category, and that's okay. Putting a name to the mental health problem just gives us a starting point to understand what's going on and how to usher you toward wellness and recovery. It's not what defines you.

So, you have a diagnosis. Now what? First, there is no need to freak out or be ashamed. For one, they are incredibly common, and for two, it's not something you took on by choice. When your provider is discussing treatment options, be sure *you* feel comfortable with the plan before proceeding with it, and feel free to get the input of a loved one if you wish.

Choose the more effective, holistic approach. It's helpful to know that most often a multipronged approach to mental health care works the best—meaning you'll likely get better faster if you take the holistic approach and support your brain and the rest of your body together.

Because you are special and unique, your plan for healing will need to be customized to you.

For example, consider meeting regularly with a mental health professional and using supportive lifestyle changes, such as sleep, physical activity, and practicing newly learned coping techniques.[2,3] Supplements may be recommended (such as omega-3 fish oil or vitamin D) or possibly adjuvant therapies (like acupuncture, light therapy, energy work, aromatherapy, or yoga).[2,3] For those of you with moderate to severe symptoms, using medication on a daily (or as-needed) basis can also be very helpful.

Recovering and truly getting back to feeling like yourself can take some time, although you may start feeling better once your treatment plan has begun. Your body has been through a lot and needs time to return to equilibrium. But the good news is you'll start noticing moments when you feel better and then not just moments but days! At this point, take care to not overcommit yourself, since it can easily be a setback. Instead, take note of the blessings and bask in the good days, allowing yourself the time you need to fully heal.

In the recovery process, you'll also have moments and even days when you don't feel so well. Don't get discouraged—this is common. Think back on your overall trajectory and be reassured when you notice you *are* improving over time. Moreover, medications and dosages can take weeks for maximal effect and may even need to be fine-tuned or switched. In the meantime, keep pursuing your mental wellness and the dream of how you wish your life to be. Every day, you're a day closer!

e. Medications in Pregnancy and While Breastfeeding

During pregnancy, or while breastfeeding, many women wonder whether they should take medications that treat mental health problems, which are called *psychotropic* or *psychiatric* medications. Please know there is no perfect or easy answer: the decision is a very personal one (possibly made together with your partner or loved one) based on your mental health history, as well as your current diagnosis and its severity.

Sometimes, we try to simplify the decision, thinking of it as a choice between either taking medication or muscling through pregnancy (and motherhood) on our own strength. But really, it's about weighing two kinds of risks for you and your baby: the potential risks of medication versus the potential risks of untreated mental health problems. If this is something you are wrestling with, remember—countless other women like you are in similar situations, trying to make the best choice for themselves and their families.

When newly pregnant, many women *mistakenly* think that the best thing to do is suddenly stop all their psychotropic medications. Please, do *not* stop taking your medication without consulting with the prescribing provider. The decision to stop such a medication must be done wisely and in the right way. If done prematurely or abruptly, you may experience significant side effects or even relapse during a time when it's important to be well. So, if you are currently taking medications, the best thing to do is connect with your pre-scriber as soon as possible to discuss their potential use in pregnancy.

The great news is there are numerous medications for perinatal mood and anxiety disorders that can be used in pregnancy and while breastfeeding, including a type called *selective serotonin reuptake inhibitors (SSRIs)* for anxiety and depression.[1-9] Over time, more medications may be included as we learn more about their safety profiles and potential risks, especially as women using them volunteer to be part of pregnancy registries.[10]

CREATIVELY SUPPORT YOUR MAMA FRIENDS

If you have mental health problems or are taking medication for your mental health, help further research on the use of psychiatric medication in pregnancy and after having a baby! Enroll in Massachusetts General Hospital's national pregnancy registry for psychiatric medications. It's designed to benefit mamas like you. Call 1-866-961-2388 or see their website in appendix C for more details.

Since there is no "best" medication, seek to make an informed decision based on the latest research. If you're worried by what you hear from friends, family, or in the media, discuss those concerns with your prescriber instead of letting them derail you. Likely you'll find the information was presented incompletely—like a sketch rather than a finished painting.

When discussing the pros and cons of continuing or starting a new medication, your healthcare provider will need to discuss (1) the medication's effects on you (benefits, side effects, and risks), and (2) any potential impact on your baby. For example, you'll want to find out what the newest research says about its use while breastfeeding, and any potential risks for miscarriage, congenital malformations, pregnancy complications, and long-term issues (like behavioral or learning problems).

Be a wise mama and listen carefully. When you're given various statistics, be sure to ask about the *absolute risk* and not just the *relative risk*. The former tells you how common a certain problem is (like 3 out of 100,000 pregnancies), while the latter tells you how many more times something occurs (like a certain side effect is twice as likely to occur). This is an important distinction because if a certain medication doubles your risk for a problem, but this problem is already very rare, a doubling of a risk still means the problem is unlikely to occur. Consider checking out the resources in appendix C if you need additional reliable information to help you decide.

Also, if an effective medication is not considered safe while breastfeeding, you may decide not to breastfeed in favor of pursuing your mental wellness. If this is you, please free yourself from guilt and think of it as avoiding breastfeeding "for medical reasons." Even share this phrase with anyone prying into your business.

Deciding to start or discontinue a psychotropic medication may be one of the best decisions of your life. By either taking the right medication(s) over time, or stopping the use of unnecessary or unhelpful ones, many women are relieved to find their symptoms improve—they feel back to themselves and can function and live life fully. This can be you!

Medications are usually started at a low dose and increased gradually until you feel well or experience ill side effects. At times, your prescriber may need to work with you on switching or replacing medications. Depending on what is prescribed, it may be taken daily or as needed and may take a few weeks to feel maximal effects. Be patient and make sure you are taking your medication(s) as prescribed. If you take a "daily" medication only occasionally, it will not work!

Reach out to your prescribing provider if you have any concerning side effects or if you're considering taking supplements or drinking alcohol, since both may affect a medication's performance and may cause significant side effects. Later in pregnancy, you may find your medication less effective due to your naturally increased blood volumes. This, too, is a time to reach out to your prescriber, since he or she may need to increase your dosage.

Last, please know that taking medication does not necessarily mean you will be on it for the rest of your life. You are unique, and your path to long-term recovery will be, too. For example, it's usually recommended to stay on SSRIs for a time after feeling well again to minimize the chance of relapse. Remember, have grace for yourself and give your body the time to stabilize and recover completely.

f. Nurturing Mental Wellness

In prior sections, we discussed the importance of your mental health and how it impacts you, your baby, and family. Here, you'll find some fun and practical ways to support your mental wellness. While the elements here have appeared in previous sections, this is a condensed version—like a bouquet of tips curated especially for you, available to enjoy at your leisure. If you're wondering, *What's leisure?* focus on one or two attainable items and explore others when you can, to see what you most enjoy.

Get adequate rest. This will make the biggest impact on your mental wellness, hands down. If you're pregnant, aim for seven to nine hours of sleep (or rest).[1] Waking up during the night? Although it can get frustrating, try to rest or fall back asleep instead of stressing over it (see "Getting Rest" in week 26 for tips).

If you're postpartum, it's vital for you to get at least five to six consecutive hours of sleep nightly, especially if mental wellness has been or continues to be a challenge. A relatively rested body and mind are game changers! To make this possible: delegate baby duty, use ear plugs or sleep in another room, and resist the urge to save the day whenever you hear your little one cry. If you're breastfeeding, this consecutive chunk of sleep may be broken up once for pumping so you can maintain your milk supply. Remember, naps are also a good way to make up for lost sleep, though the benefits you get from them are not identical to those of nighttime sleep.

Be active. Physical activity is an awesome way to decrease your stress, anxiety, or depression and can even be as effective as psychiatric medication at relieving depressive symptoms![2-5] Though the ideal type, amount, and intensity of activity needed to gain these benefits is still unknown, try to get at least the base recommendation of 30 minutes daily (for at least three days a week). With this amount, you will likely notice improvement pretty quickly. Aim for exercises that make you out of breath and a form of resistance training such as lifting weights. As always, be sure to pick something you enjoy!

> See B-2 for more on exercise in pregnancy and postpartum.

Eat well: nutritious and timely meals or snacks. Though it can be tempting to skip quality or skip a meal entirely, don't! The right fuel on time will make you feel so much better. So even if life is crazy or you don't have an appetite, eat a snack or small meal every two to three hours during the day. You'll have more energy, cope better, and have fewer mood swings.

Throughout the day, sustain your blood sugar with proteins and fiber while limiting sodas, juices, sweets, and processed foods. Two to three times a week, try low-mercury, sustainable fish like salmon, sardines, or rainbow trout, and benefit from their awesome, anti-inflammatory omega-3 fatty acids—or ask your maternity care provider about a fish oil supplement.[2,6,7] For adults, a serving size of fish is 4 oz, about the size of the palm of your hand.[7]

Stay hydrated. Dehydration can make you feel more anxious. So, drink plenty of water throughout the day—both when thirsty and if your urine is no longer clear or light yellow—and limit caffeine.

Enjoy personal space. Mamas often underestimate the intensity of mothering and feel guilty when apart from their families. However, enjoying some "you time" is a powerful way to recharge. Ask family, friends, babysitters, or local mom groups for child care support. Even taking a shower *alone* can make a difference. Try it—you won't regret it!

Become a relaxation guru. Practicing daily meditation, a type of relaxation, is wonderful for you and your baby. Tap into your body's innate calming process to counteract the fight-or-flight stress response. You can elicit this *relaxation response*, or deep relaxation, in many ways, including through yoga, progressive relaxation, hypnosis, or prayer, and even walking, swimming, or knitting.[8] Start with 1–5 minutes

HOW DO I MEDITATE?[8,11]

- Find a quiet place.
- Get comfy (whether sitting, standing, moving, or lying down).
- Pick something to focus on: an object or movement, or a sound, word, prayer, or phrase that you can repeat silently or aloud.
- Have a passive attitude. Accept when it doesn't go perfectly. In fact, when your mind is bombarded with other thoughts, don't worry. Have grace for yourself and try to refocus. It takes practice to quiet the mind.

a day and work your way up to even 20 minutes at a time.[9] Practice this regularly and also when you get stressed or anxious. If you have a history of recurrent depression, mindfulness-based cognitive behavioral therapy with a mental health professional can greatly decrease your risk of relapse![10]

Incorporate other relaxing activities. Why not make your daily life more refreshing? Check out B-3c for ideas. Some of them are quite entertaining with younger children.

Be with those you love. Friends and family can be life-giving. Spend time with those who build you up and support you. You are made for community.

Laugh. Sometimes we just need a good laugh to lighten things up. Call or hang out with those who add joy to your life, or watch, read, or listen to something that gives you a good belly laugh.

Spend time outdoors. Enjoy the fresh air, greenery, and weather. They liven the spirit and bring perspective. If you're especially tired, even opening a window or sitting outside is a great start!

Catch a few rays. Another bonus of being in the sun is it boosts your vitamin D levels—a hormone precursor essential for your body's support and immune system. In fact, if you're struggling with mental health problems, ask your healthcare provider to check your vitamin D levels, since deficiencies might be part of the cause.

Grow your spiritual side. Be sure to nurture the essence of who you are—your soul. Some ideas include reading spiritual books, listening to inspiring music or talks, going on nature walks, connecting with God/a higher power, and spending time with your spiritual community.

g. Cultivating a Healthy Relationship with Your Body

Accepting and treasuring our bodies is vital to loving and respecting ourselves. Read on for practical ways to nurture a healthy body image (courtesy of Michele Minero, MFT, and Veronica Benjamin, RD), as well as tip-offs that may indicate your relationship with your body could use a makeover.[*]

Practice daily thankfulness.[†] Answer these two questions—even on those days when your body does not look or behave perfectly.

- What are you grateful for today? (Think about all those blessings in your life, large or small.)
- In what ways is your body working for you? Write a list and post it somewhere where you'll actually see it (like the fridge door or bathroom mirror).

Reread your answers often. When your thoughts about your body are unkind or harsh, try to stop yourself and replace those thoughts with items on your list.

Practice self-compassion and empathy.[‡] Many of us forget how important it is to be loving, patient, and kind toward ourselves. Try to follow this standard for self-talk: don't say it about yourself if you wouldn't say it to someone you love.[1] Go ahead, get started today! If you're unsure how to practice self-compassion and empathy, but know you want things to be different, this is the perfect time to seek professional support. (If you're still unsure, check out how you're doing with the following litmus test.)

Take a litmus test.[§] Answering these questions can help you better assess if would benefit from a revamped relationship with your body.

---

[*] Michele Minero, MFT, personal communication July 18, 2015, and Veronica Benjamin, RD, personal communication, August 1, 2015

[†] Minero

[‡] Minero

[§] Benjamin

- Are you having trouble accepting weight gain?
- Are you fixating on things, such as what you don't like about your body, your weight, or weight gain in pregnancy?
- Are you feeling depressed or angry around your body's changes?
- Is your eating affected by your emotions or weight obsessions?
- Is your emotional state affecting your sense of well-being?

If your answer is yes to any of these, be encouraged! You don't need to go on like this. Things truly can change for you, especially if you work with a mental health professional or registered dietitian who specializes in body image or eating disorders. They can help you learn to cope with your thoughts and feelings and give you useful tools and exercises to help you have a healthy baby and an enjoyable pregnancy journey—and life! To connect to this kind of support, contact the National Eating Disorders Association helpline (see appendix C) or reach out to your health care provider.

TAKE CARE OF YOURSELF

For a holistic approach to wellness, see the guides for nurturing your mental wellness (B-4f), balanced nutrition (B-1), and getting the most out of physical activity (B-2).

h. Substance Use

Dear pregnant mama, congratulations for taking the time to learn more about how substance use may impact you and your little bundle. Please know you are not alone. Substance use (and abuse) is quite common, but the good news is there are options for support.

Although we can't get into details about every substance in this short section, we will talk about some of the research on cigarettes, alcohol, and marijuana, since they are so commonly used.[1] We will not specifically cover misused prescription drugs (like OxyContin or Xanax) or other illicit drugs (like methamphetamine or cocaine), though these also fall into the category of substances that are harmful to both you and your baby. In the second section, you'll find ideas on what to do if you have been using substances during your pregnancy and are interested in reducing or stopping your use.

Common substances and their impact

Alcohol affects your baby's brain development and can cause intellectual disabilities.[2] It can also lead to the most severe fetal alcohol spectrum disorder, Fetal Alcohol Syndrome, which includes a range of birth defects and can impair your baby's physical growth in utero.[2] As such, there is no safe amount of alcohol use in pregnancy. If you're finding it hard to suddenly quit, work on decreasing your use—it makes a difference!

If breastfeeding, remember, it's best to generally avoid alcohol since it enters your breastmilk and may decrease your milk production.[2] If you'd like to indulge in an occasional drink, right after breastfeeding, go ahead and have a standard alcoholic drink (i.e., 1.5 oz of liquor, 5 oz of wine, or 12 oz of beer).[3] You can breastfeed again once it's been at least two hours, which is how long it takes for the alcohol levels in your milk to decrease after one standard drink.[4]

Cigarette smoke, whether inhaled directly or secondhand, decreases the supply of oxygen and nutrients to your baby.[5] Cigarette smoke also increases your baby's chance of developing cleft lip or palate, being born prematurely, and having a low birth weight; it also means a greater likelihood that your baby will develop learning and behavioral problems, asthma, and lung infections later in life.[5] In pregnancy, it escalates the chance for stillbirth or developing serious problems with your placenta (your baby's lifeline), while postpartum, it increases risk of sudden infant death syndrome.[5]

The good news is it's never too late to quit! Quitting (and even decreasing) your smoking makes a huge difference to your baby! Nicotine patches, gum, lozenges, quitting with a partner, and getting good support can make quitting possible—for good.

If you're still smoking postpartum, you may still be able to breastfeed. Although nicotine enters your milk, your milk has so many amazing benefits that your healthcare provider will likely still encourage you to breastfeed.[5] Be sure to smoke outside and away from your baby while you continue to work on quitting.

Marijuana (Cannabis) can be smoked, vaped, eaten, or applied to your skin but not during pregnancy.[6] Although legal in some states, it is *not* considered safe to use in pregnancy. Yes, it is "natural," but it is made up of hundreds of chemicals and is much stronger now than it used to be.

When a mother uses cannabis products during pregnancy, her baby may be more likely to be born preterm and have a low birth weight and size—which increases the infant's chance of disabilities.[7] Moreover, marijuana harms a baby's brain development by decreasing problem-solving abilities and memory, while increasing hyperactivity and impulsivity.[7] Instead of using marijuana, check out other healthier options to relax and nurture your mental wellness (B-3c and B-4f).

If breastfeeding, it's best to avoid marijuana since the main chemical, tetrahydrocannabinol (THC), enters breastmilk and can remain there from six days to six weeks.[7,8] Because your baby's brain continues to undergo dramatic development after birth, marijuana may continue to negatively impact your little one's brain development. Marijuana may also decrease your milk production and quality.[7]

If using substances during pregnancy

Consider your relationship with substance use. Let's be honest—we begin to use substances for all sorts of reasons. Some of us use because those around us use, or we think it's a good way to relax and unwind; others of us turn to substances as a tool to cope with hardships. Many mamas who use substances are struggling with underlying issues—like untreated mental health problems, past trauma, or intimate partner violence—or they have a family history of substance use. In fact, when it comes to addiction, "[it] can be described as chronically and compulsively numbing and taking the edge off of feelings."[9]

Regardless of why or how it began, we often continue to use one or more substances to serve some purpose in our lives.[¶] It can be very hard to reduce or stop our use because of this, and the thought of quitting may cause a variety of negative feelings such as anger, sadness, or even resentment toward the baby. These feelings are completely normal and natural.

It's important to recognize your feelings about quitting but not let them dictate your behavior. You are absolutely capable of reducing or stopping your substance use to protect yourself and your baby. The right professional support can make all the difference.

Acknowledge that substance use affects your whole life. While it might be easiest to imagine physiological changes—from its impacts on your brain, heart, and lungs to potentially life-threatening overdose or withdrawals—the consequences of substance (ab)use are often more than just physiological.

Depending on the substance(s) and how often you use, you could be at greater risk for domestic violence, impaired decision-making abilities, and poor functioning at home or at work, all of which make it harder for you to enjoy your life.[6,10] Your relationship with your baby suffers from each of these, and if your functioning is impaired enough by your substance use to hurt your baby's safety and well-being, you are at risk of involvement with Child Welfare Services.[8]

Know that reducing or stopping your use is a loving act toward yourself and your baby. Most medical professionals agree that no substance use is safe for your baby during pregnancy.[11] While this is true, even reducing your use can make a difference.

Remember, regardless of what substance you are using, there is hope! If you're feeling like it's time for a change—that's wonderful! Perhaps

¶ Ann Soliday Bench, MPH, RN, PHN, personal communication, May 5, 2021

you have even realized you need real help for your mental health problems or want healing from current or past pain or trauma. With this discovery, let pregnancy or mothering be a turning point for you.

This is the perfect time to get connected with the right supportive resources that are unique to your situation, to learn healthy coping options, and to begin the process of a new life. In fact, you can take a valuable step today by starting to reduce your use. Please peruse the resources in appendix C for ideas on where to go from here, check out your local 12-step programs, or reach out to your maternity or healthcare provider if you feel safe bringing this up. For when you are well, you're giving your child one of the greatest (and most needed) gifts you could possibly give—you!

i. When Things Don't Go as Planned

Traumatic birth

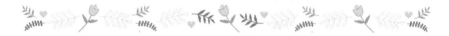

Dear friend,

If you are reading this, then your birth experience likely did not fit your hopes or expectations. Worse still, you may have felt ignored, abandoned, unsupported, uninformed, or betrayed during the labor or birthing process.[1-3] If this is you, I'm so sorry. This should have never happened.

The unfortunate truth is these experiences are all too common and can even appear alongside other, scarier circumstances that can cause a profound emotional impact. This intense impact, known as trauma, occurs when there is an actual (or perceived) threat of either serious injury or fatality for a mother or her baby.[3]

After a birth experience that was negative or traumatic, you may find that you feel down, numb, hopeless, disconnected from your baby, or have trouble sleeping. It's also common to notice birth flashbacks or distressing dreams, and you may be avoiding anything that reminds you of what you went through—even your little one.[1] Perhaps you feel guilty that you didn't somehow heroically prevent the circumstances that caused this trauma.

Please know that you are experiencing a common reaction to what you went through, and remind yourself you did the best you could in an overwhelming and scary moment.[1] Allow yourself to grieve the loss of your hoped-for birth experience and to remember it's okay to be angry with how you were let down. It's okay to cry and to ask questions—especially when talking with your maternity care provider about your labor experiences. Since we all internalize our experiences differently, unless you speak up, they may not have any idea how deeply your labor impacted you.[3] *This conversation could play a pivotal role in your healing process, while hopefully laying the groundwork for a profoundly different labor experience in the future!*

If you haven't already, please reach out for help—regardless of whether your birth trauma happened a while ago or recently. An experienced mental health professional is a wonderful resource to help you with your symptoms and usher you into a place of healing. They will have a variety of methods to help you heal, which might include the highly effective treatment called eye movement desensitization and reprocessing or EMDR.[1]

While it may be tempting to try to ignore your pain and hope you will cope with the trauma on your own, please don't. Trauma is not just about the event itself but is "also [about] the imprint left by that experience on the mind, brain and body."[4] *It affects people profoundly afterward—even causing the brain to change its alarm system, its reactions, and how it releases stress hormones.*[4] *These changes, if not treated, can negatively impact most areas of your life—including how you feel about yourself, how you bond with your baby, and even how you experience intimacy or future pregnancies.*[2]

So please, don't try to go through this alone. Reach out. You and your family deserve for you to be well, and with the right help, healing is possible!

Your friend,

Emese

Pregnancy loss

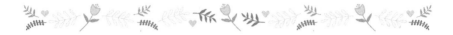

Dear friend,

When your pregnancy ends unexpectedly, it's hard to know what to do or even think. Likely, everything around you feels surreal. You may be numb and in shock, not even understanding how you got here. Ever since that moment, you may have been in utter disbelief, just going through the motions of your day. While reading this, you may be crying, noticing an ache in your heart or a void around you. Perhaps you're wondering if that heaviness will ever lift, and if you'll ever be able to laugh or feel like yourself again.

Sweet friend, how I wish I could be there with you, to help comfort you in your pain. I'd want to sit with you—even if in silence. I'd pass you fresh tissues (so you wouldn't keep reusing that same old shredded one), bring you hot tea with honey, and make you homemade chicken soup or mac 'n cheese. I'd place a nice big box of yummy chocolates on your nightstand for later—you know, for when that actually sounded good. I'd extend a hand and offer you a hug, a hair tie, and a sincere listening ear.

I hope you'd feel at ease to say whatever was on your heart. Whether anger, sadness, despair, pain, a tangle of emotions or questions, or even a string of swear words. (God knows I've used plenty of those myself.) All of that would be expected and welcomed. You're grieving, and you deserve the space to do just that—to simply be.

I know none of these things would make your pain go away, but my prayer is that you wouldn't have to go through this alone. That you'd remember how special, precious, and loved you are and would know that you were never meant to go through something like this. That's why it hurts so bad.

If I could, I'd pull back your bedroom curtains, open your window, and welcome in the fresh air and the outside sounds so they might plant within you a tiny seed of hope. Of course, you probably wouldn't notice it at the time, but this minuscule seed could still take root in your heart. Over the coming weeks to months, it would soak up your tears and slowly stretch closer to the heavens until one day, you'd marvel at how what now seems impossible—joy, beauty, and laughter—is in your life once again.

Your friend,

Emese

5. HEALTHY RELATIONSHIPS

a. Cultivate Effective Communication

> *The difference between the right word and the almost right word is*
> *the difference between lightning and a lightning bug.*
> —MARK TWAIN

So glad you've stopped by to perfect those communication skills of yours! The following content applies to all sorts of settings and relationships, so feel free to grab your partner for this section. After all, communication—the transferring of information between people—is a two-way road. The more equipped you both are, the more skillful your communication can get—even when it comes to tough topics like money, parenting, and in-laws.

And the good news? Even though effective communication can sometimes be hard and exhausting, the payout is huge. In fact, effective, considerate communication has no downsides. It not only builds friendship and intimacy but can also bring peace and satisfaction to your life. Also, it's the foundation on which you build a harmonious, joyful, and peaceful nest and haven. Your baby and family will love that.

So, what does effective communication look like? For starters, let's imagine two people salsa dancing together. Can you picture how coordinated and fluid their movements are? So impressive. Adept communication is just like this. (And don't worry, you don't have to be physically coordinated to be skilled in this.) When executed well, communication (like dancing) is smooth, freeing, and fulfilling, transforming two separate people into a unified pair.

What's tricky is that getting in sync is an art form, not a formula, and it hinges on constantly connecting with one another. Even when the partner is exhausted, sweaty, and smelly (in other words, *unlovely*).

Sure, it can be tempting to give up, but the dedicated pair presses on anyway, knowing it provides a way to not only have fun together but also to realize their goals.

To be a team, dancers (like good communicators) also need to become experts on one another, learning to both express oneself and to understand the other's verbal and nonverbal communication (like facial expressions, body language, tone of voice). That's not easy! Come to think of it, they also need to be creative, invest in learning new moves and steps, and find enough courage to practice through the awkwardness. What commitment and determination! But in the end, they'll create art in motion.

Just as a whole dance is broken into smaller steps, so, too, is the path to skilled communication. When you practice them, the following tips will help you "dance" with those close to you and prepare you to communicate with the more difficult people in your life (those with whom you'd never want to be caught dancing). So, you might ask, what are these steps to clearer communication? Check these out:

Tips for healthy communication

Be honest. Both with yourself and others. Silence is often *not* golden. In fact, it can make you fester inside, build resentment, and ultimately hurt you and others. So, if there's something needing to be said, say it, but *remember,* your words are powerful. They can stick with people for life.

Try to avoid throwing verbal daggers just to get even. Yes, it may feel so very satisfying at the time, but it will only give you more brokenness to mend in the end. Also, if you need to approach a particularly tough topic, a mediator (like a counselor) can be an invaluable resource.

Listen like a spy. Communication involves both speaking *and listening*, and one without the other is both a waste of time and a perfect recipe for a sleepless night. While people tend to be better at speaking than listening, it's important to remember we have two ears and one mouth for a reason. "The most important thing in communication," says Peter Drucker, an influential management thinker, "is hearing what isn't said."[1]

So, go ahead, take on the challenge to slow down; put down your electronic devices and listen with your eyes and heart, too. What's the person's facial expression and body language telling you? What is being said behind the words? Is the person excited, elated, hurt, disappointed, angry, ashamed, or sad?

Ask questions that take your conversation a layer deeper—while it's good to address the superficial facts about *what* happened, look beyond the *what* and try to resolve *how* it had an impact on the feelings of those involved. For instance, what do the actions or words say about how the person feels?

To get a sense for these emotions, ask clarifying questions like, "I hear you saying my parents don't give you enough space. Is that what you were trying to say?" Or "It sounds like traveling for work stresses you out. Is that right?"

If it's your turn to talk, remember, using the first person is a great way to go; it gives you the chance to say how you were affected by someone's words or actions without pointing fingers and putting the person on the defensive. Examples of first-person statements are: "I feel sad when you ___." or "When you say the soup is too salty, I feel like you don't appreciate what I do."

Express appreciation. This is equally as important as conveying pain, hurt, or frustration. Genuine affirmation is incredibly life-giving. It's what nurtures relationships and keeps them thriving. When we take time to acknowledge what we appreciate about people, the benefits are twofold. First, by focusing on the positive, we have a better outlook on life, and second, our words help others feel valued and their efforts honored. So keep your eyes peeled for what you're grateful for!

Take a break if listening well, asking good questions, and expressing appreciation are not working in the heat of the moment. Remember, you don't need to solve the problem pronto. This is especially important when difficult things are said or if your conversation is spiraling out of control.

Breathe, and get some distance. Go in another room or go for a walk. Although tempting, you don't need to storm out or slam the door; you can simply say you need some space. If you're the one hearing this from your partner, accept it. Extend grace and allow your partner to return when he or she is ready to talk.

Remember, little can be accomplished when you're so fired up that you feel like punching a hole in the wall. Do yourselves a favor and slow things down. Even 30 minutes can work wonders. This break helps re-engage the more sophisticated part of your brain (the prefrontal cortex), which helps you think more clearly (before, you were mainly operating with your emotional center, the limbic system).

Practice forgiveness. Forgiveness can free you and allow healing for both you and the relationship. Sometimes we misunderstand forgiveness and think it means being a doormat or dismissing the wrong and saying what happened was okay (when of course, it wasn't!). Really, it means we're letting go and actively choosing against unforgiveness. Remembering the wrong done and holding on to the hurt can harbor bitterness and eat us up from the inside, while forgiveness offers healing. You can even thank them for their apology if you want to go all out.[2]

As we all know, sometimes forgiveness comes fairly easy, while other times, we feel so wronged that true forgiving first involves inner work and processing. Continue in this work for your own soul's sake! When you finally do get to the point when you're ready to forgive, try saying: "I forgive you for ___." In cases where you're having a hard time forgiving, or the person continues hurting you, go ahead and talk to a counselor or therapist about how to approach your difficult situation. They can provide perspective, encouragement, and a path forward.

Practice the steps. Focus on one or two of these communication tips and add it to your repertoire. (Look at you, being all sophisticated!) Eventually, as you improve, combining all these steps will feel even more natural. To choose your first tip: Consider your home, work, or social environment. From your memory of conversations and miscommunications, which tools seem especially useful? What skill do you and your partner most need to improve to get your groove on and start dancing like the pros?

b. Explore Expectations

All of us have expectations, but most of us have no idea what they are until life exposes them. *Surprise!* Think of expectations like cracks on a sidewalk—if you're not proactive and aware, you're bound to trip over them, at some point.

However, when you discuss potential pitfalls with your partner or loved ones, you can work together to fill in those gaps, leveling the pathway between you. This process, which is much like doing construction work in your relationships, can save you both from breaking a nose, an ankle, or a friendship.

Set aside the time to chat about expectations, hopes, dreams, things that excite you, and those that worry you. Pregnancy is a journey, and a journey is a great time to reflect. Find a designated time to chat, like a lunch or walk date. To prepare for a conversation, jot down or journal your thoughts to save them for your rendezvous. If you're not quite sure where to start, check out these questions to get your ideas going.

Let the following questions launch you into an exploration of

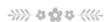

When discussing expectations, explore important topics like life with your baby, relationships, roles of mothers and fathers, childbirth, breastfeeding, going back to work, child care, and in-laws.

the thoughts and expectations related to pregnancy, labor, and parenting. Think of them like little gifts for you to open and explore with your partner, family, and friends—a process of surprising discovery. Unlike Christmas presents, though, these gifts are not meant to be opened all in one day, since that could get a tad overwhelming. Instead, pace yourself. Pick a topic that's interesting to you and run with it until you're ready for another one. You've got time.

Discussion questions

Parenting/family

- What does it mean to be a good parent?
- Do mothers and fathers have different roles, and if so, what are they?
- What did your mother and father do well and what do you want to do differently as a parent?
- Are there any cultural practices that your family expects postpartum? If so, what are they and how important are they to you? Which of these practices do you want to uphold?
- What perks and challenges do you anticipate with in-laws once your baby arrives?

Childbirth

- How do you think you'll experience labor? What are your strengths? What are your fears?
- How do you expect women and their support people to feel after labor?
- If you've given birth before, what went well then and what would you like to go differently?

New life

- What will life look like with a new baby?
- If you have other children, how do you think they'll respond to a new baby? What can you do to help them adjust and feel reassured of your love? (For some ideas, see "Helping Your Older Child Adjust" in week 39.)

- How have you seen relationships and friendships change once a baby is born?
- What method of birth control are you interested in using postpartum to safely space your pregnancies?

Logistics

- Who will help feed the baby and help change diapers?
- How do you plan to feed your baby? What do you think breastfeeding is like?
- If you breastfed before, would you like your breastfeeding experience to be any different? If so, how, specifically? (Be sure to bring these up with your maternity care provider or lactation consultant so they can help you reach your goals.)

Supporting wellness

- What kind of support do new moms need? What kind of support do new dads or partners need?
- Who are the trustworthy caregivers for your baby when you need help?
- What does postpartum depression look like for a parent?
- If you have a history of worsening postpartum mental health (like postpartum depression or anxiety), what support and strategies do you think would help you cope and decrease the risk of recurrence?

Work

- Will you go back to work postpartum, and if so, how soon?
- If breastfeeding, will you continue to breastfeed after returning to work?

c. Set Healthy Boundaries

Healthy relationships come from good, established boundaries. After all, boundaries protect, love, and keep us whole.[1] When you have them in place, they create order around you and keep you from being stomped on. Just as your uterine walls are vital for housing your baby, so boundaries protect and uphold functional relationships. They set foundational guidelines for respecting and loving others and for nurturing your family. In fact, boundaries are what will make your baby thrive and feel safe.

Empower yourself to say no—it's vital for creating healthy boundaries. Don't worry, *no* isn't a swear word or even a bad word. Use it when needed, and witness how it (ultimately) creates a positive change in your day and relationships.

Be prepared: at first, people will likely freak out, push, and try to manipulate you with all their might. Yes, this can be irritating since it takes courage to set boundaries, and instead of pushback, you truly deserve a standing ovation for making your boundaries known and holding your ground. In the face of this manipulation, stand firm like a pillar and don't back down. Why? Eventually, they will understand you mean business and this is the new you. People won't be able to control you, and you'll feel as if you just inhaled a fresh breath of mountain air.

Remember your resources. If you're still having trouble setting those much-needed boundaries or realizing where they should go, skilled counselors or therapists (expert boundary-setters) can give you valuable perspectives and practical tips. Their insight can include how to navigate difficult responses from pushy mothers-in-law, overbearing loved ones, demanding children who are acting like bosses, or bosses who are acting like children. Reach out for help! You don't have to go it alone.

Finally, congratulate yourself. By taking the time and effort to hone your communication skills, clarify expectations, and set healthy boundaries, you are proactively creating a nurturing nest for you and your family. Way to go!

d. Sex in Pregnancy

As we've discussed throughout this book, there are lots of awesome ways to cultivate your relationship with your partner. Unless your maternity care provider advised you to abstain due to pregnancy complications, sex can certainly be a great way to find pleasure and foster intimacy. However, by now you've likely realized sex while pregnant is a bit different than before. Read on to find some ideas about how to help you adjust and enjoy.

Find your inner roar. Remember, you're a sexy woman. You may not feel it, but let me remind you—you are to the rest of the world! You embody fertility and are a budding mystery from inside out. To carry a child, you're strong, unique, special, and courageous. Bask in this reality for a moment.

Embrace your changing body. Use your body to your advantage as you explore and experience new things.

Spice things up. Drape yourself in something sexy. Find lacy or leopard-print tanks and lingerie that highlight your adorable bump or your playboy-material breasts. For a splash of color, try a bold new lipstick. For a good dazzle, wear your jewelry. Make music playlists for those special moments and set the mood by pulling out the massage oil, body candy, and scented candles. Go ahead, surprise yourself and your partner by mixing it up!

Splurge on sex games or nontoxic sex toys. What a great time to try something new. Make sure the toys (like a vibrator) are phthalate-free and nontoxic. Avoid cheap toys—they're likely to have all sorts of harmful junk that could cause reproductive damage for your baby. Remember to wash them before every use.

Take some boudoir photos. Make a date with your partner for some sexy, pregnant mama pics or find a professional photographer who will help you create a little surprise for your partner.

Use props. Remember, pillows and chairs may be your new best friends.

Have fun. Pregnant mamas can never have this too much.

Slip 'n slide. Using a lubricant can work wonders if your vagina's feeling like the Sahara. However, lubes are not all created equal. Some can actually harm your vagina and vulva, making them scream, and potentially increase your chance of getting an STI.[1-4] So, make sure your lube is free of nonoxynol-9 (N-9), parabens, glycerin, propylene glycol, chlorhexidine gluconate, and polyquaternium.[1-5]

GREAT WATER-BASED LUBES[1-3]

- Good Clean Love
- AH! YES
- Pre-seed (a fertility-friendly option)

GREAT SILICONE-BASED LUBES[1-3]

- Wet Platinum
- Female Condom 2 (FC2) (pre-lubricated internal condom)

Want organic lubes? Look for an "NSF/ANSI 305" label.[6]

Remember the rules of oral and anal sex.

> **Oral sex:** Have at it, but make sure your partner doesn't blow air into your vagina. This could cause an *air embolism* (an air bubble in a blood vessel), which is dangerous to you and your baby.

> **Anal sex:** People have mixed feelings about this one. Only have anal sex if you feel comfortable with a backdoor visit. This is a very sensitive body part, and it's easy to track bacteria from the anus into the vagina. Use plenty of lubrication (designed for anal sex) and a condom if you are not absolutely sure about your partner's STI history. Never allow the penis to enter the vagina right after anal penetration. Last, if your partner is pressuring you to have sex in a way that makes you uncomfortable, please read B-5f.

Sex positions during pregnancy

Once upon a time, sex may have been more straightforward. As your cute belly grows, certain sex positions probably aren't as comfortable or as possible as before. No worries, all is not lost! Modify your positions as needed—a great opportunity to get out of your comfort zone and try something new. Here are some top contenders to consider:

Cowgirl. Partner lies down, and you sit on top, facing one another. You can control the depth of penetration.

> **Variation 1:** Same as above, except face your partner's feet.

> **Variation 2:** Partner sits in a chair, and you sit on top, facing away.

Spooning. Both lie on your right or left sides, with your partner behind you.

Doggy style. Kneel on all fours, while your partner kneels behind you.

Edge of bed. Lie face up with your legs bent, hips near the edge of the bed, and feet resting on the edge. Partner stands beside the bed.

On a chair. You sit on a chair, and your partner kneels in front of you.

e. Physical Changes That Affect Postpartum Sex

As we discussed in "Diving Back In: Sex after Childbirth" (postpartum week 6), sex postpartum may be a little different, at least for a while. On the following pages, you'll find common physical changes that can occur after birth, how long they may last, and helpful tips to try in the meantime. As always, your maternity care provider can be a great resource, as can physical therapists who specialize in the pelvic floor.

Sexual functioning. You may have decreased desire, arousal, and sexual satisfaction, and it may be more difficult to orgasm.[1-6] This is typically the hardest during the first 6 weeks postpartum, but can last longer, sometimes up to 12 months. The good news is that these tend to naturally improve each month, with a leap around 3 months postpartum.[3]

- Be patient with yourself.
- Spend time with your partner and talk about how both of you are doing.
- Be intimate in creative ways, especially if you don't want to have penetrative sex.
- Reach out to your healthcare provider. It can make all the difference to have professional support and resources.
- Remember your mental health as well as psychiatric medications and their dosages can have a profound impact. For example, sometimes selective serotonin reuptake inhibitors (SSRIs) can decrease libido and arousal or make it harder to orgasm. Healthcare providers have strategies to improve these, so don't be shy!

Breasts. While breastfeeding, your breasts are much more sensitive. They may be very tender when full or engorged and can change in size, depending on how long ago you last breastfed. You may also drip milk at unexpected times (like during orgasm, breast stimulation, or with sucking during sex). And thanks to your new bombshells, you may have an improved body image. These breast changes will continue as long as you breastfeed, though sensitivity should greatly improve after the first few weeks.

- Try having sex after breastfeeding or pumping.
- In desperate times, instate a "hands off" policy.
- Wear a supportive bra.
- Have fun with leakage during sex by keeping a cute hankie handy for clean-up. If you don't want to sprinkle, use a nursing pad in your bra.
- Of course, flaunt those babies like never before.

Nipples. If breastfeeding or pumping, your nipples can sometimes be red and sore, or may crack if your newborn is still learning to latch properly. This should greatly improve after the first few weeks of breastfeeding once this lovely latch is learned.

- Minimize touching these darlings during intimacy, as needed.
- To help with the healing, perfect your baby's latch and apply some expressed breastmilk or medical-grade lanolin cream (unless you're allergic to wool).
- If still experiencing cracking or pain, be sure to get help from a certified lactation consultant—a modern-day breastfeeding wizard.

Vagina. It probably comes as no surprise, but after pushing a baby out, vaginas can feel different—looser from childbirth, tighter from stitches, or drier from hormonal changes caused by breastfeeding.[7] Some mamas can experience painful vaginal intercourse (*dyspareunia*), which is most often mild and resolves within a few weeks to months.[3,7] It may feel more intense and last longer, however, if you had a delivery using forceps or vacuum, or trauma to your perineum.[3,6-8] These changes typically will improve with lubricant use and with time; the breastfeeding-related dryness will resolve when you stop breastfeeding.

- To help, find the right type of vaginal lubricant (see B-5d) and start out slow.
- Consider oral sex or manual stimulation before having penetrative sex.
- When ready, try positions that allow you to have more control over the depth of penetration (see B-5d).
- If experiencing the sensation of looseness, dedicate some time to the wonder exercise—Kegels! (See "recipe" in A-3c.)

Vulva. Even if you ended up having a Cesarean birth, your vulva may be swollen from labor. Or it may be painful from cuts or perineal tears. Be encouraged, though, swelling decreases within a few days to weeks, and superficial cuts heal quickly (7–10 days). Stitches reabsorb in about 3 weeks and may cause mild itching while healing. Pain in the area typically improves within 1–2 months, though in the case of a third- or fourth-degree tear or episiotomy, it may take longer.

- Wear loose clothing and avoid painful sitting positions.

- To soothe the area, try sitz baths (warm soaks in a few inches of water) for 15–20 minutes, two or three times a day, as needed.
- For additional soothing, use ice packs or witch hazel via a TUCKS pad or a DIY version. To make your own, saturate a menstrual pad with witch hazel, put it in a zip-close bag and keep it in the freezer until cold. Alternate between the ice pack and your witch hazel remedy a few times a day (for 10–15 min) as needed.
- Try ibuprofen or TYLENOL, and if the area is very painful, see your provider. A physical exam can confirm healing is progressing well, and a prescription for a topical medication can be quite glorious.

Perineum. This area may be painful from birth and may cause pain during sex. Usually this improves by about 2–3 months after delivery but can last longer for some, especially if you had a significant perineal tear or an episiotomy.[4]

- The tips for vaginal and vulvar pain also apply here.
- If bowel movements cause perineal pain, amp up the fiber and try a stool softener like Colace.

Urinary incontinence. You may find you leak urine while coughing, laughing, sneezing, or during sex. Typically, this improves within a few weeks of starting Kegels.

- Yep, time for a pelvic floor assessment. Ask your maternity- or primary care provider for a referral to a pelvic floor physical therapist if this is not their specialty.
- While practicing your prescribed pelvic floor muscle training routine, use incontinence pads instead of menstrual pads. Your skin will thank you.
- When you feel up to it, start exercising. A healthy weight helps mitigate incontinence.

Anal incontinence. As the name suggests, this is when you leak stool or have difficulty controlling gas. Recovery can take a few months, possibly longer.

- Believe it or not, Kegels can help with mild incontinence. If using Kegels for this reason, though, focus on tightening the anus, as if trying to keep stool or gas from escaping.
- If your condition is severe, talk to your maternity- or primary care provider. It's possible there is an underlying injury that wasn't obvious at delivery but can still be repaired.

f. Relationships That Hurt

In "Find Your Tribe" (week 14), we discussed how we are all made for community and healthy relationships. These are what make life meaningful, engaging, interesting, and fun, right?

However, as we may know from stories we've heard or from personal experience, healthy relationships are not always easy to find. While sometimes an *un*healthy relationship is easy to spot right away, many times it can take much longer to realize that things may not be (or are definitely *not*) right. These gut-checks can be a lifesaver and are certainly worth paying attention to.

Regardless of what we call it—whether domestic violence (DV) or intimate partner violence (IPV)—it refers to one thing: a partner intentionally using a systematic pattern of behavior to maintain power and control over another person.[1,2] It includes physical and sexual violence, threats, and emotional or even economic abuse.[2]

Unfortunately, it's incredibly common worldwide, can affect anyone, and may increase or first appear in pregnancy or postpartum.[3-5] Though frequency and severity can vary widely and the abuse may not occur every day, with DV/IPV, there is a fundamental cycle of violence that robs an intimate partner of personal freedom and forces her (or him) to do things she (or he) doesn't want to do.

Such relationships can impact a person profoundly, with effects including nutritional deficiencies, injuries, disabilities, sexually transmitted infections, chronic pain, gastrointestinal problems, depression, anxiety, post-traumatic stress disorder, and substance use and addictions.

In the case of pregnancy, DV/IPV can lead to a preterm birth, low-birth-weight baby, miscarriage, and stillbirth; postpartum, it can make it harder to bond with or breastfeed the little one or may lead to future unintended pregnancies.[5,6]

Tip-offs for this kind of relationship include these partner-specific warning signs: extreme jealousy, being critical or demeaning, discouraging or preventing spending time with others, interference with personal decision-making, use of intimidation (with weapons, threatening looks, or possible violence), pressuring to have sex or to have it in a way that makes the other feel uncomfortable, or even thwarting the use of birth control measures.[7]

When one or more partner warning signs occur regularly, talking to a healthcare provider or confidential hotlines can be life-changing. They can provide helpful information, support, and assistance with safety planning. If you know of someone who is experiencing this, please be sure to tell him or her that it's not their fault and there is help for when they're ready!

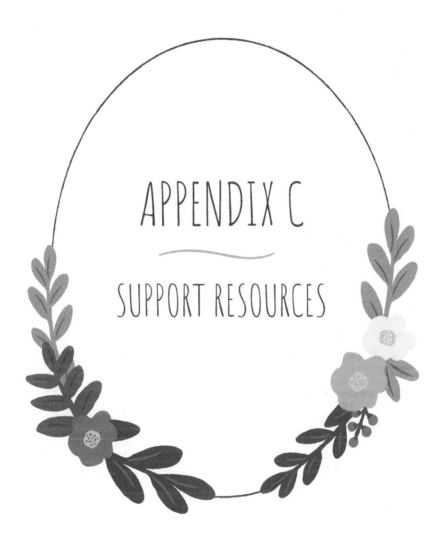

APPENDIX C

SUPPORT RESOURCES

Pregnancy/postpartum	
Childbirth and Postpartum Professional Association	Cappa.net
Childbirth Connection	Childbirthconnection.org
DONA International	Dona.org
Evidence Based Birth	Evidencebasedbirth.com
HER Foundation (Hyperemesis Education & Research Foundation)	Hyperemesis.org
Pregnant After Loss Support (PALS)	Pregnancyafterlosssupport.org
For dads	
Boot Camp for New Dads	Bootcampfornewdads.org
City Dads Group	Citydadsgroup.com
Fathering Together	Fatheringtogether.org
Mental health	
Massachusetts General Hospital's Center for Women's Mental Health	Womensmentalhealth.org
National Eating Disorder Association (NEDA)	Nationaleatingdisorders.org
National Maternal Mental Health Hotline	1-833-9-HELP4MOMS (1-833-943-5746)
988 Suicide & Crisis Lifeline	988lifeline.org 988
Postpartum Progress	Postpartumprogress.com
Postpartum Support International (PSI)	Postpartum.net
Substance Abuse and Mental Health Services Administration (SAMHSA)	Samhsa.gov
Infant feeding	
International Lactation Consultant Association (ILCA)	Ilca.org
The Fed Is Best Foundation	Fedisbest.org
United States Lactation Consultant Association (USLCA)	Uslca.org
WIC Breastfeeding Support	Wicbreastfeeding.fns.usda.gov

Medications, products, food, and environmental safety	
Environmental Working Group (EWG)	Ewg.org
InfantRisk Center	Infantrisk.com
Massachusetts General Hospital's Center for Women's Mental Health	Womensmentalhealth.org
Monterey Bay Aquarium, Seafood Watch Program	Seafoodwatch.org
MotherToBaby	Mothertobaby.org
National Pregnancy Registry for Psychiatric Medications	Womensmentalhealth.org/ research/ pregnancyregistry
Pregnant or breastfeeding at work	
A Better Balance	Abetterbalance.org
Center for WorkLife Law	Worklifelaw.org
Pregnant@Work	Pregnantatwork.org
NICU	
Graham's Foundation	Grahamsfoundation.org
Hand to Hold	Handtohold.org
March of Dimes	Marchforbabies.org
Loss	
Grief Watch	Griefwatch.com
Helping After Neonatal Death (HAND)	Handonline.org
Return to Zero: HOPE	Rtzhope.org
Other	
Bedsider (birth control support network)	Bedsider.org
National Domestic Violence Hotline	Thehotline.org 1.800.799.SAFE (7233)
Planned Parenthood	Plannedparenthood.org
Prevention and Treatment of Traumatic Childbirth (PATTCh)	Pattch.org

CREDITS

Illustrations

B-1g, The original "My Pregnancy Plate" graphic was created by Christie Naze, RD, CDE, © Oregon Health & Science University. It was re-illustrated by Ariel Garcia with permission from OHSU. Original can be found at https://www.ohsu.edu/womens-health/my-pregnancy-plate

Content

Week 13, "Parts Unknown" callout is based on "The Milk Factory" from *Making Milk 101* [Lowmilksupply.org]. Copyright © Diana Marasco and Diana West.

Week 17, "Making the Most of Your Prenatal Appointments" digging deeper questions are adapted with permission from the National Partnership for Women&Families'*MakingInformedDecisions*contentavailableathttp://www.childbirthconnection.org/maternity-caremaking-informed-decisions/

Week 18, "Dad's Impact on Child Development" digging deeper questions and recommendations are adapted with permission from *The Life of Dad: The Making of the Modern Father* by Dr. Anna Machin.

Week 19, "Knowing Your Healthcare Rights," is adapted with permission from the National Partnership for Women & Families' *The Rights of Childbearing Women* content available at https://www.nationalpart-nership.org/our-work/resources/health-care/maternity/the-rights-of-childbearing-women.pdf

Week 32, "Vaginal Births, Cesarean Births, and VBACs," is adapted with permission from the National Partnership for Women & Families' *C-section Basics* content available at http://www.childbirthconnection.org/giving-birth/c-section/basics/

Week 32, "Vaginal Births, Cesarean Births, and VBACs" digging deeper questions are adapted with permission from the National Partnership for

Women & Families' *Planning Ahead* content available at http://www.child-birthconnection.org/giving-birth/c-section/planning-ahead/

Week 33, "Connecting with Baby," and postpartum week 2, "Soothing Baby and Regaining Your Cool," content on baby cues adapted with permission from *The Secrets of Baby Behavior* by M. Jane Heinig, Jennifer Bañuelos, and Jennifer Goldbronn.

A-4c, "Decreasing Your Risk for Cesarean Birth," and A-4d, "How to Improve Your Cesarean Birth Experience," tips adapted with permission from National Partnership for Women & Families' *Planning Ahead* content available at http://www.childbirthconnection.org/giving-birth/c-section/planning-ahead/

A-5a, "Postpartum Care Plan," redeveloped by E. Parker, with permission, from content in:

"Postpartum Plan for ___ Family" by DONA International, from content available at https://www.dona.org/wp-content/uploads/2016/12/postpartum-plan-template.pdf

"The Realistic Postpartum Plan for the ___ Family" by Postpartum Support Virginia, from content available at https://www.postpartumva.org/wp-content/uploads/2013/11/The-Postpartum-Plan.pdf.

Postpartum Depression for Dummies by Shoshana S. Bennett, chapter 18 (page 320)

B-1e, "Peanut Butter Pow! Balls," recipe is adapted from Erin Dooner's *Peanut Butter Protein Balls*. Texanerin Baking. https://www.texanerin.com/peanut-butter-protein-balls/

B-1e, blueberry muffins recipe, is adapted from Ciara Attwell's *Healthy Oat & Blueberry Blender Muffins*.

Quotes

Week 15, *"Joy is what happens to . . . "* Copyright © Marianne Williamson.

Week 25, *"Before the birth of my . . . "* Copyright © Rowan Coleman.

Week 29, *"People are like stained-glass windows . . . "* Copyright © Elisabeth Kübler-Ross.

Week 30, *"What the caterpillar calls the . . . "* Excerpt from ILLUSIONS: THE ADVENTURES OF A RELUCTANT MESSIAH by Richard Bach, copyright © 1977 by Richard Bach and Leslie Parrish-Bach. Used by permission of Delacorte Press, an imprint of Random House, a division of Penguin Random House LLC. All rights reserved.

REFERENCES

FIRST TRIMESTER

WEEK 5
None.

WEEK 6
1. Landon, M. B., Galan, H. L., Jauniaux, E. R. M., Driscoll, D. A., Berghella, V., Grobman, W. A., Kilpatrick, S. J., & Cahill, A. G. (2021). Gabbe's obstetrics: Normal and problem pregnancies (8th ed.). Elsevier.
   Provides fetal measurements for weeks 6–9.
2. Committee on Practice Bulletins—Obstetrics (with S. M. Ramin). (2018). ACOG practice bulletin no. 189: Nausea and vomiting of pregnancy. Obstetrics & Gynecology, 131(1), e15-e30. https://doi.org/10.1097/AOG.0000000000002456
3. Maltepe, C. (2014). Surviving morning sickness successfully: From patient's perception to rational management. *Journal of Population Therapeutics and Clinical Pharmacology, 21*(3), e555–e564. *PubMed.* Retrieved November 11, 2021, from https://pubmed.ncbi.nlm.nih.gov/25654792/
4. London, V., Grube, S., Sherer, D. M., & Abulafia, O. (2017). Hyperemesis gravidarum: A review of recent literature. *Pharmacology, 100*(3-4), 161-171. https://doi.org/10.1159/000477853
5. Thélin, C. S., & Richter, J. E. (2020). Review article: The management of heartburn during pregnancy and lactation. *Alimentary Pharmacology & Therapeutics, 51*(4), 421-434. https://doi.org/10.1111/apt.15611
6. Thaxter Nesbeth, K. A., Samuels, L. A., Nicholson Daley, C., Gossell-Williams, M., & Nesbeth, D. A. (2016). Ptyalism in pregnancy – A review of epidemiology and practices. *European Journal of Obstetrics & Gynecology and Reproductive Biology, 198*, 47-49. https://doi.org/10.1016/j.ejogrb.2015.12.022

WEEK 7
1. Beluska-Turkan, K., Korczak, R., Hartell, B., Moskal, K., Maukonen, J., Alexander, D. E., Salem, N., Harkness, L., Ayad, W., Szaro, J., Zhang, K., & Siriwardhana, N. (2019). Nutritional gaps and supplementation in the first 1000 days. *Nutrients, 11*(12), 2891. https://doi.org/10.3390/nu11122891
2. Koletzko, B., Godfrey, K. M., Poston, L., Szajewska, H., van Goudoever, J. B., de Waard, M., Brands, B., Grivell, R. M., Deussen, A. R., Dodd, J. M., Patro-Golab, B., Zalewski, B. M., & the EarlyNutrition Project Systematic Review Group. (2019). Nutrition during pregnancy, lactation and early childhood and its implications for maternal and long-term child health: The early nutrition project recommendations. *Annals of Nutrition & Metabolism, 74*(2), 93-106. https://doi.org/10.1159/000496471
3. Danielewicz, H., Myszczyszyn, G., Dębińska, A., Myszkal, A., Boznański, A., & Hirnle, L. (2017). Diet in pregnancy—More than food. *European Journal of Pediatrics, 176*(12), 1573–1579. https://doi.org/10.1007/s00431-017-3026-5

4. Procter, S. B., & Campbell, C. G. (2014). Position of the academy of nutrition and dietetics: Nutrition and lifestyle for a healthy pregnancy outcome. *Journal of the Academy of Nutrition and Dietetics, 114*(7), 1099–1103. https://doi.org/10.1016/j.jand.2014.05.005

5. World Health Organization. (2016). Report of the commission on ending childhood obesity. https://apps.who.int/iris/handle/10665/204176

6. Hsu, M.-H., Chen, Y.-C., Sheen, J.-M., & Huang, L.-T. (2020). Maternal obesity programs offspring development and resveratrol potentially reprograms the effects of maternal obesity. *International Journal of Environmental Research and Public Health, 17*(5), 1610. https://doi.org/10.3390/ijerph17051610

7. Mennella, J. A., Jagnow, C. P., & Beauchamp, G. K. (2001). Prenatal and postnatal flavor learning by human infants. *Pediatrics, 107*(6), Article e88. https://doi.org/10.1542/peds.107.6.e88

8. Institute of Medicine & National Research Council. (2009). *Weight gain during pregnancy: Reexamining the guidelines* (K. M. Rasmussen & A. L. Yaktine, Eds.). National Academies Press. https://doi.org/10.17226/12584

9. U.S. Department of Agriculture, & U.S. Department of Health and Human Services. (2020, December). *Dietary Guidelines for Americans, 2020-2025* (9th ed.). DietaryGuidelines. https://www.dietaryguidelines.gov/sites/default/files/2021-03/Dietary_Guidelines_for_Americans-2020-2025.pdf

10. Thilaganathan, B., & Kalafat, E. (2019). Cardiovascular system in preeclampsia and beyond. *Hypertension, 73*(3), 522-531. https://doi.org/10.1161/hypertensionaha.118.11191

11. Committee on Obstetric Practice. (2013). Committee opinion no. 548: Weight gain during pregnancy. *Obstetrics & Gynecology, 121*(1), 210–212. https://doi.org/10.1097/01.aog.0000425668.87506.4c

WEEK 8
None.

WEEK 9

1. Orloff, N. C., & Hormes, J. M. (2014). Pickles and ice cream! Food cravings in pregnancy: Hypotheses, preliminary evidence, and directions for future research. *Frontiers in Psychology, 5*, Article 1076. https://doi.org/10.3389/fpsyg.2014.01076

2. Patil, C. L. (2012). Appetite sensations in pregnancy among agropastoral women in rural Tanzania. *Ecology of Food and Nutrition, 51*(5), 431–443. https://doi.org/10.1080/03670244.2012.696012

3. Blau, L. E., Lipsky, L. M., Dempster, K. W., Eisenberg Colman, M. H., Siega-Riz, A. M., Faith, M. S., & Nansel, T. R. (2020). Women's experience and understanding of food cravings in pregnancy: A qualitative study in women receiving prenatal care at the University of North Carolina–Chapel Hill. *Journal of the Academy of Nutrition and Dietetics, 120*(5), 815–824. https://doi.org/10.1016/j.jand.2019.09.020

4. Committee on Practice Bulletins—Obstetrics. (2018). ACOG practice bulletin no. 189: Nausea and vomiting of pregnancy. *Obstetrics & Gynecology*, 131(1), e15-e30. https://doi.org/10.1097/AOG.0000000000002456

5. Landon, M. B., Galan, H. L., Jauniaux, E. R. M., Driscoll, D. A., Berghella, V., Grobman, W. A., Kilpatrick, S. J., & Cahill, A. G. (2021). *Gabbe's obstetrics: Normal and problem pregnancies* (8th ed.). Elsevier.

WEEK 10

1. Miles, K. (2021, July 6). *Growth chart: Fetal length and weight, week by week.* BabyCenter. https://www.babycenter.com/pregnancy/your-body/growth-chart-fetal-length-and-weight-week-by-week_1290794

> *Provides fetal measurements for weeks 10–39. Lengths are for head to rump for weeks 10–13 and head to heel for weeks 14–39. Length measurements are rounded to the nearest quarter inch with weights rounded to the nearest ounce or (after 16 ounces) quarter pound.*

2. Reddy, U. M., Abuhamad, A. Z., Levine, D., Saade, G. R., for the Fetal Imaging Workshop Invited Participants. (2014). Fetal imaging: Executive summary of a joint *Eunice Kennedy Shriver* National Institute of Child Health and Human Development, Society for

Maternal-Fetal Medicine, American Institute of Ultrasound in Medicine, American College of Obstetricians and Gynecologists, American College of Radiology, Society for Pediatric Radiology, and Society of Radiologists in Ultrasound fetal imaging workshop. *Journal of Ultrasound in Medicine, 33*(5), 745–757. https://doi.org/10.7863/ultra.33.5.745

3. Rose, N. C., Kaimal, A. J., Dugoff, L., Norton, M. E., American College of Obstetricians and Gynecologists' Committee on Practice Bulletins—Obstetrics, Committee on Genetics & Society for Maternal-Fetal Medicine. (2020). Screening for fetal chromosomal abnormalities: ACOG practice bulletin, no. 226. *Obstetrics & Gynecology, 136*(4), e48–e69. https://doi.org/10.1097/AOG.0000000000004084

4. U.S. National Library of Medicine. (2019, October 1). *Birth defects.* MedlinePlus. https://medlineplus.gov/birthdefects.html

5. Alwan, S., & Friedman, J. M. (2018). What birth defects are common in humans? How are they diagnosed at birth? In B. Hales, A. Scialli, & M. Tassinari (Eds.), *Teratology primer* (3rd ed) [Internet book]. Society for Birth Defects Research & Prevention. https://birthdefectsresearch.org/primer/

6. Običan, S. G., Leavitt, K., & Scialli, A. R. (2018). What tests are available to screen prenatally for birth defects? In B. Hales, A. Scialli, & M. Tassinari (Eds.), *Teratology primer* (3rd ed) [Internet book]. Society for Birth Defects Research & Prevention. https://birthdefectsresearch.org/primer/

7. Centers for Disease Control and Prevention. (2020, October 26). *Data & stats on birth defects.* https://www.cdc.gov/ncbddd/birthdefects/data.html

8. Gregg, A. R., Skotko, B. G., Benkendorf, J. L., Monaghan, K. G., Bajaj, K., Best, R. G., Klugman, S., & Watson, M. S. on behalf of the ACMG Noninvasive Prenatal Screening Work Group. (2016). Noninvasive prenatal screening for fetal aneuploidy, 2016 update: A position statement of the American College of Medical Genetics and Genomics. *Genetics in Medicine, 18*(10), 1056–1065. https://doi.org/10.1038/gim.2016.97

9. Dugoff, L., for the Society for Maternal-Fetal Medicine. (2010). First-and second-trimester maternal serum markers for aneuploidy and adverse obstetric outcomes. *Obstetrics & Gynecology, 115*(5): 1052-1061. https://doi.org/10.1097/AOG.0b013e3181da93da

10. Committee on Practice Bulletins—Obstetrics, Committee on Genetics & Society for Maternal-Fetal Medicine (with M. E. Norton, & M. Jackson). (2016). Practice bulletin no. 162: Prenatal diagnostic testing for genetic disorders. *Obstetrics & Gynecology, 127*(5), e108–e122. https://doi.org/10.1097/AOG.0000000000001405

11. Fonda Allen, J., Stoll, K., & Bernhardt, B. A. (2016). Pre- and post-test genetic counseling for chromosomal and Mendelian disorders. *Seminars in Perinatology, 40*(1), 44–55. https://doi.org/10.1053/j.semperi.2015.11.007

WEEK 11
None.

WEEK 12

1. Bergbom, I., Modh, C., Lundgren, I., & Lindwall, L. (2017). First-time pregnant women's experiences of their body in early pregnancy. *Scandinavian Journal of Caring Sciences, 31*(3), 579–586. https://doi.org/10.1111/scs.12372

2. Meireles, J. F. F., Neves, C. M., de Carvalho, P. H. B., & Ferreira, M. E. C. (2015). Body dissatisfaction among pregnant women: an integrative review of the literature. *Ciência & Saúde Coletiva, 20*(7), 2091–2103. https://doi.org/10.1590/1413-81232015207.05502014

3. Hodgkinson, E. L., Smith, D. M., & Wittkowski, A. (2014). Women's experiences of their pregnancy and postpartum body image: A systematic review and meta-synthesis. *BMC Pregnancy and Childbirth*, 14, Article 330. https://doi.org/10.1186/1471-2393-14-330

4. National Eating Disorder Association. (n.d.). *Body image & eating disorders.* https://www.nationaleatingdisorders.org/body-image-eating-disorders

5. Liechty, T., Coyne, S. M., Collier, K. M., & Sharp, A. D. (2018). "It's just not very realistic": Perceptions of media among pregnant and postpartum women. *Health Communication, 33*(7), 851–859. https://doi.org/10.1080/10410236.2017.1315680

6. Claydon, E. A., Davidov, D. M., Zullig, K. J., Lilly, C. L., Cottrell, L., & Zerwas, S. C. (2018). Waking up every day in a body that is not yours: A qualitative research inquiry into the intersection between eating disorders and pregnancy. *BMC Pregnancy and Childbirth*, *18*, Article: 463. https://doi.org/10.1186/s12884-018-2105-6

7. Dryer, R., Graefin von der Schulenburg, I., & Brunton, R. (2020). Body dissatisfaction and Fat Talk during pregnancy: Predictors of distress. *Journal of Affective Disorders*, *267*, 289–296. https://doi.org/10.1016/j.jad.2020.02.031

8. Roomruangwong, C., Kanchanatawan, B., Sirivichayakul, S., & Maes, M. (2017). High incidence of body image dissatisfaction in pregnancy and the postnatal period: Associations with depression, anxiety, body mass index and weight gain during pregnancy. *Sexual & Reproductive Healthcare*, *13*, 103–109. https://doi.org/10.1016/j.srhc.2017.08.002

9. Mento, C., Le Donne, M., Crisafulli, S., Rizzo, A., & Settineri, S. (2017). BMI at early puerperium: Body image, eating attitudes and mood states. *Journal of Obstetrics and Gynaecology*, *37*(4), 428–434. https://doi.org/10.1080/01443615.2016.1250727

10. Coyne, S. M., Liechty, T., Collier, K. M., Sharp, A. D., Davis, E. J., & Kroff, S. L. (2018). The effect of media on body image in pregnant and postpartum women. *Health Communication*, *33*(7), 793–799. https://doi.org/10.1080/10410236.2017.1314853

11. Sun, W., Chen, D., Wang, J., Liu, N., & Zhang, W. (2018). Physical activity and body image dissatisfaction among pregnant women: A systematic review and meta-analysis of cohort studies. *European Journal of Obstetrics, Gynecology, and Reproductive Biology*, *229*, 38–44. https://doi.org/10.1016/j.ejogrb.2018.07.021

12. Carter-Edwards, L., Bastian, L. A., Revels, J., Durham, H., Lokhnygina, Y., Amamoo, M. A., & Ostbye, T. (2010). Body image and body satisfaction differ by race in overweight postpartum mothers. *Journal of Women's Health*, *19*(2), 305–311. https://doi.org/10.1089/jwh.2008.1238

13. Tiggemann, M. (2015). Considerations of positive body image across various social identities and special populations. *Body Image*, *14*, 168–176. https://doi.org/10.1016/j.bodyim.2015.03.002

14. Tylka, T. L., & Wood-Barcalow, N. L. (2015). The Body Appreciation Scale-2: Item refinement and psychometric evaluation. *Body Image*, *12*, 53–67. https://doi.org/10.1016/j.bodyim.2014.09.006

15. National Eating Disorder Association. (n.d.). *Pregnancy and eating disorders.* https://www.nationaleatingdisorders.org/pregnancy-and-eating-disorders

WEEK 13

1. Committee on Obstetric Practice (with M. L. Birsner, & C. Gyamfi-Bannerman). (2020). ACOG committee opinion, no. 804: Physical activity and exercise during pregnancy and the postpartum period. *Obstetrics & Gynecology*, *135*(4), e178–e188. https://doi.org/10.1097/AOG.0000000000003772

2. Bull, F. C., Al-Ansari, S. S., Biddle, S., Borodulin, K., Buman, M. P., Cardon, G., Carty, C., Chaput, J. P., Chastin, S., Chou, R., Dempsey, P. C., DiPietro, L., Ekelund, U., Firth, J., Friedenreich, C. M., Garcia, L., Gichu, M., Jago, R., Katzmarzyk, P. T., … Willumsen, J. F. (2020). World Health Organization 2020 guidelines on physical activity and sedentary behaviour. *British Journal of Sports Medicine*, *54*, 1451–1462. https://doi.org/10.1136/bjsports-2020-102955

3. Piercy, K. L., Troiano, R. P., Ballard, R. M., Carlson, S. A., Fulton, J. E., Galuska, D. A., George, S. M., & Olson, R. D. (2018). The physical activity guidelines for Americans. *JAMA*, *320*(19), 2020–2028. https://doi.org/10.1001/jama.2018.14854

4. Domenjoz, I., Kayser, B., & Boulvain, M. (2014). Effect of physical activity during pregnancy on mode of delivery. *American Journal of Obstetrics & Gynecology*, *211*(4), 401.e1-11. https://doi.org/10.1016/j.ajog.2014.03.030

5. Melzer, K., Schutz, Y., Boulvain, M., & Kayser, B. (2010). Physical activity and pregnancy: cardiovascular adaptations, recommendations and pregnancy outcomes. *Sports Medicine*, *40*(6), 493–507. https://doi.org/10.2165/11532290-000000000-00000

6. Pivarnik, J. M, Mudd, L. M., White, E. E., Schlaff, R. A., & Peyer, K. L. (2014). Physical activity during pregnancy and offspring characteristics at 8–10 years. *Journal of Sports Medicine and*

Physical Fitness, 54(5), 672–9. *PubMed.* Retrieved November 12, 2021, from https://pubmed. ncbi.nlm.nih.gov/25270788/

7. Marasco, L., & West, D. (2019). *Milk production overview: The milk factory.* LowMilkSupply https://www.lowmilksupply.org/making-milk-101

SECOND TRIMESTER

WEEK 14
None.

WEEK 15

1. Allen, S. (2018, May). *The science of gratitude* [A white paper prepared for the John Templeton Foundation]. Greater Good Science Center. https://ggsc.berkeley.edu/images/uploads/ GGSC-JTF_White_Paper-Gratitude-FINAL.pdf

2. Algoe, S. B. (2012). Find, remind, and bind: The functions of gratitude in everyday relationships. *Social and Personality Psychology Compass, 6*(6), 455–469. https://doi.org/10.1111/j.1751-9004.2012.00439.x

3. O'Connell, B. H., & Killeen-Byrt, M. (2018). Psychosocial health mediates the gratitude-physical health link. *Psychology, Health & Medicine, 23*(9), 1145–1150. https://doi.org/10.1080/13 548506.2018.1469782

4. Emmons, R. A., & Stern, R. (2013). Gratitude as a psychotherapeutic intervention. *Journal of Clinical Psychology, 69*(8), 846–855. https://doi.org/10.1002/jclp.22020

5. Mills, P. J., Redwine, L., Wilson, K., Pung, M. A., Chinh, K., Greenberg, B. H., Lunde, O., Maisel, A., Raisinghani, A., Wood, A., & Chopra, D. (2015). The role of gratitude in spiritual well-being in asymptomatic heart failure patients. *Spirituality in Clinical Practice, 2*(1), 5–17. https://doi.org/10.1037/scp0000050

6. Davis, D. E., Choe, E., Meyers, J., Wade, N., Varjas, K., Gifford, A., Quinn, A., Hook, J. N., Van Tongeren, D. R., Griffin, B. J., & Worthington, E. L., Jr. (2016). Thankful for the little things: A meta-analysis of gratitude interventions. *Journal of Counseling Psychology, 63*(1), 20–31. https://doi.org/10.1037/cou0000107

WEEK 16

1. McLellan, J. (n.d.). *What's a B belly? Let's talk about it!* Plus Size Birth. https://plussizebirth. com/whats-a-b-belly/

2. Gregg, A. R., Skotko, B. G., Benkendorf, J. L., Monaghan, K. G., Bajaj, K., Best, R. G., Klugman, S., & Watson, M. S. (2016). Noninvasive prenatal screening for fetal aneuploidy, 2016 update: A position statement of the American College of Medical Genetics and Genomics. *Genetics in Medicine, 18*(10), 1056–1065. https://doi.org/10.1038/gim.2016.97

3. American Psychiatric Association. (2013). *Diagnostic and statistical manual of mental disorders* (5th ed.). https://doi.org/10.1176/appi.books.9780890425596

WEEK 17

1. Siu, A. L., & the United States Preventive Services Task Force. (2016). Screening for depression in adults: US Preventive Services Task Force recommendation statement. *JAMA, 315*(4), 380-387. https://doi.org/10.1001/jama.2015.18392

2. Committee on Obstetric Practice. (2018). ACOG committee opinion no. 757: Screening for perinatal depression. *Obstetrics & Gynecology, 132*(5), e208–e212. https://doi.org/10.1097/ AOG.0000000000002927

3. Curry, S. J., & the United States Preventive Services Task Force. (2018). Screening for intimate partner violence, elder abuse, and abuse of vulnerable adults: US Preventive Services Task Force final recommendation statement. *JAMA, 320*(16), 1678–1687. https://doi. org/10.1001/jama.2018.14741

4. Committee on Health Care for Underserved Women. (2012). Committee opinion no. 518: Intimate partner violence. *Obstetrics & Gynecology*, *119*(2 Part 1), 412–417. https://doi.org/10.1097/AOG.0b013e318249ff74

5. Krist, A. H., & the United States Preventive Services Task Force. (2020). Screening for unhealthy drug use: US Preventive Services Task Force recommendation statement. *JAMA*. *323*(22), 2301–2309. https://doi.org/10.1001/jama.2020.8020

6. National Partnership for Women and Families. (n.d). *Making informed decisions.* Childbirth Connection. http://www.childbirthconnection.org/maternity-care/making-informed-decisions/

WEEK 18

1. Machin, A. (2018). *The life of dad: The making of the modern father.* Simon & Schuster.

2. Saxbe, D. E., Edelstein, R. S., Lyden, H. M., Wardecker, B. M., Chopik, W. J., & Moors, A. C. (2017). Fathers' decline in testosterone and synchrony with partner testosterone during pregnancy predicts greater postpartum relationship investment. *Hormones and Behavior, 90*, 39–47. https://doi.org/10.1016/j.yhbeh.2016.07.005

3. Gordon, I., Zagoory-Sharon, O., Leckman, J. F., & Feldman, R. (2010). Oxytocin and the development of parenting in humans. *Biological Psychiatry, 68*(4), 377–382. https://doi.org/10.1016/j.biopsych.2010.02.005

4. Feldman, R., Gordon, I., Schneiderman, I., Weisman, O., & Zagoory-Sharon, O. (2010). Natural variations in maternal and paternal care are associated with systematic changes in oxytocin following parent-infant contact. *Psychoneuroendocrinology, 35*(8), 1133–1141. https://doi.org/10.1016/j.psyneuen.2010.01.013

5. Kim, P., Rigo, P., Mayes, L. C., Feldman, R., Leckman, J. F., & Swain, J. E. (2014). Neural plasticity in fathers of human infants. *Social Neuroscience, 9*(5), 522–535. https://doi.org/10.1080/17470919.2014.933713

6. Malmberg, L. E., Lewis, S., West, A., Murray, E., Sylva, K., & Stein, A. (2016). The influence of mothers' and fathers' sensitivity in the first year of life on children's cognitive outcomes at 18 and 36 months. *Child: Care, Health and Development, 42*(1), 1–7. https://doi.org/10.1111/cch.12294

7. Sulik, M. J., Blair, C., Mills-Koonce, R., Berry, D., Greenberg, M., & The Family Life Project Investigators. (2015). Early parenting and the development of externalizing behavior problems: Longitudinal mediation through children's executive function. *Child Development, 86*(5), 1588–1603. https://doi.org/10.1111/cdev.12386

8. Richaud de Minzi, M. C. (2010). Gender and cultural patterns of mothers' and fathers' attachment and links with children's self-competence, depression and loneliness in middle and late childhood. *Early Child Development and Care, 180*(1-2), 193–209. https://doi.org/10.1080/03004430903415056

9. Grossmann, K., Grossmann, K. E., Fremmer-Bombik, E., Kindler, H., Scheuerer-Englisch, H., & Zimmermann, P. (2002). The uniqueness of the child-father attachment relationship: Fathers' sensitive and challenging play as a pivotal variable in a 16-year longitudinal study. *Social Development, 11*(3), 301–337. https://doi.org/10.1111/1467-9507.00202

10. Feldman, R. (2003). Infant–mother and infant–father synchrony: The coregulation of positive arousal. *Infant Mental Health Journal, 24*(1), 1–23. https://doi.org/10.1002/imhj.10041

WEEK 19

1. Agency for Healthcare Research and Quality. (2021, December). *2021 National Healthcare Quality and Disparities Report* [AHRQ Pub. No. 21 (22)-0054-EF]. Retrieved June 18, 2022, from https://www.ahrq.gov/sites/default/files/wysiwyg/research/findings/nhqrdr/2021qdr.pdf

2. National Partnership for Women and Families. (n.d.). *Rights of childbearing women.* Childbirth Connection. https://www.nationalpartnership.org/our-work/resources/health-care/maternity/the-rights-of-childbearing-women.pdf

WEEK 20

1. National Partnership for Women and Families. (2014, January). *Listening to Mothers: The experiences of expecting and new mothers in the workplace* [Data brief on the Listening to Mothers III: Pregnancy and Birth survey, 2013]. Childbirth Connection. https://www.nationalpartnership.org/our-work/resources/economic-justice/pregnancy-discrimination/listening-to-mothers-experiences-of-expecting-and-new-mothers.pdf

2. Glynn, S. J. (2019, May 10). *Breadwinning mothers continue to be the U.S. norm* [Report]. Center for American Progress. https://www.americanprogress.org/article/breadwinning-mothers-continue-u-s-norm/

3. U.S. Bureau of Labor Statistics. (2021, April). *Women in the labor force: A databook* [Report 1092]. https://www.bls.gov/opub/reports/womens-databook/2020/home.htm

4. Horowitz, J. (2019, September 12). *Despite challenges at home and work, most working moms and dads say being employed is what's best for them.* Pew Research Center. https://www.pewresearch.org/fact-tank/2019/09/12/despite-challenges-at-home-and-work-most-working-moms-and-dads-say-being-employed-is-whats-best-for-them/

5. Jackson, R. A., Gardner, S., Torres, L. N., Huchko, M. J., Zlatnik, M. G., & Williams, J. C. (2015). My obstetrician got me fired: How work notes can harm pregnant patients and what to do about it. *Obstetrics & Gynecology, 126*(2), 250–254. https://doi.org/10.1097/AOG.0000000000000971

6. Jou, J., Kozhimannil, K. B., Blewett, L. A., McGovern, P. M., & Abraham, J. M. (2016). Workplace accommodations for pregnant employees: Associations with women's access to health insurance coverage after childbirth. *Journal of Occupational and Environmental Medicine, 58*(6), 561–566. https://doi.org/10.1097/JOM.0000000000000737

WEEK 21

None.

WEEK 22

1. Sweet, L., Arjyal, S., Kuller, J. A., & Dotters-Katz, S. (2020). A review of sleep architecture and sleep changes during pregnancy. *Obstetrical & Gynecological Survey, 75*(4), 253–262. https://doi.org/10.1097/OGX.0000000000000770

WEEK 23

1. Brackett, M. (2019). *Permission to feel: Unlocking the power of emotions to help our kids, ourselves, and our society thrive.* Celadon Books.

WEEK 24

1. Stern, D. N., & Bruschweiler-Stern, N. (with Freeland, A.). (1998). *The birth of a mother: How the motherhood experience changes you forever.* Basic Books.

2. Ambrosini, A., & Stanghellini, G. (2012). Myths of motherhood. The role of culture in the development of postpartum depression. *Annali dell'Istituto Superiore di Sanità, 48*(3), 277–286. https://doi.org/10.4415/ANN_12_03_08

3. Henderson, A., Harmon, S., & Newman, H. (2016). The price mothers pay, even when they are not buying it: Mental health consequences of idealized motherhood. *Sex Roles, 74*, 512–526. https://doi.org/10.1007/s11199-015-0534-5

4. Melrose, S. (2011). Perfectionism and depression: Vulnerabilities nurses need to understand [Review article]. *Nursing Research and Practice, 2011*, Article 858497. https://doi.org/10.1155/2011/858497

WEEK 25

1. Jou, J., Kozhimannil, K. B., Abraham, J. M., Blewett, L. A., & McGovern, P. M. (2018). Paid maternity leave in the United States: Associations with maternal and infant health. *Maternal and Child Health Journal, 22*, 16–225. https://doi.org/10.1007/s10995-017-2393-x

2. Jou, J., Kozhimannil, K. B., Blewett, L. A., McGovern, P. M., & Abraham, J. M. (2016). Workplace accommodations for pregnant employees: Associations with women's access to health

insurance coverage after childbirth. *Journal of Occupational and Environmental Medicine, 58*(6), 561–566. https://doi.org/10.1097/JOM.0000000000000737

3. WORLD Policy Analysis Center. (n.d). *Is paid leave available for mothers of infants?* [2020 data]. Retrieved June 23, 2022, from https://www.worldpolicycenter.org/policies/is-paid-leave-available-for-mothers-of-infants

4. Van Niel, M. S., Bhatia, R., Riano, N. S., de Faria, L., Catapano-Friedman, L., Ravven, S., Weissman, B., Nzodom, C., Alexander, A., Budde, K., & Mangurian, C. (2020). The impact of paid maternity leave on the mental and physical health of mothers and children: A review of the literature and policy implications. *Harvard Review of Psychiatry, 28*(2), 113–126. https://doi.org/10.1097/HRP.0000000000000246

5. U.S. Department of Labor, Wage and Hour Division. (n.d.). *Family Medical Leave Act.* https://www.dol.gov/agencies/whd/fmla

6. Klerman, J. A., Daley, K., & Pozniak, A. (2014). *Family and medical leave in 2012: Technical Report* [Submitted by Abt Associates]. https://www.dol.gov/sites/dolgov/files/OASP/legacy/files/FMLA-2012-Technical-Report.pdf

7. U.S. Department of Labor, Wage and Hour Division. (2018, April). *Fact sheet #73. Break time for nursing mothers under the FLSA.* https://www.dol.gov/agencies/whd/fact-sheets/73-flsa-break-time-nursing-mothers

8. Center for WorkLife Law & A Better Balance. (2020). *Breastfeeding employees: Learn more about your workplace rights.* Pregnant@work. Retrieved June 23, 2022, from https://pregnantat-work.org/pregnant-women-pregnancy/breastfeeding-employees/

9. Declercq, E. R., Sakala, C., Corry, M. P., & Applebaum, S. (2008, August). *New mothers speak out. National survey results highlight women's postpartum experiences* [Report on *Listening to Mothers* II surveys conducted for Childbirth Connection]. National Partnership for Women and Families. https://www.nationalpartnership.org/our-work/resources/health-care/maternity/listening-to-mothers-ii-new-mothers-speak-out-2008.pdf

10. Sakala, C., Declerq, E. R., Turon, J. M., & Corry, M. P. (2018, September). *Listening to mothers in California: A population-based survey of women's childbearing experiences* [Full survey report]. National Partnership for Women and Families. https://www.chcf.org/wp-content/uploads/2018/09/ListeningMothersCAFullSurveyReport2018.pdf

WEEK 26

1. American Psychiatric Association. (n.d.). *What are sleep disorders?* https://www.psychiatry.org/patients-families/sleep-disorders/what-are-sleep-disorders

2. Sateia, M. J. (2014). International classification of sleep disorders-third edition: Highlights and modifications. *Chest, 146*(5), 1387–1394. https://doi.org/10.1378/chest.14-0970

3. Wilkerson, A. K., & Uhde, T. W. (2018). Perinatal sleep problems: Causes, complications, and management. *Obstetrics and Gynecology Clinics of North America, 45*(3), 483–494. https://doi.org/10.1016/j.ogc.2018.04.003

4. Weissbluth, M. (2015). *Healthy sleep habits, happy child: A step-by-step program for a good night's sleep* (4th ed.). Ballantine Books.

5. Hirshkowitz, M., Whiton, K., Albert, S. M., Alessi, C., Bruni, O., DonCarlos, L., Hazen, N., Herman, J., Adams Hillard, P. J., Katz, E. S., Kheirandish-Gozal, L., Neubauer, D. N., O'Donnell, A. E., Ohayon, M., Peever, J., Rawding, R., Sachdeva, R. C., Setters, B., Vitiello, M. V., & Ware, J. C. (2015). National Sleep Foundation's updated sleep duration recommendations: Final report. *Sleep Health, 1*(4), 233–243. https://doi.org/10.1016/j.sleh.2015.10.004

6. Watson, N. F., Badr, M. S., Belenky, G., Bliwise, D. L., Buxton, O. M., Buysse, D., Dinges, D. F., Gangwisch, J., Grandner, M. A., Kushida, C., Malhotra, R. K., Martin, J. L., Patel, S. R., Quan, S. F., & Tasali, E. (2015). Recommended amount of sleep for a healthy adult: A joint consensus statement of the American Academy of Sleep Medicine and Sleep Research Society. *Sleep, 38*(6), 843–844. https://doi.org/10.5665/sleep.4716

7. Grandner, M. A., Seixas, A., Shetty, S., & Shenoy, S. (2016). Sleep duration and diabetes risk: Population trends and potential mechanisms. *Current Diabetes Reports, 16*, Article 106. https://doi.org/10.1007/s11892-016-0805-8

8. Cappuccio, F. P., & Miller, M. A. (2017). Sleep and cardio-metabolic disease. *Current Cardiology Reports, 19*, Article 110. https://doi.org/10.1007/s11886-017-0916-0

9. Grandner, M. A., Jackson, N. J., Pak, V. M., & Gehrman, P. R. (2012). Sleep disturbance is associated with cardiovascular and metabolic disorders. *Journal of Sleep Research, 21*(4), 427–433. https://doi.org/10.1111/j.1365-2869.2011.00990.x

10. Christian, L. M., Carroll, J. E., Teti, D. M., & Hall, M. H. (2019). Maternal sleep in pregnancy and postpartum part I: Mental, physical, and interpersonal consequences. *Current Psychiatry Reports, 21*, Article 20. https://doi.org/10.1007/s11920-019-0999-y

11. Reichner, C. A. (2015). Insomnia and sleep deficiency in pregnancy. *Obstetric Medicine, 8*(4), 168–171. https://doi.org/10.1177/1753495X15600572

12. Moreno-Fernandez, J., Ochoa, J. J., Lopez-Frias, M., & Diaz-Castro, J. (2020). Impact of early nutrition, physical activity and sleep on the fetal programming of disease in the pregnancy: A narrative review. *Nutrients, 12*(12), Article 3900. https://doi.org/10.3390/nu12123900

13. Naghi, I., Keypour, F., Ahari, S. B., Tavalai, S. A., & Khak, M. (2011). Sleep disturbance in late pregnancy and type and duration of labour. *Journal of Obstetrics and Gynaecology: The Journal of the Institute of Obstetrics and Gynaecology, 31*(6), 489–491. https://doi.org/10.3109/014436 15.2011.579196

14. Beebe, K. R., & Lee, K. A. (2007). Sleep disturbance in late pregnancy and early labor. *The Journal of Perinatal & Neonatal Nursing, 21*(2), 103–108. https://doi.org/10.1097/01. JPN.0000270626.66369.26

15. Richter, D., Krämer, M. D., Tang, N. K. Y., Montgomery-Downs, H. E., & Lemola, S. (2019). Long-term effects of pregnancy and childbirth on sleep satisfaction and duration of first-time and experienced mothers and fathers. *Sleep, 42*(4), Article zsz015. https://doi. org/10.1093/sleep/zsz015

16. Sweet, L., Arjyal, S., Kuller, J. A., & Dotters-Katz, S. (2020). A review of sleep architecture and sleep changes during pregnancy. *Obstetrical & Gynecological Survey, 75*(4), 253–262. https:// doi.org/10.1097/OGX.0000000000000770

17. National Sleep Foundation. (2007). Summary of findings: 2007 Women and Sleep [Sleep in America Poll]. https://www.thensf.org/sleep-in-america-polls/

WEEK 27

1. Institute of Medicine & National Research Council. (2009). *Weight gain during pregnancy: Reexamining the guidelines* (K. M. Rasmussen & A. L. Yaktine, Eds.). National Academies Press. https://doi.org/10.17226/12584

2. Luke, B., Hediger, M. L., Nugent, C., Newman, R. B., Mauldin, J. G., Witter, F. R., & O'Sullivan, M. J. (2003). Body mass index—specific weight gains associated with optimal birth weights in twin pregnancies. *The Journal of Reproductive Medicine, 48*(4), 217–224. *PubMed.* Retrieved January 4, 2022, from https://pubmed.ncbi.nlm.nih.gov/12746982/

3. Landon, M. B., Galan, H. L., Jauniaux, E. R. M., Driscoll, D. A., Berghella, V., Grobman, W. A., Kilpatrick, S. J., & Cahill, A. G. (2021). *Gabbe's obstetrics: Normal and problem pregnancies* (8th ed.). Elsevier.

4. Fox, N. S. (2018). Dos and don'ts in pregnancy: Truths and myths. *Obstetrics & Gynecology, 131*(4), 713–721. https://doi.org/10.1097/AOG.0000000000002517

5. Beveridge, J. K., Vannier, S. A., & Rosen, N. O. (2018). Fear-based reasons for not engaging in sexual activity during pregnancy: Associations with sexual and relationship well-being. *Journal of Psychosomatic Obstetrics & Gynaecology, 39*(2), 138–145. https://doi.org/10.1080/01 67482X.2017.1312334

6. Ribeiro, M. C., de Tubino Scanavino, M., do Amaral, M., de Moraes Horta, A. L., & Torloni, M. R. (2017). Beliefs about sexual activity during pregnancy: A systematic review of the literature. *Journal of Sex & Marital Therapy, 43*(8), 822–832. https://doi.org/10.1080/009262 3X.2017.1305031

7. Human Reproduction Programme. (2015). Sexual health, human rights and the law. World Health Organization. https://www.who.int/publications/i/item/9789241564984

8. Division of STD Prevention & National Center for HIV, Viral Hepatitis, STD, and TB Prevention. (n.d.). *STDs during pregnancy - CDC detailed fact sheet*. Centers for Disease Control and Prevention. https://www.cdc.gov/std/pregnancy/stdfact-pregnancy-detailed.htm#details

9. Johnson, C. E. (2011). Sexual health during pregnancy and the postpartum. *The Journal of Sexual Medicine, 8*(5), 1267–1286. https://doi.org/10.1111/j.1743-6109.2011.02223.x

10. Fuchs, A., Czech, I., Sikora, J., Fuchs, P., Lorek, M., Skrzypulec-Plinta, V., & Drosdzol-Cop, A. (2019). Sexual functioning in pregnant women. *International Journal of Environmental Research and Public Health, 16*(21), Article 4216. https://doi.org/10.3390/ijerph16214216

11. Leichliter, J. S., & Aral, S. O. (2019). Pregnancy, penile-anal sex, and other sexual behaviors in the United States, 2011-2015. *Sexually Transmitted Diseases, 46*(3), e29–e31. https://doi.org/10.1097/OLQ.0000000000000927

12. Serati, M., Salvatore, S., Siesto, G., Cattoni, E., Zanirato, M., Khullar, V., Cromi, A., Ghezzi, F., & Bolis, P. (2010). Female sexual function during pregnancy and after childbirth. *The Journal of Sexual Medicine, 7*(8), 2782–2790. https://doi.org/10.1111/j.1743-6109.2010.01893.x

13. Yeniel, A. O., & Petri, E. (2014). Pregnancy, childbirth, and sexual function: Perceptions and facts. *International Urogynecology Journal, 25*(1), 5–14. https://doi.org/10.1007/s00192-013-2118-7

14. Lorenz, T., Rullo, J., & Faubion, S. (2016). Antidepressant-induced female sexual dysfunction. *Mayo Clinic Proceedings, 91*(9), 1280–1286. https://doi.org/10.1016/j.mayocp.2016.04.033

15. World Health Organization & Joint United Nations Programme on HIV/AIDS. (2007). Male circumcision: Global trends and determinants of prevalence, safety and acceptability. https://data.unaids.org/pub/report/2007/jc1360_male_circumcision_en.pdf

16. Owings, M., Uddin, S., & Williams, S. (2013). Trends in circumcision for male newborns in U.S. hospitals: 1979-2010. Centers for Disease Control and Prevention, National Center for Health Statistics. https://www.cdc.gov/nchs/data/hestat/circumcision_2013/circumcision_2013.htm

17. Decker, R. (Host). (2019, July 19). Evidence and ethics on: Circumcision (No. 88) [Text transcription of audio podcast]. Evidence Based Birth. https://evidencebasedbirth.com/evidence-and-ethics-on-circumcision/

THIRD TRIMESTER

WEEK 28

1. Meek, J. Y., Noble, L., & the Section on Breastfeeding. (2022). Policy statement: Breastfeeding and the use of human milk. *Pediatrics, 150*(1), Article e2022057988. https://doi.org/10.1542/peds.2022-057988

2. World Health Organization. (2021, June 9). *Infant and young child feeding*. https://www.who.int/news-room/fact-sheets/detail/infant-and-young-child-feeding

3. U.S. Department of Agriculture & U.S. Department of Health and Human Services. (2020, December). *Dietary Guidelines for Americans, 2020-2025* (9th ed.). DietaryGuidelines. https://www.dietaryguidelines.gov/sites/default/files/2021-03/Dietary_Guidelines_for_Americans-2020-2025.pdf

4. Reece-Stremtan, S., Marinelli, K. A., & The Academy of Breastfeeding Medicine. (2015). ABM clinical protocol #21: Guidelines for breastfeeding and substance use or substance use disorder, revised 2015. *Breastfeeding Medicine, 10*(3), 135–141. https://doi.org/10.1089/bfm.2015.9992

5. Mohrbacher, N. (2010). *Breastfeeding answers made simple: A guide for helping mothers*. Hale Publishing.

6. Hale, T. W. (2021). *Hale's medications and mothers' milk: A manual of lactational pharmacology* (19th ed.). Springer Publishing.

7. Centers for Disease Control and Prevention. (n.d.). *About breastfeeding: Why it matters*. https://www.cdc.gov/breastfeeding/about-breastfeeding/why-it-matters.html

8. U.S. Department of Health and Human Services. (n.d.). *Breastfeeding: Surgeon General's call to action fact sheet*. https://www.hhs.gov/surgeongeneral/reports-and-publications/breastfeeding/factsheet/index.html

9. Victora, C. G., Bahl, R., Barros, A. J. D., França, G. V. A., Horton, S., Krasevec, J., Murch, S., Sankar, M. J., Walker, N., & Rollins, N. C., for the Lancet *Breastfeeding Series Group*. (2016). Breastfeeding in the 21st century: Epidemiology, mechanisms, and lifelong effect. *Lancet, 387*(10017), 475–490. https://doi.org/10.1016/S0140-6736(15)01024-7

10. Bartick, M., Stehel, E. K., Calhoun, S. L., Feldman-Winter, L., Zimmerman, D., Noble, L., Rosen-Carole, C., Kair, L. R., & The Academy of Breastfeeding Medicine. (2021). Academy of Breastfeeding Medicine position statement and guideline: Infant feeding and lactation-related language and gender. *Breastfeeding Medicine, 16*(8), 587–590. https://doi.org/10.1089/bfm.2021.29188.abm

WEEK 29

1. Barha, C. K., & Galea, L. A. (2017). The maternal 'baby brain' revisited. *Nature Neuroscience, 20*(2), 134–135. https://doi.org/10.1038/nn.4473

2. Hoekzema, E., Barba-Müller, E., Pozzobon, C., Picado, M., Lucco, F., García-García, D., Soliva, J. C., Tobeña, A., Desco, M., Crone, E. A., Ballesteros, A., Carmona, S., & Vilarroya, O. (2017). Pregnancy leads to long-lasting changes in human brain structure. *Nature Neuroscience, 20*(2), 287–296. https://doi.org/10.1038/nn.4458

3. Duarte-Guterman, P., Leuner, B., & Galea, L. A. M. (2019). The long and short term effects of motherhood on the brain. *Frontiers in Neuroendocrinology, 53*, Article 100740. https://doi.org/10.1016/j.yfrne.2019.02.004

4. Kim, P., Dufford, A. J., & Tribble, R. C. (2018). Cortical thickness variation of the maternal brain in the first 6 months postpartum: Associations with parental self-efficacy. *Brain Structure & Function, 223*(7), 3267–3277. https://doi.org/10.1007/s00429-018-1688-z

5. Kim, P., Leckman, J. F., Mayes, L. C., Feldman, R., Wang, X., & Swain, J. E. (2010). The plasticity of human maternal brain: Longitudinal changes in brain anatomy during the early postpartum period. *Behavioral Neuroscience, 124*(5), 695–700. https://doi.org/10.1037/a0020884

6. Puchalski, C. M. (2001). The role of spirituality in health care. *Baylor University Medical Center Proceedings, 14*(4), 352–357. https://doi.org/10.1080/08998280.2001.11927788

7. Koenig, H. G. (2015). Religion, spirituality, and health: A review and update. *Advances in Mind-Body Medicine, 29*(3), 19–26. *PubMed*. Retrieved November 27, 2021, from https://pubmed.ncbi.nlm.nih.gov/26026153/

8. Panzini, R. G., Mosqueiro, B. P., Zimpel, R. R., Bandeira, D. R., Rocha, N. S., & Fleck, M. P. (2017). Quality-of-life and spirituality. *International Review of Psychiatry, 29*(3), 263–282. https://doi.org/10.1080/09540261.2017.1285553

9. VanderWeele, T. J., Balboni, T. A., & Koh, H. K. (2017). Health and spirituality. *JAMA, 318*(6), 519–520. https://doi.org/10.1001/jama.2017.8136

10. Benson, H. (with Klipper, M. Z.). (2000). *The relaxation response: Revised and expanded edition*. William Morrow Paperbacks. (Originally published 1975).

11. Li, S., Stampfer, M. J., Williams, D. R., & VanderWeele, T. J. (2016). Association of religious service attendance with mortality among women. *JAMA Internal Medicine, 176*(6), 777–785. https://doi.org/10.1001/jamainternmed.2016.1615

12. VanderWeele, T. J., Li, S., Tsai, A. C., & Kawachi, I. (2016). Association between religious service attendance and lower suicide rates among US women. *JAMA Psychiatry, 73*(8), 845–851. https://doi.org/10.1001/jamapsychiatry.2016.1243

13. Cohen, R., Bavishi, C., & Rozanski, A. (2016). Purpose in life and its relationship to all-cause mortality and cardiovascular events: A meta-analysis. *Psychosomatic Medicine, 78*(2), 122–133. https://doi.org/10.1097/PSY.0000000000000274

WEEK 30

1. Landon, M. B., Galan, H. L., Jauniaux, E. R. M., Driscoll, D. A., Berghella, V., Grobman, W. A., Kilpatrick, S. J., & Cahill, A. G. (2021). *Gabbe's obstetrics: Normal and problem pregnancies* (8th ed.). Elsevier.

2. Centers for Disease Control and Prevention. (n.d.). *Tdap (pertussis) vaccine and pregnancy.* https://www.cdc.gov/vaccines/pregnancy/hcp-toolkit/tdap-vaccine-pregnancy.html

3. Committee on Obstetric Practice Immunization and Emerging Infections Expert Work Group. (2017). Committee opinion no. 718: Update on immunization and pregnancy: Tetanus, diphtheria, and pertussis vaccination. *Obstetrics & Gynecology, 130*(3), e153–e157. https://doi.org/10.1097/AOG.0000000000002301

4. American College of Nurse-Midwives Division of Standards and Practice. (2018, October). Position statement: Immunization in pregnancy and postpartum. https://www.midwife.org/acnm/files/acnmlibrarydata/uploadfilename/000000000289/PS-Immunization-in-Pregnancy-and-Postpartum-FINAL-20-Nov-18.pdf

5. Johnston, D. D., & Swanson, D. H. (2003). Invisible mothers: A content analysis of motherhood ideologies and myths in magazines. *Sex Roles, 49*, 21–33. https://doi.org/10.1023/A:1023905518500

6. Constantinou, G., Varela, S., & Buckby, B. (2021). Reviewing the experiences of maternal guilt – the "Motherhood Myth" influence. *Health Care for Women International, 42*(4-6), 852–876. https://doi.org/10.1080/07399332.2020.1835917

WEEK 31

1. Herschorn, S. (2004). Female pelvic floor anatomy: The pelvic floor, supporting structures, and pelvic organs. *Reviews in Urology, 6*(Suppl. 5), S2–S10. *PubMed.* Retrieved December 2, 2021, from https://pubmed.ncbi.nlm.nih.gov/16985905/

2. Lawson, S., & Sacks, A. (2018). Pelvic floor physical therapy and women's health promotion. *Journal of Midwifery & Women's Health, 63*(4), 410–417. https://doi.org/10.1111/jmwh.12736

3. International Pelvic Pain Society. (2019, March 29). Pelvic floor dysfunction (PFD) [Informational handout]. https://www.pelvicpain.org/public/resources/educational-resources/informational-handouts

4. Jundt, K., Peschers, U., & Kentenich, H. (2015). The investigation and treatment of female pelvic floor dysfunction. *Deutsches Ärzteblatt International, 112*(33-34), 564–574. https://doi.org/10.3238/arztebl.2015.0564

5. Handa, V. L., Blomquist, J. L., Knoepp, L. R., Hoskey, K. A., McDermott, K. C., & Muñoz, A. (2011). Pelvic floor disorders 5–10 years after vaginal or Cesarean childbirth. *Obstetrics & Gynecology, 118*(4), 777–784. https://doi.org/10.1097/AOG.0b013e3182267f2f

6. Schreiner, L., Crivelatti, I., de Oliveira, J. M., Nygaard, C. C., & dos Santos, T. G. (2018). Systematic review of pelvic floor interventions during pregnancy. *International Journal of Gynecology and Obstetrics, 143*(1), 10–18. https://doi.org/10.1002/ijgo.12513

7. Woodley, S. J., Lawrenson, P., Boyle, R., Cody, J. D., Mørkved, S., Kernohan, A., & Hay-Smith, E. J. C. (2020). Pelvic floor muscle training for preventing and treating urinary and faecal incontinence in antenatal and postnatal women. *Cochrane Database of Systematic Reviews,* (5), Article CD007471. https://doi.org/10.1002/14651858.CD007471.pub4

8. Dumoulin, C., Hunter, K. F., Moore, K., Bradley, C. S., Burgio, K. L., Hagen, S., Imamura, M., Thakar, R., Williams, K., & Chambers, T. (2016). Conservative management for female urinary incontinence and pelvic organ prolapse review 2013: Summary of the 5th International Consultation on Incontinence. *Neurourology and Urodynamics, 35*(1), 15–20. https://doi.org/10.1002/nau.22677

9. Swanton, A. R., & Gormley, E. A. (2020). Prevention of urinary incontinence in women. *Current Urology Reports, 21*(10), Article 43. https://doi.org/10.1007/s11934-020-00988-x

10. Martinho, N., Friedman, T., Turel, F., Robledo, K., Riccetto, C., & Dietz, H. P. (2019). Birthweight and pelvic floor trauma after vaginal childbirth. *International Urogynecology Journal, 30*(6), 985–990. https://doi.org/10.1007/s00192-019-03882-4

WEEK 32

1. Beluska-Turkan, K., Korczak, R., Hartell, B., Moskal, K., Maukonen, J., Alexander, D. E., Salem, N., Harkness, L., Ayad, W., Szaro, J., Zhang, K., & Siriwardhana, N. (2019). Nutritional gaps and supplementation in the first 1000 days. *Nutrients, 11*(12), Article 2891. https://doi.org/10.3390/nu11122891

2. Baldassarre, M. E., Palladino, V., Amoruso, A., Pindinelli, S., Mastromarino, P., Fanelli, M., Di Mauro, A., & Laforgia, N. (2018). Rationale of probiotic supplementation during pregnancy and neonatal period. *Nutrients, 10*(11), Article 1693. https://doi.org/10.3390/nu10111693

3. Buckley, S. (2009). *Gentle birth, gentle mothering: A doctor's guide to natural childbirth and gentle early parenting choices* (foreword by I. M. Gaskin). Celestial Arts.

4. National Partnership for Women and Families. (2016). *What every pregnant woman needs to know about Cesarean birth.* https://www.nationalpartnership.org/our-work/resources/health-care/maternity/what-every-pregnant-woman-needs-to-know-about-cesarean-section.pdf

5. American College of Obstetricians and Gynecologists & Society for Maternal-Fetal Medicine (with A. B. Caughey, A. G. Cahill, J.-M. Guise, & D. J. Rouse). (2014). Safe prevention of the primary Cesarean delivery. *American Journal of Obstetrics & Gynecology, 210*(3), 179–193. https://doi.org/10.1016/j.ajog.2014.01.026

6. National Partnership for Women and Families. (n.d.). *C-section basics* [Under *Giving birth: C-section*]. Childbirth Connection. http://www.childbirthconnection.org/giving-birth/c-section/basics/

7. Childbirth Connection. (2016, August). *Why is the U.S. Cesarean section rate so high?* [Fact sheet]. National Partnership for Women and Families. https://www.nationalpartnership.org/our-work/resources/health-care/maternity/why-is-the-c-section-rate-so-high.pdf

8. Sakala, C., Declerq, E. R., Turon, J. M., & Corry, M. P. (2018, September). *Listening to mothers in California: A population-based survey of women's childbearing experiences* [Full survey report]. National Partnership for Women and Families. https://www.chcf.org/wp-content/uploads/2018/09/ListeningMothersCAFullSurveyReport2018.pdf?utm_source=National%20Partnership&utm_medium=PDF_Link&utm_campaign=Listening%20to%20Mothers

9. Committee on Practice Bulletins—Obstetrics (with W. Grobman). (2019). ACOG practice bulletin no. 205: Vaginal birth after Cesarean delivery. *Obstetrics & Gynecology, 133*(2), e110–e127. https://doi.org/10.1097/AOG.0000000000003078

10. American College of Nurse-Midwives Board of Directors. (2017, September). *Position statement: Vaginal birth after Cesarean.* https://www.midwife.org/acnm/files/ACNMLibraryData/UPLOADFILENAME/000000000090/VBAC-PS-FINAL-10-10-17.pdf

11. Centers for Disease Control and Prevention & Health Resources and Services Administration. (2017, April 20). *Healthy People 2020 mid-course review: Maternal, infant and child health (Chapter 26).* https://www.cdc.gov/nchs/data/hpdata2020/HP2020MCR-C26-MICH.pdf

12. The Leapfrog Group. (2021). *Healthy moms, healthy babies: Hospital performance on leapfrog's maternity care standards based on results of the 2020 Leapfrog Hospital Survey.* https://cdn.ymaws.com/www.perinatalqi.org/resource/resmgr/images/news/2021_Maternity_Report_Final.pdf

13. National Partnership for Women and Families. (n.d). *Planning ahead: How will I know if I need a C-section?* [Under *Giving birth: C-section*]. Childbirth Connection. http://www.childbirthconnection.org/giving-birth/c-section/planning-ahead/

WEEK 33

1. Heinig, M. J., Bañuelos, J., & Goldbronn, J. (2012). *The secrets of baby behavior.* The Regents of the University of California. https://www.amzn.com/dp/B00AP7J2G6/

2. Barr, R. G. (2006, April). Crying behaviour and its importance for psychosocial development in children. In R. E. Tremblay, M. Boivin, & R. D. Peters (Eds.), *Encyclopedia on Early Childhood Development* [Online]. Centre of Excellence for Early Childhood Development. https://www.child-encyclopedia.com/pdf/expert/crying-behaviour/according-experts/crying-behaviour-and-its-importance-psychosocial-development

3. Barr, R. G., Barr, M., Rajabali, F., Humphreys, C., Pike, I., Brant, R., Hlady, J., Colbourne, M., Fujiwara, T., & Singhal, A. (2018). Eight-year outcome of implementation of abusive head trauma prevention. *Child Abuse & Neglect, 84*, 106–114. https://doi.org/10.1016/j.chiabu.2018.07.004

4. National Center on Shaken Baby Syndrome. (n.d.). *Period of purple crying.* Purple crying. https://www.dontshake.org/purple-crying

WEEK 34

1. Department of Making Pregnancy Safer & Department of Reproductive Health and Research. (2007). *Report of a WHO technical consultation on birth spacing, Geneva, Switzerland, 13–15 June 2005.* World Health Organization. https://apps.who.int/iris/bitstream/handle/10665/69855/WHO_RHR_07.1_eng.pdf

2. Hussaini, K. S., Ritenour, D., & Coonrod, D. V. (2013). Interpregnancy intervals and the risk for infant mortality: A case control study of Arizona infants 2003-2007. *Maternal and Child Health Journal, 17*(4), 646–653. https://doi.org/10.1007/s10995-012-1041-8

3. Cofer, F. G., Fridman, M., Lawton, E., Korst, L. M., Nicholas, L., & Gregory, K. D. (2016). Interpregnancy interval and childbirth outcomes in California, 2007–2009. *Maternal and Child Health Journal, 20*(Suppl 1), 43–51. https://doi.org/10.1007/s10995-016-2180-0

4. American College of Obstetricians and Gynecologists & Society for Maternal-Fetal Medicine. (2019). Obstetric care consensus no. 8: Interpregnancy care. *Obstetrics & Gynecology, 133*(1), e51–e72. https://doi.org/10.1097/AOG.0000000000003025

5. McKinney, D., House, M., Chen, A., Muglia, L., & DeFranco, E. (2017). The influence of interpregnancy interval on infant mortality. *American Journal of Obstetrics & Gynecology, 216*(3), 316.e1–316.e9. https://doi.org/10.1016/j.ajog.2016.12.018

6. Chamberlain, L., & Levenson, R. (2013). Addressing intimate partner violence reproductive and sexual coercion: A guide for obstetric, gynecologic, and reproductive health care settings (3rd ed.) Futures Without Violence. https://www.futureswithoutviolence.org/userfiles/file/HealthCare/Reproductive%20Health%20Guidelines.pdf

7. Cottingham, J., Kismodi, E., Hilber, A. M., Lincetto, O., Stahlhofer, M., & Gruskin, S. (2010). Using human rights for sexual and reproductive health: Improving legal and regulatory frameworks. *Bulletin of the World Health Organization, 88*(7), 551–555. https://doi.org/10.2471/BLT.09.063412

8. Jackson, E., & Glasier, A. (2011). Return of ovulation and menses in postpartum nonlactating women: A systematic review. *Obstetrics & Gynecology, 117*(3), 657–662. https://doi.org/10.1097/AOG.0b013e31820ce18c

9. Hatcher, R. A., Nelson, A., Trussell, J., Cwaik, C., Cason, P., Policar, M. S., Aiken, A. R. A., Marazzo, J., & Kowal, D. (2018). *Contraceptive technology* (21st ed.). Managing Contraception.

10. Curtis, K. M., Tepper, N. K., Jatlaoui, T. C., Berry-Bibee, E., Horton, L. G., Zapata, L. B., Simmons, K. B., Pagano, H. P., Jamieson, D. J., & Whiteman, M. K. (2016). U.S. medical eligibility criteria for contraceptive use, 2016. *Morbidity and Mortality Weekly Report, 65*(RR-3), 1–104. https://doi.org/10.15585/mmwr.rr6503a1

WEEK 35

1. Beckmann, M. M., & Stock, O. M. (2013). Antenatal perineal massage for reducing perineal trauma. *Cochrane Database of Systematic Reviews,* (4), Article CD005123. https://doi.org/10.1002/14651858.CD005123.pub3

2. Dewey, K. G., Nommsen-Rivers, L. A., Heinig, M. J., & Cohen, R. J. (2003). Risk factors for suboptimal infant breastfeeding behavior, delayed onset of lactation, and excess neonatal weight loss. *Pediatrics, 112*(3), 607–619. https://doi.org/10.1542/peds.112.3.607

3. Human Milk Banking Association of North America. (2020, September). *HMBANA standards for donor human milk banking: An overview.* https://www.hmbana.org/file_download/inline/95a0362a-c9f4-4f15-b9ab-cf8cf7b7b866

4. Committee on Nutrition, Section on Breastfeeding & Committee on Fetus and Newborn. (2017). Donor human milk for the high-risk infant: Preparation, safety, and usage options in the United States. *Pediatrics.* 139(1), Article e20163440. https://doi.org/10.1542/peds.2016-3440

WEEK 36
None.

WEEK 37

1. Allen, S. M., & Hawkins, A. J. (1999). Maternal gatekeeping: Mothers' beliefs and behaviors that inhibit greater father involvement in family work. Journal of Marriage and Family, 61(1), 199-212. https://doi.org/10.2307/353894

2. Schoppe-Sullivan, S. J., Brown, G. L., Cannon, E. A., Mangelsdorf, S. C., & Sokolowski, M. S. (2008). Maternal gatekeeping, coparenting quality, and fathering behavior in families with infants. *Journal of Family Psychology, 22*(3), 389–398. https://doi.org/10.1037/0893-3200.22.3.389

3. Minnesota Fathers and Families Network. (2009, September). *Info sheet 17: Gatekeeping: Mom as a pathway to healthy father involvement.* https://www.mnfathers.org/wp-content/uploads/2013/06/InfoSheetGatekeeping-color.pdf

4. Schoppe-Sullivan, S. J., Altenburger, L. E., Settle, T. A., Kamp Dush, C. M., Sullivan, J. M., & Bower, D. J. (2014). Expectant fathers' intuitive parenting: Associations with parent characteristics and postpartum positive engagement. *Infant Mental Health Journal, 35*(5), 409–421. https://doi.org/10.1002/imhj.21468

5. Schoppe-Sullivan, S. J., Altenburger, L. E., Lee, M. A., Bower, D. J., & Kamp Dush, C. M. (2015). Who are the gatekeepers? Predictors of maternal gatekeeping. *Parenting, Science and Practice, 15*(3), 166–186. https://doi.org/10.1080/15295192.2015.1053321

6. Olsavsky, A. L., Yan, J., Schoppe-Sullivan, S. J., & Kamp Dush, C. M. (2020). New fathers' perceptions of dyadic adjustment: The roles of maternal gatekeeping and coparenting closeness. *Family Process, 59*(2), 571–585. https://doi.org/10.1111/famp.12451

WEEK 38

1. World Health Organization. (2018). *WHO recommendations: Induction of labour at or beyond term.* https://www.ncbi.nlm.nih.gov/books/NBK535795/

2. Committee on Practice Bulletins—Obstetrics (with R. Rampersad). (2014). Practice bulletin no. 146: Management of late-term and postterm pregnancies. *Obstetrics & Gynecology, 124*(2 Pt 1), 390–396. https://doi.org/10.1097/01.AOG.0000452744.06088.48

3. Landon, M. B., Galan, H. L., Jauniaux, E. R. M., Driscoll, D. A., Berghella, V., Grobman, W. A., Kilpatrick, S. J., & Cahill, A. G. (2021). *Gabbe's obstetrics: Normal and problem pregnancies* (8th ed.). Elsevier.

4. Middleton, P., Shepherd, E., & Crowther, C. A. (2018). Induction of labour for improving birth outcomes for women at or beyond term. *Cochrane Database of Systematic Reviews, 5*(5), Article CD004945. https://doi.org/10.1002/14651858.CD004945.pub4

5. American College of Nurse-Midwives, Midwives Alliance of North America & National Association of Certified Professional Midwives. (2012). Supporting healthy and normal physiologic birth: A consensus statement by ACNM, MANA, NACPM. https://doi.org/10.1891/1058-1243.22.1.14

6. Buckley, S. (2009). *Gentle birth, gentle mothering: A doctor's guide to natural childbirth and gentle early parenting choices* (foreword by I. M. Gaskin). Celestial Arts.
   "easiest transition possible—physiologically, hormonally..." [punctuation altered for clarity] p. 97

7. Amis, D. (2019). Healthy birth practice #1: Let labor begin on its own. *The Journal of Perinatal Education, 28*(2), 68–80. https://doi.org/10.1891/1058-1243.28.2.68

8. Committee on Practice Bulletins—Obstetrics (with M. Ramirez, & S. Ramin). (2009). ACOG practice bulletin no. 107: Induction of labor. *Obstetrics & Gynecology, 114*(2 Pt 1), 386–397. https://doi.org/10.1097/AOG.0b013e3181b48ef5

9. Simpson, K. R. (2020). Cervical ripening and labor induction and augmentation, 5th edition. *Nursing for Women's Health, 24*(4), S1–S41. https://doi.org/10.1016/j.nwh.2020.04.005

10. Finucane, E. M., Murphy, D. J., Biesty, L. M., Gyte, G. M. L., Cotter, A. M., Ryan, E. M., Boulvain, M., & Devane, D. (2020). Membrane sweeping for induction of labour. *Cochrane Database of Systematic Reviews, 2*(2), Article CD000451. https://doi.org/10.1002/14651858.CD000451.pub3

11. American College of Nurse-Midwives Division of Standards and Practice. (2016, September). Position statement: Induction of labor. http://midwife.org/ACNM/files/ACNMLibraryData/UPLOADFILENAME/000000000235/Induction-of-Labor-2016.pdf

12. Committee on Practice Bulletins—Obstetrics (with D. J. Rouse). (2021). Antepartum fetal surveillance: ACOG practice bulletin summary, number 229. *Obstetrics &Gynecology*, *137*(6), 1134–1136. https://doi.org/10.1097/AOG.0000000000004411

13. Hill, M. J., McWilliams, G. D., Garcia-Sur, D., Chen, B., Munroe, M., & Hoeldtke, N. J. (2008). The effect of membrane sweeping on prelabor rupture of membranes: A randomized controlled trial. *Obstetrics & Gynecology*, *111*(6), 1313–1319. https://doi.org/10.1097/AOG.0b013e31816fdcf3

WEEK 39
None.

WEEK 40
1. Landon, M. B., Galan, H. L., Jauniaux, E. R. M., Driscoll, D. A., Berghella, V., Grobman, W. A., Kilpatrick, S. J., & Cahill, A. G. (2021). *Gabbe's obstetrics: Normal and problem pregnancies* (8th ed.). Elsevier.

POSTPARTUM

WEEK 1
1. Landon, M. B., Galan, H. L., Jauniaux, E. R. M., Driscoll, D. A., Berghella, V., Grobman, W. A., Kilpatrick, S. J., & Cahill, A. G. (2021). *Gabbe's obstetrics: Normal and problem pregnancies* (8th ed.). Elsevier.

2. Mughal, S., Azhar, Y., & Siddiqui, W. (2021, July 2). *Postpartum depression* [Internet book]. StatPearls Publishing. Retrieved January 6, 2022, from https://www.ncbi.nlm.nih.gov/books/NBK519070/

3. Beck, C. T. (2006). Postpartum depression: It isn't just the blues. *The American Journal of Nursing*, *106*(5), 40–50. https://doi.org/10.1097/00000446-200605000-00020

4. Bennett, S., & Indman, P. (2019). *Beyond the blues: Understanding and treating prenatal and postpartum depression & anxiety.* Untreed Reads. (Original work published 2003)

5. Bennett, S. (2007). *Postpartum depression for dummies* (foreword by M. J. Codey). John Wiley & Sons.

6. Woody, C. A., Ferrari, A. J., Siskind, D. J., Whiteford, H. A., & Harris, M. G. (2017). A systematic review and meta-regression of the prevalence and incidence of perinatal depression. *Journal of Affective Disorders*, *219*, 86–92. https://doi.org/10.1016/j.jad.2017.05.003

WEEK 2
1. Barr, R. G. (n.d.). *The period of purple crying: Common sense and well tried soothing methods.* National Center on Shaken Baby Syndrome. http://purplecrying.info/sub-pages/soothing/common-sense-and-well-tried-soothing-methods.php

2. Heinig, M. J., Bañuelos, J., & Goldbronn, J. (2012). *The secrets of baby behavior.* The Regents of the University of California. https://www.amzn.com/dp/B00AP7J2G6/

3. Barr, R. G. (n.d.). *The period of purple crying: Common features and principles of soothing.* National Center on Shaken Baby Syndrome. http://purplecrying.info/sub-pages/soothing/common-features-and-principles-of-soothing.php

4. Esposito, G., Yoshida, S., Ohnishi, R., Tsuneoka, Y., del Carmen Rostagno, M., Yokota, S., Okabe, S., Kamiya, K., Hoshino, M., Shimizu, M., Venuti, P., Kikusui, T., Kato, T., & Kuroda, K. O. (2013). Infant calming responses during maternal carrying in humans and mice. *Current biology*, *23*(9), 739–745. https://doi.org/10.1016/j.cub.2013.03.041

5. Barr, R. G., Fairbrother, N., Pauwels, J., Green, J., Chen, M., & Brant, R. (2014). Maternal frustration, emotional and behavioural responses to prolonged infant crying. *Infant Behavior Development*, 37(4), 652-664. https://doi.org/10.1016/j.infbeh.2014.08.012

6. National Center on Shaken Baby Syndrome. (n.d.). Learn more: FAQ: How can shaken baby syndrome/abusive head trauma (AHT) be prevented? https://www.dontshake.org/learn-more#how-can-shaken-baby-syndrome-abusive-head-trauma-aht-be-prevented

7. National Center on Shaken Baby Syndrome. (n.d.). *Learn more: FAQ: What is the outcome or prognosis of victims of shaken baby syndrome/abusive head trauma (SBS/AHT)?* https://www.dontshake.org/learn-more#what-is-the-outcome-or-prognosis-of-victims-of-shaken-baby-syndrome-abusive-head-trauma-sbs-aht

8. Barr, R. G. (2006, April). Crying behaviour and its importance for psychosocial development in children. In R. E. Tremblay, M. Boivin, & R. D. Peters (Eds.), *Encyclopedia on Early Childhood Development* [Online]. Centre of Excellence for Early Childhood Development. https://www.child-encyclopedia.com/pdf/expert/crying-behaviour/according-experts/crying-behaviour-and-its-importance-psychosocial-development

9. Beck, C. T. (2004). Birth trauma: In the eye of the beholder. *Nursing Research, 53*(1), 28–35. https://doi.org/10.1097/00006199-200401000-00005

WEEK 3

1. Kim, P., Mayes, L., Feldman, R., Leckman, J. F., & Swain, J. E. (2012). Early postpartum parental preoccupation and positive parenting thoughts: Relationship with parent-infant interaction. *Infant Mental Health Journal, 34*(2), 104–116. https://doi.org/10.1002/imhj.21359

2. Phillips, J., Sharpe, L., Matthey, S., & Charles, M. (2009). Maternally focused worry. *Archives of Women's Mental Health, 12*, 409–418. https://doi.org/10.1007/s00737-009-0091-4

3. Kim, P., & Swain, J. E. (2007). Sad dads: Paternal postpartum depression. *Psychiatry* (Edgemont, PA), *4*(2), 35–47. *PubMed.* Retrieved December 20, 2021, from https://pubmed.ncbi.nlm.nih.gov/20805898/

4. Kendall-Tackett, K. A. (2017). *Depression in new mothers: Causes, consequences and treatment alternatives* (3rd ed. with foreword by P. Simkin). Routledge.

5. Rodriguez-Cabezas, L., & Clark, C. (2018). Psychiatric emergencies in pregnancy and postpartum. *Clinical Obstetrics and Gynecology, 61*(3), 615–627. https://doi.org/10.1097/GRF.0000000000000377

WEEK 4

1. Woody, C. A., Ferrari, A. J., Siskind, D. J., Whiteford, H. A., & Harris, M. G. (2017). A systematic review and meta-regression of the prevalence and incidence of perinatal depression. *Journal of Affective Disorders, 219*, 86–92. https://doi.org/10.1016/j.jad.2017.05.003

2. Sharma, V., & Mazmanian, D. (2014). The DSM-5 peripartum specifier: Prospects and pitfalls. *Archives of Women's Mental Health, 17*(2), 171–173. https://doi.org/10.1007/s00737-013-0406-3

3. Kendall-Tackett, K. A. (2017). *Depression in new mothers: Causes, consequences and treatment alternatives* (3rd ed. with foreword by P. Simkin). Routledge.

4. Grigoriadis, S., Wilton, A. S., Kurdyak, P. A., Rhodes, A. E., VonderPorten, E. H., Levitt, A., Cheung, A., & Vigod, S. N. (2017). Perinatal suicide in Ontario, Canada: A 15-year population-based study. *Canadian Medical Association Journal, 189*(34), E1085–E1092. https://doi.org/10.1503/cmaj.170088

5. Ramchandani, P., Stein, A., Evans, J., O'Connor, T. G., & the ALSPAC study team (2005). Paternal depression in the postnatal period and child development: A prospective population study. *Lancet, 365*(9478), 2201–2205. https://doi.org/10.1016/S0140-6736(05)66778-5

6. Davé, S., Petersen, I., Sherr, L., & Nazareth, I. (2010). Incidence of maternal and paternal depression in primary care: A cohort study using a primary care database. *Archives of Pediatrics & Adolescent Medicine, 164*(11), 1038–1044. *PubMed.* Retrieved December 20, 2021, from https://pubmed.ncbi.nlm.nih.gov/20819960/

7. Bauman, B. L., Ko, J. Y., Cox, S., D'Angelo, D. V., Warner, L., Folger, S., Tevendale, H. D., Coy, K. C., Harrison, L., & Barfield, W. D. (2020). *Vital signs*: Postpartum depressive symptoms and provider discussions about perinatal depression - United States, 2018. *Morbidity and Mortality Weekly Report, 69*(19), 575–581. https://doi.org/10.15585/mmwr.mm6919a2

8. Paulson, J. F., & Bazemore, S. D. (2010). Prenatal and postpartum depression in fathers and its association with maternal depression: A meta-analysis. *JAMA*, *303*(19), 1961–1969. https://doi.org/10.1001/jama.2010.605

9. Kim, P., & Swain, J. E. (2007). Sad dads: Paternal postpartum depression. *Psychiatry* (Edgemont, PA), *4*(2), 35–47. *PubMed*. Retrieved December 20, 2021, from https://pubmed.ncbi.nlm.nih.gov/20805898/

10. Ko, J. Y., Rockhill, K. M., Tong, V. T., Morrow, B., & Farr, S. L. (2017). Trends in postpartum depressive symptoms – 27 states, 2004, 2008, and 2012. *Morbidity and Mortality Weekly Report*, *66*(6), 153–158. https://doi.org/10.15585/mmwr.mm6606a1

11. Stuart-Parrigon, K., & Stuart, S. (2014). Perinatal depression: An update and overview. *Current Psychiatry Reports*, *16*(9), Article 468. https://doi.org/10.1007/s11920-014-0468-6

12. Rao, W.-W., Zhu, X.-M., Zong, Q.-Q., Zhang, Q., Hall, B. J., Ungvari, G. S., & Xiang, Y.-T. (2020). Prevalence of prenatal and postpartum depression in fathers: A comprehensive meta-analysis of observational surveys. *Journal of Affective Disorders*, *263*, 491–499. https://doi.org/10.1016/j.jad.2019.10.030

13. Wisner, K. L., Sit, D. K. Y., McShea, M. C., Rizzo, D. M., Zoretich, R. A., Hughes, C. L., Eng, H. F., Luther, J. F., Wisniewski, S. R., Costantino, M. L., Confer, A. L., Moses-Kolko, E. L., Famy, C. S., & Hanusa, B. H. (2013). Onset timing, thoughts of self-harm, and diagnoses in postpartum women with screen-positive depression findings. *JAMA Psychiatry*, *70*(5), 490–498. https://doi.org/10.1001/jamapsychiatry.2013.87

14. Beck, C. T. (2006). Postpartum depression: It isn't just the blues. *The American Journal of Nursing*, *106*(5), 40–50. https://doi.org/10.1097/00000446-200605000-00020

15. Beck, C. T. (2001). Predictors of postpartum depression: An update. *Nursing Research*, *50*(5), 275–285. https://doi.org/10.1097/00006199-200109000-00004
    "thief that steals motherhood" p. 40

16. Bennett, S. (2007). *Postpartum depression for dummies* (foreword by M. J. Codey). John Wiley & Sons.

17. Beck, C. T., & Indman, P. (2005). The many faces of postpartum depression. *Journal of Obstetric, Gynecologic, and Neonatal Nursing*, *34*(5), 569–576. https://doi.org/10.1177/0884217505279995

18. Rochlen, A. B., Paterniti, D. A., Epstein, R. M., Duberstein, P., Willeford, L., & Kravitz, R. L. (2010). Barriers in diagnosing and treating men with depression: A focus group report. *American Journal of Men's Health*, *4*(2), 167–175. https://doi.org/10.1177/1557988309335823

19. Singley, D. B. (2017, November 16). *Paternal perinatal mental health: Yes, it exists and what to do about it* [Webinar conference session]. The Center for Men's Excellence, San Diego, CA, United States and Postpartum Support International.

WEEK 5

1. Withers, M., Kharazmi, N., & Lim, E. (2018). Traditional beliefs and practices in pregnancy, childbirth and postpartum: A review of the evidence from Asian countries. *Midwifery*, *56*, 158–170. https://doi.org/10.1016/j.midw.2017.10.019

2. U.S. Department of Agriculture & U.S. Department of Health and Human Services. (2020, December). *Dietary Guidelines for Americans, 2020-2025* (9th ed.). DietaryGuidelines. https://www.dietaryguidelines.gov/sites/default/files/2021-03/Dietary_Guidelines_for_Americans-2020-2025.pdf

3. Foong, S. C., Tan, M. L., Foong, W. C., Marasco, L. A., Ho, J. J., & Ong, J. H. (2020). Oral galactagogues (natural therapies or drugs) for increasing breast milk production in mothers of non-hospitalised term infants. *Cochrane Database of Systematic Reviews*, *5*(5), Article CD011505. https://doi.org/10.1002/14651858.CD011505.pub2

WEEK 6

1. DeMaria, A. L., Delay, C., Sundstrom, B., Wakefield, A. L., Avina, A., & Meier, S. (2019). Understanding women's postpartum sexual experiences. *Culture, Health & Sexuality*, *21*(10), 1162–1176. https://doi.org/10.1080/13691058.2018.1543802

2. Wallwiener, S., Müller, M., Doster, A., Kuon, R. J., Plewniok, K., Feller, S., Wallwiener, M., Reck, C., Matthies, L. M., & Wallwiener, C. (2017). Sexual activity and sexual dysfunction

of women in the perinatal period: A longitudinal study. *Archives of Gynecology and Obstetrics*, *295*(4), 873–883. https://doi.org/10.1007/s00404-017-4305-0

3. Jawed-Wessel, S., & Sevick, E. (2017). The impact of pregnancy and childbirth on sexual behaviors: A systematic review. *Journal of Sex Research*, *54*(4-5), 411–423. https://doi.org/10.1080/00224499.2016.1274715

4. Lagaert, L., Weyers, S., Van Kerrebroeck, H., & Elaut, E. (2017). Postpartum dyspareunia and sexual functioning: A prospective cohort study. *The European Journal of Contraception & Reproductive Health Care*, *22*(3), 200–206. https://doi.org/10.1080/13625187.2017.1315938

5. Alp Yılmaz, F., Şener Taplak, A., & Polat, S. (2019). Breastfeeding and sexual activity and sexual quality in postpartum women. *Breastfeeding Medicine*, *14*(8), 587–591. https://doi.org/10.1089/bfm.2018.0249

6. O'Malley, D., Higgins, A., Begley, C., Daly, D., & Smith, V. (2018). Prevalence of and risk factors associated with sexual health issues in primiparous women at 6 and 12 months postpartum; A longitudinal prospective cohort study (the MAMMI study). *BMC Pregnancy and Childbirth*, *18*(1), Article 196. https://doi.org/10.1186/s12884-018-1838-6

7. Zhang, Q., Shen, M., Zheng, Y., Jiao, S., Gao, S., Wang, X., Zou, L., & Shen, M. (2021). Sexual function in Chinese women from pregnancy to postpartum: A multicenter longitudinal prospective study. *BMC Pregnancy and Childbirth*, *21*(1), Article 65. https://doi.org/10.1186/s12884-021-03546-6

8. Faisal-Cury, A., Menezes, P. R., Quayle, J., Matijasevich, A., & Diniz, S. G. (2015). The relationship between mode of delivery and sexual health outcomes after childbirth. *The Journal of Sexual Medicine*, *12*(5), 1212–1220. https://doi.org/10.1111/jsm.12883

9. McDonald, E. A., & Brown, S. J. (2013). Does method of birth make a difference to when women resume sex after childbirth? *BJOG: An International Journal of Obstetrics and Gynaecology*, *120*(7), 823–830. https://doi.org/10.1111/1471-0528.12166

10. Dennis, C. L., Fung, K., Grigoriadis, S., Robinson, G. E., Romans, S., & Ross, L. (2007). Traditional postpartum practices and rituals: A qualitative systematic review. *Women's Health*, *3*(4), 487–502. https://doi.org/10.2217/17455057.3.4.487

11. Shabangu, Z., & Madiba, S. (2019). The role of culture in maintaining post-partum sexual abstinence of Swazi women. *International Journal of Environmental Research and Public Health*, *16*(14), Article 2590. https://doi.org/10.3390/ijerph16142590

12. Ahlborg, T., Rudeblad, K., Linnér, S., & Linton, S. (2008). Sensual and sexual marital contentment in parents of small children—a follow-up study when the first child is four years old. *Journal of Sex Research*, *45*(3), 295–304. https://doi.org/10.1080/00224490802204423

13. Hansson, M., & Ahlborg, T. (2012). Quality of the intimate and sexual relationship in first-time parents – A longitudinal study. *Sexual & Reproductive Healthcare*, *3*(1), 21–29. https://doi.org/10.1016/j.srhc.2011.10.002

14. Gommesen, D., Nøhr, E., Qvist, N., & Rasch, V. (2019). Obstetric perineal tears, sexual function and dyspareunia among primiparous women 12 months postpartum: A prospective cohort study. *BMJ Open*, *9*(12), Article we032368. https://doi.org/10.1136/bmjopen-2019-032368

WEEK 7
None.

WEEK 8

1. Committee on Obstetric Practice (with M. L. Birsner, & C. Gyamfi-Bannerman). (2020). Physical activity and exercise during pregnancy and the postpartum period: ACOG committee opinion, number 804. *Obstetrics & Gynecology*, *135*(4), e178–e188. https://doi.org/10.1097/AOG.0000000000003772

2. Grigoriadis, S., Erlick Robinson, G., Fung, K., Ross, L. E., Chee, C. (Y. I.), Dennis, C.-L., & Romans, S. (2009). Traditional postpartum practices and rituals: Clinical implications. *Canadian Journal of Psychiatry*, *54*(12), 834–840. https://doi.org/10.1177/070674370905401206

3. Amorim Adegboye, A. R., & Linne, Y. M. (2013). Diet or exercise, or both, for weight reduction in women after childbirth. *Cochrane Database of Systematic Reviews*, (7), Article CD005627. https://doi.org/10.1002/14651858.CD005627.pub3

4. Piercy, K. L., Troiano, R. P., Ballard, R. M., Carlson, S. A., Fulton, J. E., Galuska, D. A., George, S. M., & Olson, R. D. (2018). The physical activity guidelines for Americans. *JAMA*, *320*(19), 2020–2028. https://doi.org/10.1001/jama.2018.14854

5. Bull, F. C., Al-Ansari, S. S., Biddle, S., Borodulin, K., Buman, M. P., Cardon, G., Carty, C., Chaput, J.-P., Chastin, S., Chou, R., Dempsey, P. C., DiPietro, L., Ekelund, U., Firth, J., Friedenreich, C. M., Garcia, L., Gichu, M., Jago, R., Katzmarzyk, P. T., ... Willumsen, J. F. (2020). World Health Organization 2020 guidelines on physical activity and sedentary behaviour. *British Journal of Sports Medicine*, *54*(24), 1451–1462. https://doi.org/10.1136/bjsports-2020-102955

WEEK 9

1. Prinds, C., Nikolajsen, H., & Folmann, B. (2020). Yummy mummy — The ideal of not looking like a mother. *Women and Birth*, *33*(3), e266–e273. https://doi.org/10.1016/j.wombi.2019.05.009

2. Hodgkinson, E. L., Smith, D. M., & Wittkowski, A. (2014). Women's experiences of their pregnancy and postpartum body image: A systematic review and meta-synthesis. *BMC Pregnancy and Childbirth*, *14*, Article 330. https://doi.org/10.1186/1471-2393-14-330

WEEK 10

1. Cigna & Ipsos. (2018, May). *Cigna U.S. loneliness index: Survey of 20,000 Americans examining behaviors driving loneliness in the United States.* https://www.cigna.com/assets/docs/newsroom/loneliness-survey-2018-full-report.pdf
   "there are people who really . . . " p. 4

2. Action for Children & Jo Cox Loneliness. (2017). *It starts with hello: A report looking into the impact of loneliness in children, young people and families.* British Association of Social Workers. https://www.basw.co.uk/system/files/resources/basw_94738-5_0.pdf
   "an unwelcome subjective feeling of . . . " p. 4
   "there is [still] a mismatch . . . " p. 4

3. Junttila, N., Ahlqvist-Björkroth, S., Aromaa, M., Rautava, P., Piha, J., & Räihä, H. (2015). Intercorrelations and developmental pathways of mothers' and fathers' loneliness during pregnancy, infancy and toddlerhood–STEPS study. *Scandinavian Journal of Psychology*, *56*(5), 482–488. https://doi.org/10.1111/sjop.12241

4. Nowland, R., Thomson, G., McNally, L., Smith, T., & Whittaker, K. (2021). Experiencing loneliness in parenthood: A scoping review. *Perspectives in Public Health*, *141*(4), 214–225. https://doi.org/10.1177/17579139211018243

5. Yang, K., & Victor, C. (2011). Age and loneliness in 25 European nations. *Ageing and Society*, *31*(8), 1368-1388. https://doi.org/10.1017/S0144686X1000139X

6. Griffin, J. (2010). *The lonely society?* [Report]. Mental Health Foundation. https://www.bl.uk/collection-items/lonely-society

7. Hawkley, L. C., & Cacioppo, J. T. (2010). Loneliness matters: A theoretical and empirical review of consequences and mechanisms. *Annals of Behavioral Medicine*, *40*(2), 218–227. https://doi.org/10.1007/s12160-010-9210-8

8. Lee, K., Vasileiou, K., & Barnett, J. (2019). 'Lonely within the mother': An exploratory study of first-time mothers' experiences of loneliness. *Journal of Health Psychology*, *24*(10), 1334–1344. https://doi.org/10.1177/1359105317723451

9. Luoma, I., Korhonen, M., Puura, K., & Salmelin, R. K. (2019). Maternal loneliness: Concurrent and longitudinal associations with depressive symptoms and child adjustment. *Psychology, Health & Medicine*, *24*(6), 667–679. https://doi.org/10.1080/13548506.2018.1554251

WEEK 11

1. Benschop, L., Duvekot, J. J., & Roeters van Lennep, J. E. (2019). Future risk of cardiovascular disease risk factors and events in women after a hypertensive disorder of pregnancy. *Heart* (British Cardiovascular Society), *105*(16), 1273–1278. https://doi.org/10.1136/heartjnl-2018-313453

2. Zhu, Y., & Zhang, C. (2016). Prevalence of gestational diabetes and risk of progression to type 2 diabetes: A global perspective. *Current Diabetes Reports*, *16*(1), Article 7. https://doi.org/10.1007/s11892-015-0699-x

3. McKinley, M. C., Allen-Walker, V., McGirr, C., Rooney, C., & Woodside, J. V. (2018). Weight loss after pregnancy: Challenges and opportunities. *Nutrition Research Reviews*, *31*(2), 225–238. https://doi.org/10.1017/S0954422418000070

4. Amorim Adegboye, A. R., & Linne, Y. M. (2013). Diet or exercise, or both, for weight reduction in women after childbirth. *Cochrane Database of Systematic Reviews*, (7), Article CD005627. https://doi.org/10.1002/14651858.CD005627.pub3

WEEK 12

1. Rotkirch, A., & Janhunen, K. (2010). Maternal guilt. *Evolutionary Psychology*, *8*(1), 90–106. https://doi.org/10.1177/147470491000800108

2. Caldwell, J., Meredith, P., Whittingham, K., & Ziviani, J. (2021). Shame and guilt in the postnatal period: A systematic review. *Journal of Reproductive and Infant Psychology*, *39*(1), 67–85. https://doi.org/10.1080/02646838.2020.1754372

3. Constantinou, G., Varela, S., & Buckby, B. (2021). Reviewing the experiences of maternal guilt – the "Motherhood Myth" influence. *Health Care for Women International*, *42*(4-6), 852–876. https://doi.org/10.1080/07399332.2020.1835917

4. Brown, B. (2010). *The gifts of imperfection: Let go of who you think you're supposed to be and embrace who you are: Your guide to a wholehearted life.* Hazelden Publishing.

> *"the intensely painful feeling or . . . " from "The Things That Get in the Way: Shame Resilience 101," paragraph 6.*
> *"metastasizes" from "Courage, Compassion, and Connection: The Gifts of Imperfection: The Gun-for-hire Shame Storm" paragraph 17.*
> *"healthy achievement and growth," from "GUIDEPOST #2: Cultivating Self-Compassion: Letting Go of Perfectionism," paragraph 7.*
> *"Perfectionism is the belief that . . . " from "GUIDEPOST #2: Cultivating Self-Compassion: Letting Go of Perfectionism," paragraph 7.*

5. Winnicot, D. W. (2006). *Playing and reality* (2nd ed.). Routledge.

6. Shloim, N., Lans, O., Brown, M., Mckelvie, S., Cohen, S., & Cahill, J. (2020). "Motherhood is like a roller coaster... lots of ups, then downs, something chaotic...": UK & Israeli women's experiences of motherhood 6-12 months postpartum. *Journal of Reproductive and Infant Psychology*, *38*(5), 523–545. https://doi.org/10.1080/02646838.2019.1631448

7. Cooper, G., Hoffman, K., Powell, B., & Circle of Security International. (2018). *(Almost) everything I need to know about supporting security in 25 words or less.* https://www.circleofsecurity-international.com/wp-content/uploads/COS_25wordsorless-1.pdf

> *"Always be: bigger, stronger, wiser . . . "*

WEEK 13

1. Healthcare.gov. (n.d.). *Preventative care benefits for women.* Retrieved January 10, 2022, from https://www.healthcare.gov/preventive-care-women/

2. Committee on Gynecologic Practice (with C. Witkop). (2018). ACOG committee opinion no. 755: Well-woman visit. *Obstetrics & Gynecology*, *132*(4), e181–e186. https://doi.org/10.1097/AOG.0000000000002897

3. Gavin, L., Moskosky, S., Carter, M., Curtis, K., Glass, E., Godfrey, E., Marcell, A., Mautone-Smith, N., Pazol, K., Tepper, N., Zapata, L., & Centers for Disease Control and Prevention. (2014). *Providing quality family planning services: Recommendations of CDC and the U.S. Office of Population Affairs. Morbidity and Mortality Weekly Report*, *63*(RR-04), 1–54. *PubMed* Retrieved January 29, 2022, from https://pubmed.ncbi.nlm.nih.gov/24759690/

4. Committee on Gynecologic Practice (with C. Cansino, & L. Chohan). (2018). ACOG committee opinion no. 754: The utility of and indications for routine pelvic examination. *Obstetrics & Gynecology*, *132*(4), e174–e180. https://doi.org/10.1097/AOG.0000000000002895

5. Guirguis-Blake, J. M., Henderson, J. T., & Perdue, L. A. (2017). Periodic screening pelvic examination: Evidence report and systematic review for the US Preventive Services Task Force. *JAMA*, *317*(9), 954–966. https://doi.org/10.1001/jama.2016.12819

6. U.S. Preventive Services Task Force. (n.d.). *A and B recommendations.* Retrieved January 10, 2022, from https://www.uspreventiveservicestaskforce.org/uspstf/recommendation-topics/uspstf-and-b-recommendations

7. Perkins, R. B., Guido, R. S., Castle, P. E., Chelmow, D., Einstein, M. H., Garcia, F., Huh, W. K., Kim, J. J., Moscicki, A.-B., Nayar, R., Saraiya, M., Sawaya, G. F., Wentzensen, N., Schiffman, M., for the 2019 ASCCP Risk-Based Management Consensus Guidelines Committee. (2020). 2019 ASCCP Risk-Based Management Consensus Guidelines for abnormal cervical cancer screening tests and cancer precursors. *Journal of Lower Genital Tract Disease, 24*(2), 102–131. https://doi.org/10.1097/LGT.0000000000000525

8. American Cancer Society. (2020, July 30). *Cervical cancer early detection, diagnosis and staging.* https://www.cancer.org/content/dam/CRC/PDF/Public/8601.00.pdf

9. American College of Obstetricians and Gynecologists. (2022). *Cervical cancer screening.* https://www.acog.org/womens-health/infographics/cervical-cancer-screening

10. U.S. Preventive Services Task Force. (2018, August 21). *Cervical cancer: Screening.* https://www.uspreventiveservicestaskforce.org/uspstf/recommendation/cervical-cancer-screening

11. Committee on Practice Bulletins-Gynecology (with M. Pearlman, M. Jeudy, & D. Chelmow). (2017). Practice bulletin number 179: Breast cancer risk assessment and screening in average-risk women. *Obstetrics & Gynecology, 130*(1), e1–e16. https://doi.org/10.1097/AOG.0000000000002158

WEEK 14

1. Merriam-Webster. (n.d.). Legacy. *Merriam-Webster.com dictionary.* Retrieved April 10, 2022, from https://www.merriam-webster.com/dictionary/legacy

WEEK 15
None.

APPENDIX A

1. PREGNANCY ROADMAP

1. Rose, N. C., Kaimal, A. J., Dugoff, L., Norton, M. E., American College of Obstetricians and Gynecologists' Committee on Practice Bulletins—Obstetrics, Committee on Genetics & Society for Maternal-Fetal Medicine. (2020). ACOG practice bulletin, no. 226: Screening for fetal chromosomal abnormalities. *Obstetrics & Gynecology, 136*(4), e48–e69. https://doi.org/10.1097/AOG.0000000000004084

2. MacDonald, L. A., Waters, T. R., Napolitano, P. G., Goddard, D. E., Ryan, M. A., Nielsen, P., & Hudock, S. D. (2013). Clinical guidelines for occupational lifting in pregnancy: Evidence summary and provisional recommendations. *American Journal of Obstetrics & Gynecology, 209*(2), 80–88. https://doi.org/10.1016/j.ajog.2013.02.047.

3. U.S. Preventive Services Task Force (with K. W. Davidson). (2021). US Preventive Services Task Force Recommendation Statement: Screening for gestational diabetes. *JAMA, 326*(6), 531–538. https://doi.org/10.1001/jama.2021.11922

4. Committee on Practice Bulletins—Obstetrics (with A. B. Caughey, & M. Turrentine). (2018). ACOG practice bulletin no. 190: Gestational diabetes mellitus. *Obstetrics & Gynecology, 131*(2), e49–e64. https://doi.org/10.1097/AOG.0000000000002501

5. U.S. Preventive Services Task Force (with D. K. Owens). (2019). US Preventive Services Task Force Recommendation Statement: Screening for asymptomatic bacteriuria in adults. *JAMA, 322*(12), 1188–1194. https://doi.org/10.1001/jama.2019.13069

6. Landon, M. B., Galan, H. L., Jauniaux, E. R. M., Driscoll, D. A., Berghella, V., Grobman, W. A., Kilpatrick, S. J., & Cahill, A. G. (2021). *Gabbe's obstetrics: Normal and problem pregnancies* (8th ed.). Elsevier.

7. Centers for Disease Control and Prevention. (n.d.). *Tdap (pertussis) vaccine and pregnancy.* https://www.cdc.gov/vaccines/pregnancy/hcp-toolkit/tdap-vaccine-pregnancy.html

8. Committee on Obstetric Practice & Immunization and Emerging Infections Expert Work Group (with R. Beigi). (2017). Committee opinion no. 718: Update on immunization and pregnancy: Tetanus, diphtheria, and pertussis vaccination. *Obstetrics & Gynecology, 130*(3), e153–e157. https://doi.org/10.1097/AOG.0000000000002301

9. American College of Nurse-Midwives Division of Standards and Practice. (2018, August). *Position statement: Immunization in pregnancy and postpartum.* https://www.midwife.org/ acnm/files/acnmlibrarydata/uploadfilename/000000000289/PS-Immunization-in-Pregnancy-and-Postpartum-FINAL-20-Nov-18.pdf

10. U.S. Preventive Services Task Force. (2004). *Rh (D) incompatibility: Screening.* https://www. uspreventiveservicestaskforce.org/uspstf/recommendation/rh-d-incompatibility-screening

11. American College of Obstetricians and Gynecologists. (2020). ACOG committee opinion, number 797: Prevention of group b streptococcal early-onset disease in newborns. *Obstetrics & Gynecology, 135*(2), e51–e72. https://doi.org/10.1097/AOG.0000000000003668

12. Filkins, L., Hauser, J. R., Robinson-Dunn, B., Tibbetts, R., Boyanton, B. L., & Revell, P., on behalf of the American Society for Microbiology Clinical and Public Health Microbiology Committee, Subcommittee on Laboratory Practices. (2020). American Society for Microbiology provides 2020 guidelines for detection and identification of group b *Streptococcus. Journal of Clinical Microbiology, 59*(1), e01230-20. https://doi.org/10.1128/JCM.01230-20

13. American College of Nurse-Midwives Division of Standards and Practice. (2019, September). *Position statement: Prevention of group b streptococcal infection in the newborn.* https://www. midwife.org/acnm/files/acnmlibrarydata/uploadfilename/000000000319/PS%20Prevention%20of%20Group%20B%20Streptococcal%20Disease%20in%20the%20Newborn%20 190927.pdf

14. Presidential Task Force on Redefining the Postpartum Visit & Committee on Obstetric Practice (with A. Stuebe, T. Auguste, & M. Gulati). (2018). ACOG committee opinion no. 736: Optimizing postpartum care. *Obstetrics & Gynecology, 131*(5), e140–e150. https://doi. org/10.1097/AOG.0000000000002633

15. Centers for Disease Control and Prevention. (2021). *Influenza (flu): Pregnancy.* https://www. cdc.gov/flu/highrisk/pregnant.htm

16. Immunization and Emerging Infections Expert Work Group & Committee on Obstetric Practice (with N. S., Silverman, & R. Beigi). (2018, April). *Influenza vaccination during pregnancy* [Reaffirmed 2021]. American College of Obstetricians and Gynecologists. https:// www.acog.org/clinical/clinical-guidance/committee-opinion/articles/2018/04/influenza-vaccination-during-pregnancy

2. WHEN TO SEEK PROFESSIONAL HELP
None.

3. PREGNANCY TIPS

a. Getting Started

1. U.S. Preventive Services Task Force (with K. Bibbins-Domingo). (2017). Folic acid supplementation for the prevention of neural tube defects: US Preventive Services Task Force recommendation statement. *JAMA. 317*(2), 183-189. http://doi.org/10.1001/jama.2016.19438

2. National Institutes of Health, Office of Dietary Supplements. (2021, March 29). *Folate.* https:// ods.od.nih.gov/factsheets/Folate-HealthProfessional/

3. Procter S. B., & Campbell, C. G. (2014). Position of the Academy of Nutrition and Dietetics: Nutrition and lifestyle for a healthy pregnancy outcome. *Journal of the Academy of Nutrition and Dietetics, 114*(7), 1099-1103. https://doi.org/10.1016/j.jand.2014.05.0054.

4. FIGO Working Group on Best Practice in Maternal-Fetal Medicine. (2015). Best practice in maternal-fetal medicine. *International Journal of Gynaecology and Obstetrics, 128*(1), 80–82. https://doi.org/10.1016/j.ijgo.2014.10.011

5. Crider, K. S., Bailey, L. B., & Berry, R. J. (2011). Folic acid food fortification—Its history, effect, concerns, and future directions. *Nutrients, 3*(3), 370–384. https://doi.org/10.3390/ nu3030370

6. Centers for Disease Control and Prevention. (n.d.). *Recommendations: Women and folic acid.* https://www.cdc.gov/ncbddd/folicacid/recommendations.html

7. Mousa, A., Naqash, A., & Lim, S. (2019). Macronutrient and micronutrient intake during pregnancy: An overview of recent evidence. *Nutrients, 11*(2), Article 443. https://doi.org/10.3390/nu11020443

8. Valentin, M., Coste Mazeau, P., Zerah, M., Ceccaldi, P. F., Benachi, A., & Luton, D. (2018). Acid folic and pregnancy: A mandatory supplementation. *Annales d'Endocrinologie, 79*(2), 91–94. https://doi.org/10.1016/j.ando.2017.10.001

9. Chitayat, D., Matsui, D., Amitai, Y., Kennedy, D., Vohra, S., Rieder, M., & Koren, G. (2016). Folic acid supplementation for pregnant women and those planning pregnancy: 2015 update. *The Journal of Clinical Pharmacology, 56*(2), 170–5. https://doi.org/10.1002/jcph.616

10. Ferrazzi, E., Tiso, G., & Di Martino, D. (2020). Folic acid versus 5- methyl tetrahydrofolate supplementation in pregnancy. *European Journal of Obstetrics, Gynecology, and Reproductive Biology, 253,* 312–319. https://doi.org/10.1016/j.ejogrb.2020.06.012

11. Henderson, J. T., Vesco, K. K., Senger, C. A., Thomas, R. G., & Redmond, N. (2021). Aspirin use to prevent preeclampsia and related morbidity and mortality: Updated evidence report and systematic review for the US Preventive Services Task Force. *JAMA, 326*(12), 1192–1206. https://doi.org/10.1001/jama.2021.8551

12. U.S. Food and Drug Administration. (2014, December 3). *Pregnancy and lactation labeling (drugs) final rule* [Current as of 2021, March 5]. https://www.fda.gov/drugs/labeling-information-drug-products/pregnancy-and-lactation-labeling-drugs-final-rule

13. Mosley, J. F., II, Smith, L. L., & Dezan, M. D. (2015). An overview of upcoming changes in pregnancy and lactation labeling information. *Pharmacy Practice, 13*(2), Article 605. https://doi.org/10.18549/pharmpract.2015.02.605

14. Pernia, S., & DeMaagd, G. (2016). The new pregnancy and lactation labeling rule. *Pharmacy & Therapeutics, 41*(11), 713–715. *PubMed.* Retrieved January 13, 2022, from https://www.ncbi.nlm.nih.gov/pmc/articles/PMC5083079/

b. Managing Symptoms

1. Matthews, A., Haas, D. M., O'Mathúna, D. P., & Dowswell, T. (2015). Interventions for nausea and vomiting in early pregnancy. *Cochrane Database of Systematic Reviews,* (9), Article CD007575. https://doi.org/10.1002/14651858.CD007575.pub4

2. Landon, M. B., Galan, H. L., Jauniaux, E. R. M., Driscoll, D. A., Berghella, V., Grobman, W. A., Kilpatrick, S. J., & Cahill, A. G. (2021). *Gabbe's obstetrics: Normal and problem pregnancies* (8th ed.). Elsevier.

3. Maltepe, C. (2014). Surviving morning sickness successfully: From patient's perception to rational management. *Journal of Population Therapeutics and Clinical Pharmacology, 21*(3), Article e555-564. *PubMed.* Retrieved November 12, 2021, from https://pubmed.ncbi.nlm.nih.gov/25654792/

4. Committee on Practice Bulletins—Obstetrics (with S. M. Ramin). (2018). ACOG practice bulletin no. 189: Nausea and vomiting of pregnancy. *Obstetrics & Gynecology, 131*(1), e15-e30. https://doi.org/10.1097/aog.0000000000002456

5. Anh, N. H., Kim, S. J., Long, N. P., Min, J. E., Yoon, Y. C., Lee, E. G., Kim, M., Kim, T. J., Yang, Y. Y., Son, E. Y., Yoon, S. J., Diem, N. C., Kim, H. M., & Kwon, S. W. (2020). Ginger on human health: A comprehensive systematic review of 109 randomized controlled trials. *Nutrients, 12*(1), Article 157. https://doi.org/10.3390/nu12010157

6. Koren, G., Clark, S., Hankins, G. D. V., Caritis, S. N., Umans, J. G., Miodovnik, M., Mattison, D. R., & Matok, I. (2015). Maternal safety of the delayed-release doxylamine and pyridoxine combination for nausea and vomiting of pregnancy; a randomized placebo controlled trial. *BMC Pregnancy and Childbirth, 15,* Article 59. https://doi.org/10.1186/s12884-015-0488-1

7. Thaxter Nesbeth, K. A., Samuels, L. A., Nicholson Daley, C., Gossell-Williams, M., & Nesbeth, D. A. (2016). Ptyalism in pregnancy – A review of epidemiology and practices. *European Journal of Obstetrics & Gynecology and Reproductive Biology, 198,* 47-49. https://doi.org/10.1016/j.ejogrb.2015.12.022

8. Rungsiprakarn, P., Laopaiboon, M., Sangkomkamhang, U. S., Lumbiganon, P., & Pratt, J. J. (2015). Interventions for treating constipation in pregnancy. *Cochrane Database of Systematic Reviews*, (9), Article CD011448. https://doi.org/10.1002/14651858.CD011448.pub2

9. Vazquez, J. C. (2010). Constipation, haemorrhoids, and heartburn in pregnancy. *BMJ Clinical Evidence*, Article 1411. *PubMed*. Retrieved November 12, 2021, from https://pubmed.ncbi. nlm.nih.gov/21418682/

10. Institute of Medicine. (2006). Summary tables, dietary reference intakes: Recommended dietary allowances and adequate intakes, total water and macronutrients. In J. J. Otten, J. Pitzi Hellwig, & L. D. Meyers (Eds.), *Dietary reference intakes: The essential guide to nutrient requirements* (pp. 529-542). The National Academies Press. https://nap.nationalacademies. org/read/11537/chapter/59

11. American College of Obstetricians and Gynecologists. (2020, October). *Ask ACOG: How much water should I drink during pregnancy?* https://www.acog.org/womens-health/experts-and-stories/ask-acog/how-much-water-should-i-drink-during-pregnancy

12. Sheyholislami, H., & Connor, K. L. (2021). Are probiotics and prebiotics safe for use during pregnancy and lactation? A systematic review and meta-analysis. *Nutrients, 13*(7), Article 2382. https://doi.org/10.3390/nu13072382

13. Baldassarre, M. E., Palladino, V., Amoruso, A., Pindinelli, S., Mastromarino, P., Fanelli, M., Di Mauro, A., & Laforgia, N. (2018). Rationale of probiotic supplementation during pregnancy and neonatal period. *Nutrients, 10*(11), Article 1693. https://doi.org/10.3390/nu10111693

14. Mirghafourvand, M., Homayouni Rad, A., Mohammad Alizadeh Charandabi, S., Fardiazar, Z., & Shokri, K. (2016). The effect of probiotic yogurt on constipation in pregnant women: A randomized controlled clinical trial. *Iranian Red Crescent Medical Journal, 18*(11), Article e39870. https://doi.org/10.5812/ircmj.39870

15. Trottier, M., Erebara, A., & Bozzo, P. (2012). Treating constipation during pregnancy. *Canadian Family Physician, 58*(8), 836–838. *PubMed*. Retrieved November 11, 2021, from https:// pubmed.ncbi.nlm.nih.gov/22893333/

16. de Milliano, I., Tabbers, M. M., van der Post, J. A., & Benninga, M. A. (2012). Is a multispecies probiotic mixture effective in constipation during pregnancy? 'A pilot study.' *Nutrition Journal*, (11), Article 80. https://doi.org/10.1186/1475-2891-11-80

17. MotherToBaby. (2020, March 1). *Docusate sodium* [Fact sheet]. https://mothertobaby.org/factsheets/docusate-sodium-pregnancy/pdf/

18. Servey, J., & Chang, J. (2014). Over-the-counter medications in pregnancy. *American Family Physician. 90*(8), 548-555. *PubMed*. Retrieved November 11, 2021, from https://pubmed. ncbi.nlm.nih.gov/25369643/

19. Phupong, V, & Hanprasertpong, T. (2015). Interventions for heartburn in pregnancy. *Cochrane Database of Systematic Reviews*, (9), Article CD011379. https://doi.org/10.1002/14651858. CD011379.pub2

20. Thélin, C. S., & Richter, J. E. (2020). Review article: The management of heartburn during pregnancy and lactation. *Alimentary Pharmacology & Therapeutics, 51*(4), 421-434. https://doi. org/10.1111/apt.15611

21. Narayan, B., & Nelson-Piercy, C. (2016). Medical problems in pregnancy. *Clinical Medicine Journal, 16*(Suppl 6), s110–s116. https://doi.org/10.7861/clinmedicine.16-6-s110

22. Lucas, S. (2019). Migraine and other headache disorders: ACOG clinical updates in women's health care primary and preventive care review summary volume XVIII, number 4. *Obstetrics & Gynecology, 134*(1), 211. https://doi.org/10.1097/AOG.0000000000003322

23. Hainer, B. L., & Matheson, E. M. (2013). Approach to acute headache in adults. American Family Physician, 87(10), 682–687. PubMed. Retrieved November 11, 2021, from https:// pubmed.ncbi.nlm.nih.gov/23939446/

24. American Migraine Foundation. (2017, July 27). *The American Migraine Foundation's guide to triggers & how to manage them: Tips for managing the 10 most common migraine triggers.* https://americanmigrainefoundation.org/resource-library/top-10-migraine-triggers/

25. Hirshkowitz, M., Whiton, K., Albert, S. M., Alessi, C., Bruni, O., DonCarlos, L., Hazen, N., Herman, J., Katz, E. S., Kheirandish-Gozal, L., Neubauer, D. N., O'Donnell, A. E., Ohayon, M., Peever, J., Rawding, R., Sachdeva, R. C., Setters, B., Vitiello, M. V., Catesby Ware, J., &

Adams Hillard, P. J. (2015). National Sleep Foundation's sleep time duration recommendations: Methodology and results summary. *Sleep, 1*(1), 40-43. https://doi.org/10.1016/j.sleh.2014.12.010

26. Linde, K., Allais, G., Brinkhaus, B., Fei, Y., Mehring, M., Vertosick, E. A., Vickers, A., & White, A. R. (2016). Acupuncture for the prevention of episodic migraine. *Cochrane Database of Systematic Reviews*, (6), Article CD001218. https://doi.org/10.1002/14651858.CD001218.pub3

27. Gregory, D. S., Wu, V., & Tuladhar, P. (2018). The pregnant patient: Managing common acute medical problems. American Family Physician, 98(9), 595-602. PubMed. Retrieved November 11, 2021, from https://pubmed.ncbi.nlm.nih.gov/30325641/

c. Pelvic Floor Health for Pregnancy and Beyond

1. Lawson, S., & Sacks, A. (2018). Pelvic floor physical therapy and women's health promotion. *Journal of Midwifery & Women's Health, 63*(4), 410–417. https://doi.org/10.1111/jmwh.12736

2. Jundt, K., Peschers, U., & Kentenich, H. (2015). The investigation and treatment of female pelvic floor dysfunction. *Deutsches Arzteblatt International, 112*, 564–574. https://doi.org/10.3238/arztebl.2015.0564

3. Woodley, S. J., Lawrenson, P., Boyle, R., Cody, J. D., Mørkved, S., Kernohan, A., & Hay-Smith, J. E. (2020). Pelvic floor muscle training for preventing and treating urinary and faecal incontinence in antenatal and postnatal women. *Cochrane Database of Systematic Reviews*, (5), Article CD007471. https://doi.org/10.1002/14651858.CD007471.pub4

4. Dumoulin, C., Hunter, K. F., Moore, K., Bradley, C. S., Burgio, K. L., Hagen, S., Imamura, M., Thakar, R., Williams, K., & Chambers, T. (2016). Conservative management for female urinary incontinence and pelvic organ prolapse review 2013: Summary of the 5th International Consultation on Incontinence. *Neurourology and Urodynamics, 35*(1), 15–20. https://doi.org/10.1002/nau.22677

5. Sobhgol, S. S., Priddis, H., Smith, C. A., & Dahlen, H. G. (2019). The effect of pelvic floor muscle exercise on female sexual function during pregnancy and postpartum: A systematic review. *Sexual Medicine Reviews, 7*(1), 13–28. https://doi.org/10.1016/j.sxmr.2018.08.002

d. Selecting a Maternity Care Provider and Practice
None.

e. Prenatal Screening and Testing Options

1. U.S. National Library of Medicine. (2019, October 1). *Birth defects.* MedlinePlus. https://medlineplus.gov/birthdefects.html

2. MotherToBaby. (2021, March 1). *Critical Periods of Development* [Fact sheet]. https://mothertobaby.org/fact-sheets/critical-periods-development/pdf/

3. Alwan, S., & Friedman, J. M. (2018). What birth defects are common in humans? How are they diagnosed at birth? In B. Hales, A. Scialli, & M. Tassinari (Eds.), *Teratology primer* (3rd ed) [Internet book]. Society for Birth Defects Research & Prevention. https://birthdefectsresearch.org/primer/

4. Shaw, G. M., & Finnell, R. H. (2018). How do gene-environment interactions affect the risk of birth defects? In B. Hales, A. Scialli, & M. Tassinari (Eds.), *Teratology primer* (3rd ed) [Internet book]. Society for Birth Defects Research & Prevention. https://birthdefectsresearch.org/primer/

5. Rose, N. C., Kaimal, A. J., Dugoff, L., Norton, M. E., American College of Obstetricians and Gynecologists' Committee on Practice Bulletins—Obstetrics, Committee on Genetics & Society for Maternal-Fetal Medicine. (2020). Screening for fetal chromosomal abnormalities: ACOG practice bulletin, number 226. *Obstetrics & Gynecology, 136*(4), e48–e69. https://doi.org/10.1097/AOG.0000000000004084

6. Gregg, A. R., Skotko, B. G., Benkendorf, J. L., Monaghan, K. G., Bajaj, K., Best, R. G., Klugman, S., & Watson, M. S. on behalf of the ACMG Noninvasive Prenatal Screening Work Group. (2016). Noninvasive prenatal screening for fetal aneuploidy, 2016 update: A position

statement of the American College of Medical Genetics and Genomics. *Genetics in Medicine,* *18*(10), 1056–1065. https://doi.org/10.1038/gim.2016.97

7. Society for Maternal-Fetal Medicine (with M. E. Norton, J. R. Biggio, J. A. Kuller, & S. C. Blackwell). (2017). The role of ultrasound in women who undergo cell-free DNA screening. *American Journal of Obstetrics & Gynecology, 216*(3), B2–B7. https://doi.org/10.1016/j.ajog.2017.01.005

8. Committee on Practice Bulletins—Obstetrics, Committee on Genetics & Society for Maternal-Fetal Medicine (with M. E. Norton, & M. Jackson). (2016). Practice bulletin no. 162: Prenatal diagnostic testing for genetic disorders. *Obstetrics & Gynecology, 127*(5), e108–e122. https://doi.org/10.1097/AOG.0000000000001405

9. Akolekar, R., Beta, J., Picciarelli, G., Ogilvie, C., & D'Antonio, F. (2015). Procedure-related risk of miscarriage following amniocentesis and chorionic villus sampling: A systematic review and meta-analysis. *Ultrasound in Obstetrics and Gynecology, 45*(1), 16-26. *PubMed.* Retrieved November 11, 2021, from https://pubmed.ncbi.nlm.nih.gov/25042845/

10. Committee on Genetics (with B. Rink, S. Romero, J. R. Biggio, Jr., D. N. Saller, Jr., & R. Giardine). (2017). Committee opinion no. 691: Carrier screening for genetic conditions. (2017). *Obstetrics & Gynecology, 129*(3), e41–e55. https://doi.org/10.1097/AOG.0000000000001952

11. Committee on Genetics (with S. Romero, B. Rink, J. R. Biggio, Jr., & D. N. Saller, Jr.). (2017). Committee opinion no. 690: Carrier screening in the age of genomic medicine. *Obstetrics & Gynecology, 129*(3), e35–e40. https://doi.org/10.1097/AOG.0000000000001951

12. Prior, T. W., for the Professional Practice and Guidelines Committee. (2008). Carrier screening for spinal muscular atrophy. *Genetics in Medicine, 10*(11), 840–842. https://doi.org/10.1097/GIM.0b013e318188d069

13. Gross, S. J., Pletcher, B. A., & Monaghan, K. G., for the Professional Practice and Guidelines Committee. (2008). Carrier screening in individuals of Ashkenazi Jewish descent. *Genetics in Medicine, 10*(1): 54-56. https://doi.org/10.1097/GIM.0b013e31815f247c

14. Fonda Allen, J., Stoll, K., & Bernhardt, B. A. (2016). Pre- and post-test genetic counseling for chromosomal and Mendelian disorders. *Seminars in Perinatology, 40*(1), 44–55. https://doi.org/10.1053/j.semperi.2015.11.007

f. Weight Gain Recommendations

1. Institute of Medicine & National Research Council. (2009). Determining optimal weight gain. In K. M. Rasmussen, & A. L. Yaktine (Eds.), *Weight gain during pregnancy: Reexamining the guidelines.* National Academies Press. https://doi.org/10.17226/

2. Martínez-Hortelano, J. A., Cavero-Redondo, I., Álvarez-Bueno, C., Garrido-Miguel, M., Soriano-Cano, A., & Martínez-Vizcaíno, V. (2020). Monitoring gestational weight gain and prepregnancy BMI using the 2009 IOM guidelines in the global population: A systematic review and meta-analysis. *BMC Pregnancy and Childbirth, 20*(1), Article 649. https://doi.org/10.1186/s12884-020-03335-7

3. Centers for Disease Control and Prevention. (2016, October 14). QuickStats: Gestational weight gain* among women with full-term, singleton births, compared with recommendations — 48 States and the District of Columbia, 2015. *Morbidity and Mortality Weekly Report, 65*(40), Article 1121. https://doi.org/10.15585/mmwr.mm6540a10

4. Mameli, C., Mazzantini, S., & Zuccotti, G. V. (2016). Nutrition in the first 1000 days: The origin of childhood obesity. *International Journal of Environmental Research and Public Health, 13*(9), Article 838. https://doi.org/10.3390/ijerph13090838

5. Rogozińska, E., Zamora, J., Marlin, N., Betrán, A. P., Astrup, A., Bogaerts, A., Cecatti, J. G., Dodd, J. M., Facchinetti, F., Geiker, N. R. W., Haakstad, L. A. H., Hauner, H., Jensen, D. M., Kinnunen, T. I., Mol, B. W. J., Owens, J., Phelan, S., Renault, K. M., Salvesen, K. Å., … Thangaratinam, S., for the International Weight Management in Pregnancy (i-WIP) Collaborative Group. (2019). Gestational weight gain outside the Institute of Medicine recommendations and adverse pregnancy outcomes: Analysis using individual participant data from randomised trials. *BMC Pregnancy and Childbirth, 19*, Article 322. https://doi.org/10.1186/s12884-019-2472-7

6. Siega-Riz, A. M., Viswanathan, M., Moos, M.-K., Deierlein, A., Mumford, S., Knaack, J., Thieda, P., Lux, L. J., & Lohr, K. N. (2009). A systematic review of outcomes of maternal weight

gain according to the Institute of Medicine recommendations: Birthweight, fetal growth, and postpartum weight retention. *American Journal of Obstetrics & Gynecology, 201*(4), 339. E1-E14. https://doi.org/10.1016/j.ajog.2009.07.002

7. American Pregnancy Association. (n.d.). *Pregnancy weight gain: Is how much weight you gain during pregnancy important?* https://americanpregnancy.org/healthy-pregnancy/pregnancy-health-wellness/pregnancy-weight-gain/

g. Tips for Working While Pregnant

1. Jackson, R. A., Gardner, S., Torres, L. N., Huchko, M. J., Zlatnik, M. G., & Williams, J. C. (2015). My obstetrician got me fired: How work notes can harm pregnant patients and what to do about it. *Obstetrics & Gynecology, 126*(2), 250–254. https://doi.org/10.1097/AOG.0000000000000971

2. Karkowsky, C. E., & Morris, L. (2016). Pregnant at work: Time for prenatal care providers to act. *American Journal of Obstetrics & Gynecology, 215*(3), 306.e1–306.e5. https://doi.org/10.1016/j.ajog.2016.05.036

3. Morris, L. (2020). *Please don't fire my patient: How to support your pregnant patients' ability to earn income and stay healthy on the job* [Video]. Pregnant@Work. https://pregnantatwork.org/please-dont-fire-my-patient/

4. U.S. Department of Labor, Wage and Hour Division. (n.d.). *Family and Medical Leave Act.* https://www.dol.gov/agencies/whd/fmla

5. *Paid family and medical leave (PFML) overview and benefits: Learn more about Massachusetts's Paid Family and Medical Leave (PFML), including how to apply, leave benefits, and approval timelines.* (n.d.). Mass.gov. https://www.mass.gov/info-details/paid-family-and-medical-leave-pfml-fact-sheet

6. State of California Employment Development Department. (n.d.). *Fact sheet: California Paid Family Leave.* https://www.edd.ca.gov/pdf_pub_ctr/de8714cf.pdf

7. A Better Balance. (2022, July 1). *Comparative chart of paid family and medical leave laws in the United States.* https://www.abetterbalance.org/resources/paid-family-leave-laws-chart/

h. Baby Naming
None.

i. Nesting Tips

1. United States Environmental Protection Agency. (n.d.). *Non-durable goods: Product-specific data: Disposable diapers.* Retrieved July 24, 2022, from https://www.epa.gov/facts-and-figures-about-materials-waste-and-recycling/nondurable-goods-product-specific-data#Disposable-Diapers

2. Ajmeri, J. R., & Ajmeri, C. J. (2016). Development in the use of nonwovens for disposable hygiene products. In G. Kellie (Ed.), *Woodhead publishing series in textiles: No. 181. Advances in technical nonwovens* (1st ed., pp. 473-496). Woodhead Publishing. https://doi.org/10.1016/B978-0-08-100575-0.00018-8

3. Moon, R. Y., Carlin, R. F., Hand, I., American Academy of Pediatrics Task Force on Sudden Infant Death Syndrome & American Academy of Pediatrics Committee on Fetus and Newborn. (2022). Sleep-related infant deaths: Updated 2022 recommendations for reducing infant deaths in the sleep environment. *Pediatrics, 150*(1), Article e2022057990. https://doi.org/10.1542/peds.2022-057990

4. Children's Environmental Health Network. (2018, October 10). *Eco-healthy Child Care: Safer food packaging: BPA* [FAQ series]. https://cehn.org/wp-content/uploads/2019/10/BPA.FAQNewTemplate-Oct-2018-FINAL-1.pdf

5. Environmental Working Group. (2013, October 28). *Dirty dozen endocrine disrupters: 12 hormone-altering chemicals and how to avoid them.* https://www.ewg.org/consumer-guides/dirty-dozen-endocrine-disruptors

6. American Cancer Society. (2019, August 14). *Known and probable human carcinogens* [General information about carcinogens]. https://www.cancer.org/cancer/cancer-causes/general-info/known-and-probable-human-carcinogens.html

7. American Cancer Society. (2014, May 23). *Formaldehyde.* https://www.cancer.org/content/dam/CRC/PDF/Public/7671.pdf

8. United States Environmental Protection Agency. (2022, May 26). *Lead: Protect your family from sources of lead.* https://www.epa.gov/lead/protect-your-family-sources-lead#sl-home

9. Children's Environmental Health Network. (2019, October 16). *Eco-healthy Child Care: Safer food packaging: PVC/phthalates* [FAQ series]. https://cehn.org/wp-content/uploads/2019/10/PVCPhthalates-FAQ-10.16.19-1.pdf

10. Children's Environmental Health Network. (2019, October 16). *Eco-healthy Child Care: PVC dolls* [FAQ series]. https://cehn.org/wp-content/uploads/2019/10/PVC-dolls-FAQ-10.16.19-2.pdf

11. Children's Environmental Health Network (2019, October 16). *Eco-healthy Child Care: Safer food packaging: PFAS* [FAQ series]. https://cehn.org/wp-content/uploads/2020/01/PFAS.FAQ_.1.10.20.pdf

12. American Lung Association. (2020, February 12). *Volatile organic compounds.* https://www.lung.org/clean-air/at-home/indoor-air-pollutants/volatile-organic-compounds

13. National Institute of Environmental Health Sciences. (2016, July). *Flame retardants* [Fact sheet]. U.S. Department of Health and Human Services, National Institutes of Health. https://www.niehs.nih.gov/health/materials/flame_retardants_508.pdf

14. Boor, B. E., Spilak, M. P., Laverge, J., Novoselac, A., & Xu, Y. (2017). Human exposure to indoor air pollutants in sleep microenvironments: A literature review. *Building and Environment, 125,* 528-555. https://doi.org/10.1016/j.buildenv.2017.08.050

j. Twenty Ways to Pass the Time Before Birth

1. Carbone, L., De Vivo, V., Saccone, G., D'Antonio, F., Mercorio, A., Raffone, A., Arduino, B., D'Alessandro, P., Sarno, L., Conforti, A., Maruotti, G. M., Alviggi, C., & Zullo, F. (2019). Sexual intercourse for induction of spontaneous onset of labor: A systematic review and meta-analysis of randomized controlled trials. *The Journal of Sexual Medicine, 16*(11), 1787-1795. https://doi.org/10.1016/j.jsxm.2019.08.002

2. Castro, C., Afonso, M., Carvalho, R., Clode, N., & Graça, L. M. (2014). Effect of vaginal intercourse on spontaneous labor at term: A randomized controlled trial. *Archives of Gynecology and Obstetrics, 290,* 1121-1125. https://doi.org/10.1007/s00404-014-3343-0

3. Kavanagh, J., Kelly, A. J., & Thomas, J. (2001). Sexual intercourse for cervical ripening and induction of labour. *Cochrane Database of Systematic Reviews,* (2), Article CD003093. https://doi.org/10.1002/14651858.CD003093

4. BIRTHING TIPS

a. Preparing for Labor

1. Bohren, M. A., Hofmeyr, G. J., Sakala, C., Fukuzawa, R. K., & Cuthbert, A. (2017). Continuous support for women during childbirth. *Cochrane Database of Systematic Reviews,* (7), Article CD003766. https://doi.org/10.1002/14651858.CD003766.pub6

2. Committee on Obstetric Practice (with A. S. Bryant, & A. E. Borders). (2019). ACOG committee opinion no. 766: Approaches to limit intervention during labor and birth. (2019). *Obstetrics & Gynecology, 133*(2), e164-e173. https://doi.org/10.1097/AOG.0000000000003074

3. Fortier, J. H., & Godwin, M. (2015). Doula support compared with standard care: Meta-analysis of the effects on the rate of medical interventions during labour for low-risk women delivering at term. *Canadian Family Physician, 61*(6), e284-e292.

4. Landon, M. B., Galan, H. L., Jauniaux, E. R. M., Driscoll, D. A., Berghella, V., Grobman, W. A., Kilpatrick, S. J., & Cahill, A. G. (2021). *Gabbe's obstetrics: Normal and problem pregnancies* (8th ed.). Elsevier.

5. National Partnership for Women and Families. (n.d.). *Labor pain basics* [Under *Giving birth: Labor pain*]. Childbirth Connection. http://www.childbirthconnection.org/giving-birth/labor-pain/basics/

6. American College of Nurse-Midwives, Division of Standards and Practice, Clinical Documents Section. (2014). *Position statement: Hydrotherapy during labor and birth.* https://www.midwife.

org/acnm/files/ACNMLibraryData/UPLOADFILENAME/000000000286/Hydrothera-py-During-Labor-and-Birth-April-2014.pdf

7. National Partnership for Women and Families. (n.d.). *Comfort measures for labor pain relief* [Under *Giving birth: Labor pain*]. Childbirth Connection. http://www.childbirthconnection.org/giving-birth/labor-pain/comfort-relief/

8. Nanji, J. A., & Carvalho, B. (2020). Pain management during labor and vaginal birth. *Best Practice & Research, Clinical Obstetrics & Gynaecology, 67*, 100–112. https://doi.org/10.1016/j.bpobgyn.2020.03.002

9. Anim-Somuah, M., Smyth, R., Cyna, A. M., & Cuthbert, A. (2018). Epidural versus non-epidural or no analgesia for pain management in labour. *Cochrane Database of Systematic Reviews*, (5), Article CD000331. https://doi.org/10.1002/14651858.CD000331.pub4

10. DONA International. (n.d.). *What is a doula?* https://www.dona.org/what-is-a-doula/

b. Illustrated Labor Positions
None.

c. Decreasing Your Risk for Cesarean Birth

1. National Partnership for Women and Families. (2021). *Planning ahead* [Under *Giving birth: C-section*]. Childbirth Connection. http://www.childbirthconnection.org/giving-birth/c-section/planning-ahead/

2. Bohren, M. A., Hofmeyr, G. J., Sakala, C., Fukuzawa, R. K., & Cuthbert, A. (2017). Continuous support for women during childbirth. *Cochrane Database of Systematic Reviews*, (7), Article CD003766. https://doi.org/10.1002/14651858.CD003766.pub6

3. Committee on Obstetric Practice (with A. S. Bryant, & A. E. Borders). (2019). ACOG committee opinion no. 766: Approaches to limit intervention during labor and birth. *Obstetrics & Gynecology, 133*(2), e164–e173. https://doi.org/10.1097/AOG.0000000000003074

4. Alfirevic, Z., Gyte, G. M. L., Cuthbert, A., & Devane, D. (2017). Continuous cardiotocography (CTG) as a form of electronic fetal monitoring (EFM) for fetal assessment during labour. *Cochrane Database of Systematic Reviews*, (2), Article CD006066. https://doi.org/10.1002/14651858.CD006066.pub3

5. American College of Nurse-Midwives Division of Standards and Practice, Clinical Standards and Documents Section. (2015). Intermittent auscultation for intrapartum fetal heart rate surveillance: American College of Nurse-Midwives. *Journal of Midwifery & Women's Health, 60*(5), 626–632. https://doi.org/10.1111/jmwh.12372

6. Committee on Practice Bulletins (with G. A. Macones). (2009). ACOG practice bulletin no. 106: Intrapartum fetal heart rate monitoring: Nomenclature, interpretation, and general management principles. (2009). *Obstetrics & Gynecology, 114*(1), 192–202. https://doi.org/10.1097/AOG.0b013e3181aef106

d. How to Improve Your Cesarean Birth Experience

1. National Partnership for Women and Families. (2021). *Planning ahead* [Under *Giving birth: C-section*]. Childbirth Connection. http://www.childbirthconnection.org/giving-birth/c-section/planning-ahead/

e. Prepping Your Support
None.

f. Perineal Massage

1. Beckmann, M. M., & Stock, O. M. (2013). Antenatal perineal massage for reducing perineal trauma. *Cochrane Database of Systematic Reviews*, (4), Article CD005123. https://doi:10.1002/14651858.CD005123.pub3

g. Birth Plan (Wish List)

1. Committee on Obstetric Practice (with M. A. Mascola, T. F. Porter, & T. T.-M. Chao). (2017). Committee opinion no. 684: Delayed umbilical cord clamping after birth. *Obstetrics & Gynecology, 129*(1), e5-e10. https://doi.org/10.1097/AOG.0000000000001860

2. American College of Nurse-Midwives Division of Standards and Practice, Clinical Standards and Documents Section. (2021, July). *Position statement: Optimal management of the umbilical cord at the time of birth.* https://www.midwife.org/acnm/files/acnmlibrarydata/uploadfilename/000000000290/Optimal%20Management%202021_Final.pdf

3. Raju, T. N. K., & Singhal, N. (2012). Optimal timing for clamping the umbilical cord after birth. *Clinics in Perinatology, 39*(4), 889-900. https://doi.org/10.1016/j.clp.2012.09.006

h. Hospital Bag Checklist

None.

5. POSTPARTUM TIPS

a. Postpartum Care Plan

1. DONA International. (n.d.). *Postpartum plan for _____ family.* https://www.dona.org/wp-content/uploads/2016/12/postpartum-plan-template.pdf

2. Postpartum Support Virginia. (2014). *The realistic postpartum plan for the ___ family: Plan for adjusting to life with a new baby.* https://www.postpartumva.org/wp-content/uploads/2013/11/The-Postpartum-Plan.pdf

3. Bennett, S. (2007). *Postpartum depression for dummies* (foreword by M. J. Codey) [Chapter 18: Deciding whether to have another baby: Planning ahead if you decide to pass go: Surveying the elements of a postpartum plan, pp. 320]. John Wiley & Sons.

b. Birth Control Options

1. Hatcher, R. A., Nelson, A., Trussell, J., Cwaik, C., Cason, P., Policar, M. S., Aiken, A. R. A., Marazzo, J., & Kowal, D. (2018). *Contraceptive technology* (21st ed.). Managing Contraception.

2. White, K., Teal, S. B., & Potter, J. E. (2015). Contraception after delivery and short interpregnancy intervals among women in the United States. *Obstetrics & Gynecology, 125*(6), 1471-1477. https//doi.org/10.1097/AOG.0000000000000841

3. Thiel de Bocanegra, H., Chang, R., Howell, M., & Darney, P. (2014). Interpregnancy intervals: Impact of postpartum contraceptive effectiveness and coverage. *American Journal of Obstetrics & Gynecology, 210*(4), 311.e1–311.e8. https://doi.org/10.1016/j.ajog.2013.12.020

4. Curtis, K. M., Tepper, N. K., Jatlaoui, T. C., Berry-Bibee, E., Horton, L. G., Zapata, L. B., Simmons, K. B., Pagano, H. P., Jamieson, D. J., & Whiteman, M. K. (2016). U.S. medical eligibility criteria for contraceptive use, 2016. *Morbidity and Mortality Weekly Report, 65*(RR-3), 1–104. https://doi.org/10.15585/mmwr.rr6503a1

5. Sundström-Poromaa, I., Comasco, E., Sumner, R., & Luders, E. (2020). Progesterone – Friend or foe? *Frontiers in Neuroendocrinology, 59*, Article 100856. https://doi.org/10.1016/j.yfrne.2020.100856

6. Robakis, T., Williams, K. E., Nutkiewicz, L., & Rasgon, N. L. (2019). Hormonal contraceptives and mood: Review of the literature and implications for future research. *Current Psychiatry Reports, 21*, Article 57. https://doi.org/10.1007/s11920-019-1034-z

7. Hall, K. S., Steinberg, J. R., Cwiak, C. A., Allen, R. H., & Marcus, S. M. (2015). Contraception and mental health: A commentary on the evidence and principles for practice. *American Journal of Obstetrics & Gynecology, 212*(6), 740–746. https://doi.org/10.1016/j.ajog.2014.12.010

8. Lundin, C., Danielsson, K. G., Bixo, M., Moby, L., Bengtsdotter, H., Jawad, I., Marions, L., Brynhildsen, J., Malmborg, A., Lindh, I., & Sundström Poromaa, I. (2017). Combined oral contraceptive use is associated with both improvement and worsening of mood in the different phases of the treatment cycle – A double-blind, placebo-controlled randomized trial. *Psychoneuroendocrinology, 76*, 135–143. https://doi.org/10.1016/j.psyneuen.2016.11.033

9. McCloskey, L. R., Wisner, K. L., Cattan, M. K., Betcher, H. K., Stika, C. S., & Kiley, J. W. (2021). Contraception for women with psychiatric disorders. *The American Journal of Psychiatry, 178*(3), 247–255. https://doi.org/10.1176/appi.ajp.2020.20020154

10. Weschler, T. (2015). *Taking charge of your fertility* (20th ed.). William Morrow.

11. Bahamondes, L., Bahamondes, M. V., Modesto, W., Tilley, I. B., Magalhães, A., Pinto e Silva, J. L., Amaral, E., & Mishell, D. R., Jr. (2013). Effect of hormonal contraceptives during breastfeeding on infant's milk ingestion and growth. *Fertility and Sterility, 100*(2), 445–450. https://doi.org/10.1016/j.fertnstert.2013.03.039

12. Tepper, N. K., Phillips, S. J., Kapp, N., Gaffield, M. E., & Curtis, K. M. (2016). Combined hormonal contraceptive use among breastfeeding women: An updated systematic review. *Contraception, 94*(3), 262–274. https://doi.org/10.1016/j.contraception.2015.05.006

13. Mohrbacher, N. (2010). *Breastfeeding answers made simple: A guide for helping mothers.* Hale Publishing.

14. Curtis, K. M., Jatlaoui, T. C., Tepper, N. K., Zapata, L. B., Horton, L. G., Jamieson, D. J., & Whiteman, M. K. (2016). U.S. selected practice recommendations for contraceptive use, 2016. *Morbidity and Mortality Weekly Report, 65*(4), 1-66. http://dx.doi.org/10.15585/mmwr.rr6504a1

15. Guttmacher Institute. (2022, July 1). *State laws and policies: Emergency contraception.* https://www.guttmacher.org/state-policy/explore/emergency-contraception

16. Micks, E. A., & Jensen, J. T. (2020). A technology evaluation of Annovera: A segesterone acetate and ethinyl estradiol vaginal ring used to prevent pregnancy for up to one year. *Expert Opinion on Drug Delivery, 17*(6), 743–752. https://doi.org/10.1080/17425247.2020.1764529

17. Ali, M., Akin, A., Bahamondes, L., Brache, V., Habib, N., Landoulsi, S., & Hubacher, D., for the WHO study group on subdermal contraceptive implants for women. (2016). Extended use up to 5 years of the etonogestrel-releasing subdermal contraceptive implant: Comparison to levonorgestrel-releasing subdermal implant. *Human Reproduction* (Oxford, England), *31*(11), 2491–2498. https://doi.org/10.1093/humrep/dew222

18. Bayer. (n.d.). *Mirena IUD | Official HCP website.* https://www.mirenahcp.com/

19. McNicholas, C., Swor, E., Wan, L., & Peipert, J. F. (2017). Prolonged use of the etonogestrel implant and levonorgestrel intrauterine device: 2 years beyond Food and Drug Administration-approved duration. *American Journal of Obstetrics & Gynecology, 216*(6), 586.e1–586.e6. https://doi.org/10.1016/j.ajog.2017.01.036

20. AbbVie and Medicines360. (n.d.). *Liletta.* https://www.liletta.com/

c. Bonding with Baby

1. McClure, V. (2017). *Infant massage: A handbook for loving parents* (4th ed.). Bantam Books.

2. International Association of Infant Massage. (n.d.). *Massage your baby: Benefits.* https://www.iaim.net/massage-your-baby/benefits/

3. Meek, J. Y., Noble, L., & the Section on Breastfeeding. (2022). Policy statement: Breastfeeding and the use of human milk. *Pediatrics, 150*(1), Article e2022057988. https://doi.org/10.1542/peds.2022-057988

4. American College of Nurse-Midwives. (2013). Promoting skin-to-skin contact. *Journal of Midwifery & Women's Health, 58*(3), 359-360. https://doi.org/10.1111/jmwh.12034

d. Feeding Your Milk Monster

1. American Academy of Pediatrics. (2021, July 6). *Infant food and feeding.* https://www.aap.org/en/patient-care-pages-in-progress/healthy-active-living-for-families/infant-food-and-feeding/ https://www.aap.org/en/patient-care/healthy-active-living-for-families/infant-food-and-feeding/

2. Centers for Disease Control and Prevention. (n.d.). *Nutrition: How much and how often to feed infant formula* [Last reviewed 2021, July 23]. https://www.cdc.gov/nutrition/infantandtoddlernutrition/formula-feeding/how-much-how-often.html

3. U.S. Department of Agriculture & U.S. Department of Health and Human Services. (2020, December). *Dietary Guidelines for Americans, 2020-2025* (9th ed.). DietaryGuidelines. https://www.dietaryguidelines.gov/sites/default/files/2021-03/Dietary_Guidelines_for_Americans-2020-2025.pdf

4. Mohrbacher, N. (2010). *Breastfeeding answers made simple: A guide for helping mothers.* Hale Publishing.

5. Dennis, C. L., Jackson, K., & Watson, J. (2014). Interventions for treating painful nipples among breastfeeding women. *Cochrane Database of Systematic Reviews*, (12), Article CD007366. https://doi.org/10.1002/14651858.CD007366.pub2

6. Jackson, K. T., & Dennis, C. L. (2017). Lanolin for the treatment of nipple pain in breastfeeding women: A randomized controlled trial. *Maternal & Child Nutrition, 13*, Article e12357. https://doi.org/10.1111/mcn.12357

7. Dennis, C. L., Schottle, N., Hodnett, E., & McQueen, K. (2012). An all-purpose nipple ointment versus lanolin in treating painful damaged nipples in breastfeeding women: A randomized controlled trial. *Breastfeeding Medicine, 7*(6), 473–479. https://doi.org/10.1089/bfm.2011.0121

8. U.S. National Library of Medicine. (2021, October 18). *Lanolin.* In *Drugs and Lactation Database (LactMed)* [Internet]. https://www.ncbi.nlm.nih.gov/books/NBK501842/

9. Wiessinger, D., West, D., & Pitman, T. (2010). *The womanly art of breastfeeding* (8th ed.). Ballantine Books.

10. Le Leche League International. (2019, January). *Bottles and other tools: Ideas for introducing a bottle to a breastfed baby.* https://www.llli.org/breastfeeding-info/bottles/

11. Heinig, M. J., Bañuelos, J., & Goldbronn, J. (2012). *The secrets of baby behavior.* The Regents of the University of California. https://www.amzn.com/dp/B00AP7J2G6/

e. Child-Care Provider Tips
None.

f. Tips for Returning to Work or School

1. Wiessinger, D., West, D., & Pitman, T. (2010). *The womanly art of breastfeeding* (8th ed.). Ballantine Books.

2. Le Leche League International. (2019, January). *Bottles and other tools.* https://www.llli.org/breastfeeding-info/bottles/

APPENDIX B

1. NUTRITION

1. U.S. Department of Agriculture & U.S. Department of Health and Human Services. (2020, December). *Dietary Guidelines for Americans, 2020-2025* (9th ed.). DietaryGuidelines. https://www.dietaryguidelines.gov/sites/default/files/2021-03/Dietary_Guidelines_for_Americans-2020-2025.pdf

2. Pollan, M. (2009). *Food rules: An eater's manual.* Penguin Books.

3. Harvard T. H. Chan School of Public Health. (n.d.). *The nutrition source: Healthy eating plate.* http://www.hsph.harvard.edu/nutritionsource/healthy-eating-plate/

4. Culinary Institute of America & Harvard T. H. Chan School of Public Health, Department of Nutrition. (2020). *Menus of Change Initiative: Plant-forward by the numbers.* https://www.ciaprochef.com/MOC/PFbytheNumbers.pdf/

5. Food and Agriculture Organization of the United Nations. (2021). *Key facts and findings* [Of the "Tackling climate change through livestock: A global assessment of emissions and mitigation opportunities" report]. https://www.fao.org/news/story/en/item/197623/icode/

6. Monterey Bay Aquarium. (n.d.). *Seafood watch.* https://www.seafoodwatch.org/

a. Eating for Two While Pregnant

1. Baroni, L., Goggi, S., Battaglino, R., Berveglieri, M., Fasan, I., Filippin, D., Griffith, P., Rizzo, G., Tomasina, C., Tosatti, M. A., & Battino, M. A. (2019). Vegan nutrition for mothers and children: Practical tools for healthcare providers. *Nutrients, 11*(1), Article 5. https://doi.org/10.3390/nu11010005

2. Danielewicz, H., Myszczyszyn, G., Dębińska, A., Myszkal, A., Boznański, A., & Hirnle, L. (2017). Diet in pregnancy—More than food. *European Journal of Pediatrics, 176,* 1573–1579. https://doi.org/10.1007/s00431-017-3026-5

3. American Heart Association. (n.d.). *Eat more color infographic.* https://www.heart.org/en/healthy-living/healthy-eating/add-color/eat-more-color

4. Landon, M. B., Galan, H. L., Jauniaux, E. R. M., Driscoll, D. A., Berghella, V., Grobman, W. A., Kilpatrick, S. J., & Cahill, A. G. (2021). *Gabbe's obstetrics: Normal and problem pregnancies* (8th ed.). Elsevier.

5. U.S. Department of Agriculture & U.S. Department of Health and Human Services. (2020, December). *Dietary Guidelines for Americans, 2020-2025* (9th ed.). DietaryGuidelines. https://www.dietaryguidelines.gov/sites/default/files/2021-03/Dietary_Guidelines_for_Americans-2020-2025.pdf

6. U.S. Food and Drug Administration. (2022, June). *Advice about eating fish: For those who might become or are pregnant or breastfeeding and children ages 1 - 11 years.* https://www.fda.gov/food/consumers/advice-about-eating-fish

7. U.S. Department of Agriculture. (2019, March). *Organic 101: What the USDA organic label means.* https://www.usda.gov/media/blog/2012/03/22/organic-101-what-usda-organic-label-means

8. Environmental Working Group. (2022). *Dirty dozen: EWG's 2022 shopper's guide to pesticides in produce.* https://www.ewg.org/foodnews/dirty-dozen.php

9. American College of Obstetricians and Gynecologists. (2020, October). *Ask ACOG: How much water should I drink during pregnancy?* https://www.acog.org/womens-health/experts-and-stories/ask-acog/how-much-water-should-i-drink-during-pregnancy

10. Denny, L., Coles, S., & Blitz, R. (2017). Fetal alcohol syndrome and fetal alcohol spectrum disorders. *American Family Physician, 96*(8), 515–522. *PubMed.* Retrieved January 29, 2022, from https://pubmed.ncbi.nlm.nih.gov/29094891/

11. Committee on Health Care for Underserved Women. (2011). Committee opinion no. 496: At-risk drinking and alcohol dependence: Obstetric and gynecologic implications. *Obstetrics & Gynecology, 118*(2 Pt 1), 383–388. https://doi.org/10.1097/AOG.0b013e31822c9906

12. Kominiarek, M. A., & Rajan, P. (2016). Nutrition recommendations in pregnancy and lactation. *Medical Clinics of North America, 100*(6), 1199–1215. https://doi.org/10.1016/j.mcna.2016.06.004

13. American College of Obstetricians and Gynecologists. (2021, February). *FAQs: Multiple pregnancy.* https://www.acog.org/womens-health/faqs/multiple-pregnancy

b. Choosing Healthier Options

1. Committee on Obstetric Practice. (2010, August). Committee opinion no. 462: Moderate caffeine consumption during pregnancy [Reaffirmed 2020]. *Obstetrics & Gynecology, 116*(2 Pt 1), 467–468. https://doi.org/10.1097/AOG.0b013e3181eeb2a1

2. Center for Science in the Public Interest. (n.d.). *Caffeine chart.* https://cspinet.org/eating-healthy/ingredients-of-concern/caffeine-chart
    Quantities rounded to the nearest 0.5 mg, in the cases where the serving size was not 8 oz.

c. Navigating Cravings and Food Aversions
None.

d. After Childbirth

1. U.S. Preventive Services Task Force (with K. Bibbins-Domingo). (2017). Folic acid supplementation for the prevention of neural tube defects: US Preventive Services Task Force recommendation statement. *JAMA. 317*(2), 183-189. http://doi.org/10.1001/jama.2016.19438.

2. World Health Organization. (2005). *Report of a WHO technical consultation on birth spacing: Geneva, Switzerland: 13–15 June 2005.* https://apps.who.int/iris/bitstream/handle/10665/69855/WHO_RHR_07.1_eng.pdf

3. McKinney, D., House, M., Chen, A., Muglia, L., & DeFranco, E. (2017). The influence of interpregnancy interval on infant mortality. *American Journal of Obstetrics & Gynecology, 216*(3), 316.e1–316.e9. https://doi.org/10.1016/j.ajog.2016.12.018

4. American College of Obstetricians and Gynecologists & Society for Maternal-Fetal Medicine (with J. Marie Louis, A. Bryant, D. Ramos, A. Stuebe, & S. C. Blackwell). (2019). Obstetric care consensus no. 8: Interpregnancy care. *Obstetrics & Gynecology, 133*(1), e51–e72. https://doi.org/10.1097/AOG.0000000000003025

5. U.S. Department of Agriculture & U.S. Department of Health and Human Services. (2020, December). *Dietary Guidelines for Americans, 2020-2025* (9th ed.). DietaryGuidelines. https://www.dietaryguidelines.gov/sites/default/files/2021-03/Dietary_Guidelines_for_Americans-2020-2025.pdf

6. Kominiarek, M. A., & Rajan, P. (2016). Nutrition recommendations in pregnancy and lactation. *Medical Clinics of North America, 100*(6), 1199–1215. https://doi.org/10.1016/j.mcna.2016.06.004

7. American College of Obstetrics & Gynecologists. (2021, May). *FAQs: Breastfeeding your baby.* https://www.acog.org/womens-health/faqs/breastfeeding-your-baby

8. Sears, W., & Sears, M. (with R. Sears & J. Sears). (2014). *The baby book: Everything you need to know about your baby from birth to age two* (Revised and updated ed.). Little Brown and Company.

9. Mohrbacher, N. (2010). *Breastfeeding answers made simple: A guide for helping mothers.* Hale Publishing.

10. Brodribb, W. (2018). ABM clinical protocol #9: Use of galactogogues in initiating or augmenting maternal milk production, second revision 2018. *Breastfeeding Medicine, 13*(5), 307-314. http://doi.org/10.1089/bfm.2018.29092.wjb

11. Hale, T. H. (2021). *Medications and mother's milk* (19th ed.). Springer Publishing.

12. U. S. National Library of Medicine. (2022, June 20). Caffeine. In *Drugs and Lactation Database (LactMed)* [Internet]. https://www.ncbi.nlm.nih.gov/books/NBK501467/

e. Tasty Snacks and Recipes

1. Dooner, E. (2017, January 16). *Peanut butter protein balls.* Texanerin Baking. https://www.texanerin.com/peanut-butter-protein-balls/

2. Attwell, C. (2021, December 7). *Healthy oat & blueberry blender muffins.* https://www.myfussyeater.com/healthy-oat-blueberry-blender-muffins/

f. Nitty-Gritty Nutrition

1. Institute of Medicine. (2006). Summary tables, dietary reference intakes: Recommended dietary allowances and adequate intakes: Vitamins; Elements; Total Water and Macronutrients. In J. J. Otten, J. Pitzi Hellwig, & L. D. Meyers (Eds.), *Dietary reference intakes: The essential guide to nutrient requirements* (pp. 532-536). The National Academies Press. https://nap.nationalacademies.org/read/11537/chapter/59

2. Perinatology.com. (2010). *Daily dietary reference Intakes** during pregnancy.* Focus Information Technology. https://perinatology.com/Reference/RDApregnancy.html

3. Institute of Medicine. (2006). *Dietary reference intakes: The essential guide to nutrient requirements.* National Academies. https://www.nap.edu/catalog/11537/dietary-reference-intakes-the-essential-guide-to-nutrient-requirements

4. Dietary Guidelines for Americans. (n.d.). *Food sources of select nutrients.* https://www.dietaryguidelines.gov/resources/2020-2025-dietary-guidelines-online-materials/food-sources-select-nutrients

5. National Institute of Health. (2022, April 28). *Iodine: Fact sheet for health care professionals.* https://ods.od.nih.gov/factsheets/Iodine-HealthProfessional/

6. National Institute of Health. (2021, March 26). *Selenium: Fact sheet for health care professionals.* https://ods.od.nih.gov/factsheets/Selenium-HealthProfessional/

7. National Institute of Health. (2021, March 26). *Phosphorous: Fact sheet for healthcare professionals.* https://ods.od.nih.gov/factsheets/Phosphorus-HealthProfessional/

8. National Institute of Health. (2022, June 2). *Choline: Fact sheet for health care professionals.* https://ods.od.nih.gov/factsheets/Choline-HealthProfessional/

9. National Institute of Health. (2022, June 2). *Omega 3 fatty acids: Fact sheets for health care professionals.* https://ods.od.nih.gov/factsheets/Omega3FattyAcids-HealthProfessional/

g. My Pregnancy Plate

1. Oregon Health Sciences University Center for Women's Health. (2015). *My pregnancy plate.* https://www.ohsu.edu/sites/default/files/2020-10/CWH%203051517%20Pregnancy%20Plate%20FLY%202019.pdf

2. PHYSICAL ACTIVITY

1. Piercy, K. L., Troiano, R. P., Ballard, R. M., Carlson, S. A., Fulton, J. E., Galuska, D. A., George, S. M., & Olsen, R. D. (2018). The physical activity guidelines for Americans. *JAMA, 320*(19), 2020–2028. http://doi.org/10.1001/jama.2018.14854

2. Bull, F. C., Al-Ansari, S. S., Biddle, S., Borodulin, K., Buman, M. P., Cardon, G., Carty, C., Chaput, J. P., Chastin, S., Chou, R., Dempsey, P. C., DiPietro, L., Ekelund, U., Firth, J., Friedenreich, C. M., Garcia, L., Gichu, M., Jago, R., Katzmarzyk, P. T., … Willumsen, J. F. (2020). World Health Organization 2020 guidelines on physical activity and sedentary behaviour. *British Journal of Sports Medicine, 54*(24), 1451–1462. https://doi.org/10.1136/bjsports-2020-102955

a. General Activity Guidelines

1. Piercy, K. L., Troiano, R. P., Ballard, R. M., Carlson, S. A., Fulton, J. E., Galuska, D. A., George, S. M., & Olsen, R. D. (2018). The physical activity guidelines for Americans. *JAMA, 320*(19), 2020–2028. http://doi.org/10.1001/jama.2018.14854

2. Bull, F. C., Al-Ansari, S. S., Biddle, S., Borodulin, K., Buman, M. P., Cardon, G., Carty, C., Chaput, J. P., Chastin, S., Chou, R., Dempsey, P. C., DiPietro, L., Ekelund, U., Firth, J., Friedenreich, C. M., Garcia, L., Gichu, M., Jago, R., Katzmarzyk, P. T., … Willumsen, J. F. (2020). World Health Organization 2020 guidelines on physical activity and sedentary behaviour. *British Journal of Sports Medicine, 54*(24), 1451–1462. https://doi.org/10.1136/bjsports-2020-102955

b. Move That Pregnant Bod

1. Committee on Obstetric Practice (with M. L. Birsner, & C. Gyamfi-Bannerman). (2020). Physical activity and exercise during pregnancy and the postpartum period: ACOG committee opinion, number 804. *Obstetrics & Gynecology, 135*(4), e178–e188. https://doi.org/10.1097/AOG.0000000000003772

2. American College of Obstetrics and Gynecology. (2022, March). *FAQs: Exercise during pregnancy.* https://www.acog.org/womens-health/faqs/exercise-during-pregnancy

3. Piercy, K. L., Troiano, R. P., Ballard, R. M., Carlson, S. A., Fulton, J. E., Galuska, D. A., George, S. M., & Olsen, R. D. (2018). The physical activity guidelines for Americans. *JAMA, 320*(19), 2020–2028. http://doi.org/10.1001/jama.2018.14854

4. Bull, F. C., Al-Ansari, S. S., Biddle, S., Borodulin, K., Buman, M. P., Cardon, G., Carty, C., Chaput, J. P., Chastin, S., Chou, R., Dempsey, P. C., DiPietro, L., Ekelund, U., Firth, J., Friedenreich, C. M., Garcia, L., Gichu, M., Jago, R., Katzmarzyk, P. T., … Willumsen, J. F. (2020). World Health Organization 2020 guidelines on physical activity and sedentary behaviour. *British Journal of Sports Medicine, 54*(24), 1451–1462. https://doi.org/10.1136/bjsports-2020-102955

5. Artal, R. (2016). Exercise in pregnancy: Guidelines. *Clinical Obstetrics & Gynecology, 59*(3), 639–644. https://doi.org/10.1097/GRF.0000000000000223

6. MacDonald, L. A., Waters, T. R., Napolitano, P. G., Goddard, D. E., Ryan, M. A., Nielsen, P., & Hudock, S. D. (2013). Clinical guidelines for occupational lifting in pregnancy: Evidence summary and provisional recommendations. *American Journal of Obstetrics & Gynecology, 209*(2), 80–88. https://doi.org/10.1016/j.ajog.2013.02.047

c. Activity Postpartum

1. Committee on Obstetric Practice (with M. L. Birsner, & C. Gyamfi-Bannerman). (2020). ACOG committee opinion, no. 804: Physical activity and exercise during pregnancy and the postpartum period. *Obstetrics & Gynecology, 135*(4), e178–e188. https://doi.org/10.1097/AOG.0000000000003772

2. Sperstad, J. B., Tennfjord, M. K., Hilde, G., Ellström-Engh, M., & Bø, K. (2016). Diastasis recti abdominis during pregnancy and 12 months after childbirth: Prevalence, risk factors and report of lumbopelvic pain. *British Journal of Sports Medicine, 50*(17), 1092–1096. https://doi.org/10.1136/bjsports-2016-096065

3. Fernandes da Mota, P. G., Pascoal, A. G., Carita, A. I., & Bø, K. (2015). Prevalence and risk factors of diastasis recti abdominis from late pregnancy to 6 months postpartum, and relationship with lumbo-pelvic pain. Manual Therapy, 20(1), 200–205. https://doi.org/10.1016/j.math.2014.09.002

3. REST AND RELAXATION

a. Sleeping Tips for Pregnancy

1. National Sleep Foundation. (2018). *Sleep in America poll: 2018: Sleep & effectiveness are linked, but few plan their sleep.* https://www.sleepfoundation.org/wp-content/uploads/2018/03/Sleep-in-America-2018_prioritizing-sleep_1.pdf?x88683

2. National Sleep Foundation. (2020, May 5). *10 tips for a better night's sleep.* https://www.thensf.org/10-sleep-tips-sleep-quality/

3. Chinoy, E. D., Duffy, J. F., & Czeisler, C. A. (2018). Unrestricted evening use of light-emitting tablet computers delays self-selected bedtime and disrupts circadian timing and alertness. *Physiological Reports, 6*(10), Article e13692. https://doi: 10.14814/phy2.13692

4. Chang, A. M., Aeschbach, D., Duffy, J. F., & Czeisler, C. A. (2014). Evening use of light-emitting ereaders negatively affects sleep, circadian timing, and next-morning alertness. *Proceedings of the National Academy of Sciences of the United States of America, 112*(4), 1232–1237. https://doi.org/10.1073/pnas.1418490112

5. Christensen, M. A., Bettencourt, L., Kaye, L., Moturu, S. T., Nguyen, K. T., Olgin, J. E., Pletcher, M. J., & Marcus, G. M. (2016). Direct measurements of smartphone screen-time: Relationships with demographics and sleep. *PLOS ONE, 11*(11), Article e0165331. https://doi.org/10.1371/journal.pone.0165331

6. Conrad, P. (2019). *Women's health aromatherapy.* Singing Dragon.

7. Allen, R. E., & Kirby, K. A. (2012). Nocturnal leg cramps. *American Family Physician, 86*(4), 350–355. *PubMed.* Retrieved November 23, 2021 from https://pubmed.ncbi.nlm.nih.gov/22963024/

8. Grover, A., Clark-Bilodeau, C., & D'Ambrosio, C. M. (2015). Restless leg syndrome in pregnancy. *Obstetric Medicine, 8*(3), 121–125. https://doi.org/10.1177/1753495X15587452

9. Trotti, L. M., & Becker, L. A. (2019). Iron for the treatment of restless legs syndrome. *Cochrane Database of Systematic Reviews,* (1), Article CD007834. https://doi.org/10.1002/14651858.CD007834.pub3

10. Dominguez, J. E., Krystal, A. D., & Habib, A. S. (2018). Obstructive sleep apnea in pregnant women: A review of pregnancy outcomes and an approach to management. *Anesthesia and Analgesia, 127*(5), 1167–1177. https://doi.org/10.1213/ANE.0000000000003335

11. Louis, J. M., Mogos, M. F., Salemi, J. L., Redline, S., & Salihu, H. M. (2014). Obstructive sleep apnea and severe maternal-infant morbidity/mortality in the United States, 1998-2009. *Sleep, 37*(5), 843–849. https://doi.org/10.5665/sleep.3644

12. Terzioğlu Bebitoğlu, B. (2020). Frequently used herbal teas during pregnancy – Short update. *Medeniyet Medical Journal, 35*(1), 55–61. https://doi.org/10.5222/MMJ.2020.69851

13. Illamola, S. M., Amaeze, O. U., Krepkova, L. V., Birnbaum, A. K., Karanam, A., Job, K. M., Bortnikova, V. V., Sherwin, C. M. T., & Enioutina, E. Y. (2020). Use of herbal medicine by pregnant women: What physicians need to know. *Frontiers in Pharmacology*, *10*, Article 1483. https://doi.org/10.3389/fphar.2019.01483

14. Therapeutic Research Center. (2020, November 11). Strawberry [Current through 2020, September 18]. *Natural Medicines Database.*

15. Therapeutic Research Center. (2022, February 14). Blueberry [Current through 2021, December 15]. *Natural Medicines Database.*

16. Therapeutic Research Center. (2022, May 16). *Peppermint* [Current through 2022, March 18]. *Natural Medicines Database.*

17. Therapeutic Research Center. (2022, June 11). *Cranberry* [Current through 2022, April 20]. *Natural Medicines Database.*

18. Therapeutic Research Center. (2022, April 27). *Ginger* [Current through 2022, March 18]. *Natural Medicines Database.*

19. Therapeutic Research Center. (2022, May 24). *Red raspberry* [Current through 2022, June 28]. *Natural Medicines Database.*

20. Therapeutic Research Center. (2022, April 14). *Green Tea* [Current through 2021, December 17]. *Natural Medicines Database.*

21. Therapeutic Research Center. (2022, July 8). *Oolong Tea* [Current through 2021, December 15]. *Natural Medicines Database.*

22. Therapeutic Research Center. (2022, February 9). *Black Tea* [Current through 2021, December 15]. *Natural Medicines Database.*

23. Therapeutic Research Center. (2022, March 31). *Echinacea* [Current through 2022, February 18]. *Natural Medicines Database.*

24. Therapeutic Research Center. (2022, March 31). *German Chamomile* [Current through 2022, June 28]. *Natural Medicines Database.*

25. Therapeutic Research Center. (2022, March 25). *Roman Chamomile* [Current through 2022, January 14]. *Natural Medicines Database.*

26. Therapeutic Research Center. (2022, July 1). *Licorice* [Current through 2022, April 20]. *Natural Medicines Database.*

27. Therapeutic Research Center. (2021, November 10). *Hibiscus* [Current through 2022, May 25]. *Natural Medicines Database.*

28. Therapeutic Research Center. (2021, August 11). *Rose Hip* [Current through 2022, January 14]. *Natural Medicines Database.*

29. Therapeutic Research Center. (2022, March 29). *Passionflower* [Current through 2021, February 20]. *Natural Medicines Database.*

30. Therapeutic Research Center. (2022, April 7). *Yerba Mate* [Current through 2021, December 15]. *Natural Medicines Database.*

31. Therapeutic Research Center. (2021, December 29). *Ephedra* [Current through 2022, June 28]. *Natural Medicines Database.*

32. Therapeutic Research Center. (2022, March 14). *Ginkgo* [Current through 2022, May 25]. *Natural Medicines Database.*

33. Therapeutic Research Center. (2021, September 17). *Lemon Balm* [Current through 2021, January 15]. *Natural Medicines Database.*

34. Therapeutic Research Center. (2020, December 3). *Rooibos* [Current through 2021, October 23]. *Natural Medicines Database.*

b. Sleeping Tips for Postpartum

1. Weissbluth, M. (2015). *Healthy sleep habits, happy child: A step-by-step program for a good night's sleep* (4th ed.). Ballantine Books.

2. Heinig, M. J., Bañuelos, J., & Goldbronn, J. (2012). *The secrets of baby behavior.* The Regents of the University of California. https://www.amzn.com/dp/B00AP7J2G6/

3. International Hip Dysplasia Institute. (n.d.). *Hip healthy swaddling* [Brochure]. https://hipdysplasia.org/wp-content/uploads/2020/05/HipHealthySwaddlingBrochure.pdf

4. Clarke, N. M. P. (2014). Swaddling and hip dysplasia: An orthopaedic perspective. *Archives of Disease in Childhood*, *99*(1), 5–6. https://doi.org/10.1136/archdischild-2013-304143

5. Moon, R. Y., Carlin, R. F., Hand, I., American Academy of Pediatrics Task Force on Sudden Infant Death Syndrome & American Academy of Pediatrics Committee on Fetus and Newborn. (2022). Sleep-related infant deaths: Updated 2022 recommendations for reducing infant deaths in the sleep environment. *Pediatrics*, *150*(1), Article e2022057990. https://doi.org/10.1542/peds.2022-057990

6. American College of Nurse-Midwives Division of Standards and Practice, Clinical Practice and Documents Section. (2017, September). *Position statement: Safe infant sleep practice.* https://www.midwife.org/acnm/files/acnmlibrarydata/uploadfilename/000000000312/Safe-Infant-Sleep-Practices-PS-12-11-17.pdf

c. Relaxation Tips for Pregnancy and Beyond
None.

4. MENTAL HEALTH

a. Mental Wellness in Pregnancy and Beyond

1. Mentalhealth.gov. (2022, February 28). *What is mental health?* https://www.mentalhealth.gov/basics/what-is-mental-health

2. World Health Organization Regional Office for Europe. (2019). *Mental health: Fact Sheet.* https://www.euro.who.int/__data/assets/pdf_file/0004/404851/MNH_FactSheet_ENG.pdf?ua=1

3. Galderisi, S., Heinz, A., Kastrup, M., Beezhold, J., & Sartorius, N. (2015). Toward a new definition of mental health. *World Psychiatry*, *14*(2), 231–233. https://doi.org/10.1002/wps.20231

4. Substance Abuse and Mental Health Services Administration. (n.d.). Section 8: Adult mental health tables – 8.1 to 8.70. In *2019 National Survey on Drug Use and Health [NSDUH] detailed tables.* U.S. Department of Health and Human Services. https://www.samhsa.gov/data/sites/default/files/reports/rpt29394/NSDUHDetailedTabs2019/NSDUHDetTabsSect8pe2019.htm

5. Substance Abuse and Mental Health Services Administration. (n.d.). Section 9: Youth mental health tables –9.1 to 9.11. In *2019 National Survey on Drug Use and Health [NSDUH] detailed tables.* U.S. Department of Health and Human Services. https://www.samhsa.gov/data/sites/default/files/reports/rpt29394/NSDUHDetailedTabs2019/NSDUHDetTabsSect9pe2019.htm

6. Substance Abuse and Mental Health Services Administration. (n.d.). Section 10: Adult mental health trend tables – 10.1 to 10.43 [Table 10.1B]. In *2019 National Survey on Drug Use and Health [DSDUH] detailed tables.* U.S. Department of Health and Human Services. https://www.samhsa.gov/data/sites/default/files/reports/rpt29394/NSDUHDetailedTabs2019/NSDUHDetTabsSect10pe2019.htm

7. Gaynes, B. N., Gavin, N., Meltzer-Brody, S., Lohr, K. N., Swinson, T., Gartlehner, G., Brody, S., & Miller, W. C. (2005). Perinatal depression: Prevalence, screening accuracy, and screening outcomes. *Evidence Report Technology Assessment (Summary)*, (119), 1–8. https://doi.org/10.1037/e439372005-001

8. Kendall-Tackett, K. A. (2017). *Depression in new mothers: Causes, consequences and treatment alternatives* (3rd ed. with foreword by P. Simkin). Routledge.

9. Glasser, S., & Lerner-Geva, L. (2019). Focus on fathers: Paternal depression in the perinatal period. *Perspectives in Public Health*, *139*(4), 195–198. https://doi.org/10.1177/1757913918790597

10. Aktar, E., Qu, J., Lawrence, P. J., Tollenaar, M. S., Elzinga, B. M., & Bögels, S. M. (2019). Fetal and infant outcomes in the offspring of parents with perinatal mental disorders: Earliest influences. *Frontiers in Psychiatry*, *10*, Article 391. https://doi.org/10.3389/fpsyt.2019.00391

11. Fairbrother, N., Janssen, P., Antony, M. M., Tucker, E., & Young, A. H. (2016). Perinatal anxiety disorder prevalence and incidence. *Journal of Affective Disorders*, *200*, 148–155. https://doi.org/10.1016/j.jad.2015.12.082

12. Dadi, A. F., Miller, E. R., Bisetegn, T. A., & Mwanri, L. (2020). Global burden of antenatal depression and its association with adverse birth outcomes: An umbrella review. *BMC Public Health*, *20*, Article 173. https://doi.org/10.1186/s12889-020-8293-9

13. Glover, V. (2014). Maternal depression, anxiety and stress during pregnancy and child outcome; What needs to be done. *Best Practice & Research Clinical Obstetrics & Gynaecology*, *28*(1), 25–35. https://doi.org/10.1016/j.bpobgyn.2013.08.017

14. Babenko, O., Kovalchuk, I., & Metz, G. A. S. (2015). Stress-induced perinatal and transgenerational epigenetic programming of brain development and mental health. *Neuroscience & Biobehavioral Reviews*, *48*, 70–91. https://doi.org/10.1016/j.neubiorev.2014.11.013

15. Woody, C. A., Ferrari, A. J., Siskind, D. J., Whiteford, H. A., & Harris, M. G. (2017). A systematic review and meta-regression of the prevalence and incidence of perinatal depression. *Journal of Affective Disorders*, *219*, 86–92. https://doi.org/10.1016/j.jad.2017.05.003

16. Kim, P., Mayes, L., Feldman, R., Leckman, J. F., & Swain, J. E. (2013). Early postpartum parental preoccupation and positive parenting thoughts: Relationship with parent-infant interaction. *Infant Mental Health Journal*, *34*(2), 104–116. https://doi.org/10.1002/imhj.21359

17. McKee, K., Admon, L. K., Winkelman, T. N. A., Muzik, M., Hall, S., Dalton, V. K., & Zivin, K. (2020). Perinatal mood and anxiety disorders, serious mental illness, and delivery-related health outcomes, United States, 2006-2015. *BMC Women's Health*, *20*, Article 150. https://doi.org/10.1186/s12905-020-00996-6

18. Grote, N. K., Bridge, J. A., Gavin, A. R., Melville, J. L., Iyengar, S., & Katon, W. J. (2010). A meta-analysis of depression during pregnancy and the risk of preterm birth, low birth weight, and intrauterine growth restriction. *Archives of General Psychiatry*, *67*(10), 1012–1024. https://doi.org/10.1001/archgenpsychiatry.2010.111

19. Hobel, C. J., Goldstein, A., & Barrett, E. S. (2008). Psychosocial stress and pregnancy outcome. *Clinical Obstetrics & Gynecology*, *51*(2), 333–348. https://doi.org/10.1097/GRF.0b013e31816f2709

20. Stein, A., Pearson, R. M., Goodman, S. H., Rapa, E., Rahman, A., McCallum, M., Howard, L. M., & Pariante, C. M. (2014). Effects of perinatal mental disorders on the fetus and child. *Lancet* (London, England), *384*(9956), 1800–1819. https://doi.org/10.1016/S0140-6736(14)61277-0

21. Alder, J., Fink, N., Bitzer, J., Hösli, I., & Holzgreve, W. (2007). Depression and anxiety during pregnancy: A risk factor for obstetric, fetal and neonatal outcome? A critical review of the literature. *The Journal of Maternal-Fetal & Neonatal Medicine*, *20*(3), 189–209. https://doi.org/10.1080/14767050701209560

22. Fraser, A., Macdonald-Wallis, C., Tilling, K., Boyd, A., Golding, J., Davey Smith, G., Henderson, J., Macleod, J., Molloy, L., Ness, A., Ring, S., Nelson, S. M., & Lawlor, D. A. (2013). Cohort profile: The Avon Longitudinal Study of Parents and Children: ALSPAC mothers cohort. *International Journal of Epidemiology*, *42*(1), 97–110. https://doi.org/10.1093/ije/dys066

23. Lautarescu, A., Craig, M. C., & Glover, V. (2020). Prenatal stress: Effects on fetal and child brain development. *International Review of Neurobiology*, *150*, 17–40. https://doi.org/10.1016/bs.irn.2019.11.002

24. Witt, W. P., Wisk, L. E., Cheng, E. R., Hampton, J. M., Creswell, P. D., Hagen, E. W., Spear, H. A., Maddox, T., & Deleire, T. (2011). Poor prepregnancy and antepartum mental health predicts postpartum mental health problems among US women: A nationally representative population-based study. *Women's Health Issues*, *21*(4), 304–313. https://doi.org/10.1016/j.whi.2011.01.002

25. Wisner, K. L., Sit, D. K. Y., McShea, M. C., Rizzo, D. M., Zoretich, R. A., Hughes, C. L., Eng, H. F., Luther, J. F., Wisniewski, S. R., Costantino, M. L., Confer, A. L., Moses-Kolko, E. L., Famy, C. S., & Hanusa, B. H. (2013). Onset timing, thoughts of self-harm, and diagnoses in postpartum women with screen-positive depression findings. *JAMA Psychiatry*, *70*(5), 490–498. https://doi.org/10.1001/jamapsychiatry.2013.87

26. Thorsness, K. R., Watson, C., & LaRusso, E. M. (2018). Perinatal anxiety: Approach to diagnosis and management in the obstetric setting. *American Journal of Obstetrics & Gynecology*, *219*(4), 326–345. https://doi.org/10.1016/j.ajog.2018.05.017

27. Viguera, A. C., Tondo, L., Koukopoulos, A. E., Reginaldi, D., Lepri, B., & Baldessarini, R. J. (2011). Episodes of mood disorders in 2,252 pregnancies and postpartum periods. *The American Journal of Psychiatry, 168*(11), 1179–1185. https://doi.org/10.1176/appi. ajp.2011.11010148

28. Pawluski, J. L., Lonstein, J. S., & Fleming, A. S. (2017). The neurobiology of postpartum anxiety and depression. *Trends in Neurosciences, 40*(2), 106–120. https://doi.org/10.1016/j. tins.2016.11.009

29. Hoffman, C., Dunn, D. M., & Njoroge, W. F. M. (2017). Impact of postpartum mental illness upon infant development. *Current Psychiatry Reports, 19*(12), 100. https://doi.org/10.1007/ s11920-017-0857-8

30. Bennett, S. (2007). *Postpartum depression for dummies* (foreword by M. J. Codey). John Wiley & Sons.

31. American Psychiatric Association. (2013). *Diagnostic and statistical manual of mental disorders* (5th ed.). https://doi.org/10.1176/appi.books.9780890425596

32. Rodriguez-Cabezas, L., & Clark, C. (2018). Psychiatric emergencies in pregnancy and postpartum. *Clinical Obstetrics & Gynecology, 61*(3), 615–627. https://doi.org/10.1097/ GRF.0000000000000377

b. Self Check-in

1. Postpartum Support International. (n.d.). *Perinatal mental health discussion tool.* https://www. postpartum.net/resources/discussion-tool/

c. Find the Right Professional Help

1. Bennett, S., & Indman, P. (2019). *Beyond the blues: Understanding and treating prenatal and postpartum depression & anxiety.* Untreed Reads. (Original work published 2003)

d. Diagnosis and Treatment

1. American Psychiatric Association. (2013). *Diagnostic and statistical manual of mental disorders* (5th ed.). https://doi.org/10.1176/appi.books.9780890425596

2. Kendall-Tackett, K. A. (2017). *Depression in new mothers: Causes, consequences and treatment alternatives* (3rd ed. with foreword by P. Simkin). Routledge.

3. Bennett, S. (2007). *Postpartum depression for dummies* (foreword by M. J. Codey). John Wiley & Sons.

e. Medications in Pregnancy and While Breastfeeding

1. Kendall-Tackett, K. A. (2017). *Depression in new mothers: Causes, consequences and treatment alternatives* (3rd ed. with foreword by P. Simkin). Routledge.

2. Malm, H., Sourander, A., Gissler, M., Gyllenberg, D., Hinkka-Yli-Salomäki, S., McKeague, I. W., Artama, M., & Brown, A. S. (2015). Pregnancy complications following prenatal exposure to SSRIs or maternal psychiatric disorders: Results from population-based national register data. *The American Journal of Psychiatry, 172*(12), 1224–1232. https://doi.org/10.1176/ appi.ajp.2015.14121575

3. ACOG Committee on Practice Bulletins—Obstetrics (with Z. N. Stowe, & K. Ragan). (2008). ACOG practice bulletin no. 92: Use of psychiatric medications during pregnancy and lactation. *Obstetrics & Gynecology, 111*(4), 1001–1020. https://doi.org/10.1097/ AOG.0b013e31816fd910

4. Huybrechts, K. F., Palmsten, K., Avorn, J., Cohen, L. S., Holmes, L. B., Franklin, J. M., Mogun, H., Levin, R., Kowal, M., Setoguchi, S., & Hernández-Díaz, S. (2014). Antidepressant use in pregnancy and the risk of cardiac defects. *The New England Journal of Medicine, 370*(25), 2397–2407. https://doi.org/10.1056/NEJMoa1312828

5. Raffi, E. R., Nonacs, R., & Cohen, L. S. (2019). Safety of psychotropic medications during pregnancy. *Clinics in Perinatology, 46*(2), 215–234. https://doi.org/10.1016/j.clp.2019.02.004

6. Cohen, L. S., & Nonacs, R. (2016). Neurodevelopmental implications of fetal exposure to selective serotonin reuptake inhibitors and untreated maternal depression: Weighing relative risks. *JAMA Psychiatry, 73*(11), 1170–1172. https://doi.org/10.1001/jamapsychiatry.2016.2705

7. Gao, S. Y., Wu, Q. J., Sun, C., Zhang, T. N., Shen, Z. Q., Liu, C. X., Gong, T. T., Xu, X., Ji, C., Huang, D. H., Chang, Q., & Zhao, Y. H. (2018). Selective serotonin reuptake inhibitor use during early pregnancy and congenital malformations: A systematic review and meta-analysis of cohort studies of more than 9 million births. *BMC Medicine, 16*, Article 205. https://doi.org/10.1186/s12916-018-1193-5

8. Viguera, A. C., Freeman, M. P., Góez-Mogollón, L., Sosinsky, A. Z., McElheny, S. A., Church, T. R., Young, A. V., Caplin, P. S., Chitayat, D., Hernández-Díaz, S., & Cohen, L. S. (2021). Reproductive safety of second-generation antipsychotics: Updated data from the Massachusetts General Hospital National Pregnancy Registry for atypical antipsychotics. *The Journal of Clinical Psychiatry, 82*(4), Article 20m13745. https://doi.org/10.4088/JCP.20m13745

9. Freeman, M. P., Góez-Mogollón, L., McInerney, K. A., Davies, A. C., Church, T. R., Sosinsky, A. Z., Noe, O. B., Viguera, A. C., & Cohen, L. S. (2018). Obstetrical and neonatal outcomes after benzodiazepine exposure during pregnancy: Results from a prospective registry of women with psychiatric disorders. *General Hospital Psychiatry, 53*, 73–79. https://doi.org/10.1016/j.genhosppsych.2018.05.010

10. MGH Center for Women's Mental Health Reproductive Psychiatry Resource and Information Center. (n.d.). *National pregnancy registry for psychiatric medications.* https://womensmentalhealth.org/research/pregnancyregistry/

f. Nurturing Mental Wellness

1. Hirshkowitz, M., Whiton, K., Albert, S. M., Alessi, C., Bruni, O., DonCarlos, L., Hazen, N., Herman, J., Adams Hillard, P. J., Katz, E. S., Kheirandish-Gozal, L., Neubauer, D. N., O'Donnell, A. E., Ohayon, M., Peever, J., Rawding, R., Sachdeva, R. C., Setters, B., Vitiello, M. V., & Ware, J. C. (2015). National Sleep Foundation's updated sleep duration recommendations: Final report. *Sleep Health, 1*(4), 233–243. https://doi.org/10.1016/j.sleh.2015.10.004

2. Kendall-Tackett, K. A. (2017). *Depression in new mothers: Causes, consequences and treatment alternatives* (3rd ed. with foreword by P. Simkin). Routledge.

3. American Psychological Association. (2019, Feburary). *APA clinical practice guideline for the treatment of depression across three age cohorts.* https://www.apa.org/depression-guideline/guideline.pdf

4. Cooney, G. M., Dwan, K., Greig, C. A., Lawlor, D. A., Rimer, J., Waugh, F. R., McMurdo, M., & Mead, G. E. (2013). Exercise for depression. *Cochrane Database of Systematic Reviews*, (9), Article CD004366. https://doi.org/10.1002/14651858.CD004366.pub6

5. Saeed, S. A., Cunningham, K., & Bloch, R. M. (2019). Depression and anxiety disorders: Benefits of exercise, yoga, and meditation. *American Family Physician, 99*(10), 620–627. *PubMed.* Retrieved December 15, 2021, from https://pubmed.ncbi.nlm.nih.gov/31083878/

6. Environmental Working Group. (2014, September 18). *EWG's consumer guide to seafood.* https://www.ewg.org/consumer-guides/ewgs-consumer-guide-seafood

7. U.S. Food and Drug Administration. (2021, October). *Advice about eating fish: For those who might become pregnant or are pregnant or breastfeeding and children ages 1-11 years* [Content current as of 2022, June]. https://www.fda.gov/food/consumers/advice-about-eating-fish

8. Benson, H. (with Klipper, M. Z.). (2000). *The relaxation response: Revised and expanded edition.* William Morrow Paperbacks. (Originally published 1975)

9. Cettina, L. A. (2018). Meditation, not medication, to relieve anxiety. *Nursing, 48*(9), 44–47. https://doi.org/10.1097/01.NURSE.0000541390.29234.0b

10. Kabat-Zinn, J. (2013). *Full catastrophe living: Using the wisdom of your body and mind to face stress, pain, and illness* (Revised and updated ed. with preface by T. Nhat Hanh). Bantam Books Trade Paperbacks. (Original work published 1990)

11. Benson-Henry Institute. (2016, July 15). *HerbertBensonRelaxationResponse2016* [Video]. YouTube. https://www.youtube.com/watch?v=HR0bUf2jwOg&t=1s

g. Cultivating a Healthy Relationship with Your Body

1. Bennett, S. (2007). *Postpartum depression for dummies* (foreword by M. J. Codey). John Wiley & Sons.

h. Substance Use

1. Substance Abuse and Mental Health Services Administration. (2020, September). *2019 National survey on drug use and health: Women* [PowerPoint]. https://www.samhsa.gov/data/sites/default/files/reports/rpt31102/2019NSDUH-Women/Women%202019%20NSDUH.pdf

2. MotherToBaby. (2020, August 1). *Alcohol* [Fact sheet]. https://mothertobaby.org/fact-sheets/alcohol-pregnancy/pdf/

3. National Institute on Alcohol Abuse and Alcoholism. (n.d.). *What is a standard drink?* National Institutes of Health. https://www.niaaa.nih.gov/alcohols-effects-health/overview-alcohol-consumption/what-standard-drink

4. Meek, J. Y., Noble, L., & the Section on Breastfeeding. (2022). Policy statement: Breastfeeding and the use of human milk. *Pediatrics, 150*(1), Article e2022057988. https://doi.org/10.1542/peds.2022-057988

5. MotherToBaby. (2020, October 1). *Cigarette smoke* [Fact sheet]. https://mothertobaby.org/fact-sheets/cigarette-smoking-pregnancy/pdf/

6. National Institute on Drug Abuse. (2020, January 22). *Substance use in women DrugFacts.* National Institutes of Health. https://nida.nih.gov/download/19238/substance-use-in-women-drugfacts.pdf?v=8e3444077b0c0e237d1413403790818a

7. MotherToBaby. (2021, July 1). *Marijuana (Cannabis)* [Fact sheet]. https://mothertobaby.org/fact-sheets/marijuana-pregnancy/pdf/

8. Ryan, S. A., Ammerman, S. D., O'Connor, M. E., Committee on Substance Use and Prevention & Section on Breastfeeding (2018). Marijuana use during pregnancy and breastfeeding: Implications for neonatal and childhood outcomes. *Pediatrics, 142*(3), Article e20181889. https://doi.org/10.1542/peds.2018-1889

9. Brown, B. (2010). *The gifts of imperfection: Let go of who you think you're supposed to be and embrace who you are: Your guide to a wholehearted life* [ebook]. Hazelden Publishing.
   "[it] can be described as chronically . . . " Guidepost #3, "numbing and taking the edge off" section, paragraph 4

10. World Health Organization. (2014, November 19). *Guidelines for the identification and management of substance use disorders in pregnancy.* https://www.who.int/publications/i/item/9789241548731

11. American College of Obstetricians and Gynecologists. (2020, June). *FAQs: Tobacco, alcohol, drugs, and pregnancy.* https://www.acog.org/womens-health/faqs/tobacco-alcohol-drugs-and-pregnancy

i. When Things Don't Go as Planned

1. Kendall-Tackett, K. A. (2017). *Depression in new mothers: Causes, consequences and treatment alternatives* (3rd ed. with foreword by P. Simkin). Routledge.

2. Simpson, M., & Catling, C. (2016). Understanding psychological traumatic birth experiences: A literature review. *Women and Birth, 29*(3), 203–207. https://doi.org/10.1016/j.wombi.2015.10.009

3. Beck, C. T. (2004). Birth trauma: In the eye of the beholder. *Nursing Research, 53*(1), 28–35. https://doi.org/10.1097/00006199-200401000-00005

4. van der Kolk, B. A. (2015). *The body keeps the score: Brain, mind, and body in the healing of trauma.* Penguin Books. (Original work published 2014)
   "also [about] the imprint left . . . " p. 21

5. HEALTHY RELATIONSHIPS

a. Cultivate Effective Communication

1. Moyers, B. (Host). (1988, November 17). *Peter Drucker: Father of modern management* [April 2, 2015, transcript of TV interview]. In J. Sameth (Executive Producer), *A World of Ideas with Bill Moyers.* CBS. https://billmoyers.com/content/peter-drucker/

2. Lerner, H. (2017). *Why won't you apologize? Healing big betrayals and everyday hurts.* Gallery Books.

b. Explore Expectations
None.

c. Set Healthy Boundaries

1. Cloud, H., & Townsend, J. (2017). *Boundaries: When to say yes, how to say no to take control of your life* (Updated and expanded ed.). Zondervan. (Original work published 1992)

d. Sex in Pregnancy

1. Dezzutti, C. S., Brown, E. R., Moncla, B., Russo, J., Cost, M., Wang, L., Uranker, K., Kunjara Na Ayudhya, R. P., Pryke, K., Pickett, J., Leblanc, M. A., & Rohan, L. C. (2012). Is wetter better? An evaluation of over-the-counter personal lubricants for safety and anti-HIV-1 activity. *PLOS ONE, 7*(11), Article e48328. https://doi.org/10.1371/journal.pone.0048328

2. Adriaens, E., & Remon, J. P. (2008). Mucosal irritation potential of personal lubricants relates to product osmolality as detected by the slug mucosal irritation assay. *Sexually Transmitted Diseases, 35*(5), 512–516. https://doi.org/10.1097/OLQ.0b013e3181644669

3. Wilkinson, E. M., Łaniewski, P., Herbst-Kralovetz, M. M., & Brotman, R. M. (2019). Personal and clinical vaginal lubricants: Impact on local vaginal microenvironment and implications for epithelial cell host response and barrier function. *The Journal of Infectious Diseases, 220*(12), 2009–2018. https://doi.org/10.1093/infdis/jiz412

4. World Health Organization. (2012). *Use and procurement of additional lubricants for male and female condoms: WHO/UNFPA/FHI360 advisory note.* https://apps.who.int/iris/bitstream/handle/10665/76580/WHO_RHR_12.33_eng.pdf?

5. Desmedt, B., Vanhamme, M., Vanhee, C., Rogiers, V., & Deconinck, E. (2019). Consumer protection provided by the European medical device and cosmetic legislation for condoms and lubricants. *Regulatory Toxicology and Pharmacology, 103*, 106–112. https://doi.org/10.1016/j.yrtph.2019.01.022

6. NSF. (n.d.). *Organic personal care standards.* https://www.nsf.org/standards-development/standards-portfolio/organic-personal-care-standards

e. Physical Changes That Affect Postpartum Sex

1. DeMaria, A. L., Delay, C., Sundstrom, B., Wakefield, A. L., Avina, A., & Meier, S. (2019). Understanding women's postpartum sexual experiences. *Culture, Health & Sexuality, 21*(10), 1162–1176. https://doi.org/10.1080/13691058.2018.1543802

2. Wallwiener, S., Müller, M., Doster, A., Kuon, R. J., Plewniok, K., Feller, S., Wallwiener, M., Reck, C., Matthies, L. M., & Wallwiener, C. (2017). Sexual activity and sexual dysfunction of women in the perinatal period: A longitudinal study. *Archives of Gynecology and Obstetrics, 295*(4), 873–883. https://doi.org/10.1007/s00404-017-4305-0

3. Jawed-Wessel, S., & Sevick, E. (2017). The impact of pregnancy and childbirth on sexual behaviors: A systematic review. *Journal of Sex Research, 54*(4-5), 411–423. https://doi.org/10.1080/00224499.2016.1274715

4. O'Malley, D., Higgins, A., Begley, C., Daly, D., & Smith, V. (2018). Prevalence of and risk factors associated with sexual health issues in primiparous women at 6 and 12 months postpartum; A longitudinal prospective cohort study (the MAMMI study). *BMC Pregnancy and Childbirth, 18*, Article 196. https://doi.org/10.1186/s12884-018-1838-6

5. Hansson, M., & Ahlborg, T. (2012). Quality of the intimate and sexual relationship in first-time parents – A longitudinal study. *Sexual & Reproductive Healthcare, 3*(1), 21–29. https://doi.org/10.1016/j.srhc.2011.10.002

6. Alp Yılmaz, F., Şener Taplak, A., & Polat, S. (2019). Breastfeeding and sexual activity and sexual quality in postpartum women. *Breastfeeding Medicine, 14*(8), 587–591. https://doi.org/10.1089/bfm.2018.0249

7. Lagaert, L., Weyers, S., Van Kerrebroeck, H., & Elaut, E. (2017). Postpartum dyspareunia and sexual functioning: A prospective cohort study. *The European Journal of Contraception & Reproductive Health Care, 22*(3), 200–206. https://doi.org/10.1080/13625187.2017.1315938

8. Gutzeit, O., Levy, G., & Lowenstein, L. (2020). Postpartum female sexual function: Risk factors for postpartum sexual dysfunction. *Sexual Medicine*, *8*(1), 8–13. https://doi.org/10.1016/j.esxm.2019.10.005

f. Relationships That Hurt

1. National Domestic Violence Hotline. (n.d.). *Understand relationship abuse* [Under *Identify abuse*]. https://www.thehotline.org/identify-abuse/understand-relationship-abuse/

2. National Institute of Corrections. (2018, February). *DV/IPV: Domestic violence/intimate partner violence* [NICIC Annotated Bibliography series]. U.S. Department of Justice, Federal Bureau of Prisons. https://nicic.gov/sites/default/files/031384_0.pdf

3. National Coalition against Domestic Violence. (n.d.). *Domestic violence* [Fact sheet]. https://assets.speakcdn.com/assets/2497/domestic_violence-2020080709350855.pdf?

4. Smith, S. G., Zhang, X., Basile, K. C., Merrick, M. T., Wang, J., Kresnow, M., & Chen, J. (2018, November). *The National Intimate Partner and Sexual Violence Survey (NISVS): 2015 Data brief – Updated release.* Centers for Disease Control and Prevention, National Center for Injury Prevention and Control, Division of Violence Prevention. https://www.cdc.gov/violenceprevention/pdf/2015data-brief508.pdf

5. World Health Organization. (2011). *Intimate partner violence during pregnancy* [Information sheet]. https://apps.who.int/iris/bitstream/handle/10665/70764/WHO_RHR_11.35_eng.pdf

6. Alhusen, J. L., Ray, E., Sharps, P., & Bullock, L. (2015). Intimate partner violence during pregnancy: Maternal and neonatal outcomes. *Journal of Women's Health*, *24*(1), 100–106. https://doi.org/10.1089/jwh.2014.4872

7. National Domestic Violence Hotline. (n.d.). *Warning signs of abuse* [Under *Identify abuse*]. https://www.thehotline.org/identify-abuse/domestic-abuse-warning-signs/

INDEX

hemorrhoids 397, 563
illicit drugs and 10, 195
in pregnancy 25, 392, 533–536
labeling 394
labor/delivery 436
over-the-counter (OTC), pain
  399–400, 404, 563
psychiatric/psychotropic 191, 393,
  533–536, 561
risks/safety 535, 569
sleeping pills 517, 521
stool softeners/laxatives 397, 563
supplements 25, 395, 490, 532
meditation 538
membrane sweeping 273
mementos/keepsakes 138–141, 158
menstrual cycles 339, 389, 460, 462
mental health. *See also* self-care
anxiety 50, **95–97**, 290, 454, 524–528
baby blues 299–300, 389
bipolar disorder 524, 526–527
birth control and 461
body image **61–64**, 342, 540–541, 561
depression **299–300**, 314–317, 389,
  524, 528
eating disorders 25, 63, 352, 393, 486,
  541, 568
emergencies 455, 529, 568
emotions 41, 43, 332, 526
fear 50, 95, 290, 356, 528
guilt 356
hallucinations 527
help for 391, 410, 528–533
loneliness 346
mental wellness 55–56, 523, 529–531,
  536–539
nutrition 537
obsessive-compulsive disorder (OCD)
  96, 310–311
paranoia 527
perinatal mood and anxiety disorders
  (PMADs) 454, 524–526
physical activity 537
postpartum depression 299–300,
  314–317, 389, 524, 528
pregnancy/postpartum wellness 454,
  523–532
psychosis 527
PTSD (post-traumatic stress disorder)
  524, 564

sleep and 537
stigma 525
stress 151, 206, 399, 538
support resources 456, 534, 556, 568
tips for 454, 536–539
migraines 399
milk banks 250
mindfulness 9, 352, 483
minerals. *See* vitamins/minerals
miscarriages 548–549, 568–569
monitoring baby 106, 275, 386
moodiness 43, 300, 316, 528
morning sickness 9, 11, 16, 22, 394
motherhood myths 212, 299–300, 347
mothers. *See also* work/school
advice vs. intuition 370
caregiver jealousy 333
expectations 170, 346, 355, 368
momsters 168–169
motherhood 163, 212, 363, 376
"natural" mothers 170–171
protective 265–267
reflections 372
mucus plug 166, 184, 391
multiple markers screenings 387, 414.
  See also screenings
musculoskeletal assessments 401

N

names 423–424
naps 516. *See also* sleep
nausea 9, 11, **16**, 22, 390, 394–396
neonatal intensive care unit (NICU)
  569
nesting 147, 425–431
neurological warnings 390
newborns. *See also* baby gear; crying
aromatherapy 521
baby classes 455
bathing 464
bed sharing 428
bonding with 442, 457, 464
child care 333, 455, 471–473
circumcision 186, 448
clothes 426
communicating 237, 338, 360, 467
comparing 369
concerns about 310
cues 237, 467